Psychiatry as a Neuroscience

Psychiatry as a Neuroscience

Edited by

Juan José López-Ibor
Complutense University of Madrid, Spain

Wolfgang Gaebel
University of Düsseldorf, Germany

Mario Maj
University of Naples, Italy

Norman Sartorius
University of Geneva, Switzerland

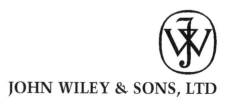

JOHN WILEY & SONS, LTD

Other Wiley Editorial Offices

John Wiley & Sons, Inc., 605 Third Avenue,
New York, NY 10158-0012, USA

WILEY-VCH Verlag GmbH, Pappelallee 3,
D-69469 Weinheim, Germany

John Wiley & Sons Australia, Ltd., 33 Park Road, Milton,
Queensland 4064, Australia

John Wiley & Sons (Asia) Pte Ltd., 2 Clementi Loop #02-01,
Jin Xing Distripark, Singapore 129809

John Wiley & Sons (Canada), Ltd., 22 Worcester Road,
Rexdale, Ontario M9W IL1, Canada

British Library Cataloguing in Publication Data

A catalogue record for this book is available from the British Library

ISBN 0-471-49656-1

Typeset in 10/12pt Palatino by Kolam Information Services Pvt Ltd, Pondicherry, India
Printed and bound in Great Britain by T J International Ltd, Padstow, Cornwall
This book is printed on acid-free paper responsibly manufactured from sustainable forestry,
in which at least two trees are planted for each one used for paper production.

Contributors

Francine M. Benes Laboratories for Structural Neuroscience, McLean Hospital, 115 Mill Street, Belmont, MA 02478, USA

Silvana Galderisi Department of Psychiatry, University of Naples SUN, Largo Madonna delle Grazie, 80138 Naples, Italy

John H. Gruzelier Department of Cognitive Neuroscience and Behaviour, Imperial College of Science, Technology and Medicine, St. Dunstan's Road, London W6 8RF, United Kingdom

David A. Gutman Department of Psychiatry and Behavioral Sciences, Emory University School of Medicine, 1639 Pierce Drive, Suite 4000, Atlanta, GA 30322-4990, USA

Simon Lovestone Departments of Old Age Psychiatry and Neuroscience, Institute of Psychiatry, De Crespigny Park, London, SE5 8AF, United Kingdom

Peter McGuffin SGDP Research Centre, Institute of Psychiatry, De Crespigny Park, Denmark Hill, London, SE5 8AF, United Kingdom

Charles B. Nemeroff Department of Psychiatry and Behavioral Sciences, Emory University School of Medicine, 1639 Pierce Drive, Suite 4000, Atlanta, GA 30322-4990, USA

Alexander B. Niculescu III Neuroscience Education Institute and Department of Psychiatry, University of California at San Diego, 9500 Gilman Drive, La Jolla, CA 92093-0603, USA

Stefan Pauli Department of Clinical Neuroscience, Karolinska Institute and Hospital, 171 76 Stockholm, Sweden

Marcus Richards MRC National Survey of Health and Development, University College Medical School, 1–19 Torrington Place, London WC1E 6BT, United Kingdom

Karen Ritchie EPI 9930 INSERM, Bâtiment Recherche, CRLC Val d'Aurelle, Parc Euromedecine, 326 rue des Apothicaires, 34298 Montpellier Cedex 5, France

Göran Sedvall Department of Clinical Neuroscience, Karolinska Institute and Hospital, 171 76 Stockholm, Sweden

Ravi Singareddy Department of Psychiatry and Behavioral Neurosciences, School of Medicine, Wayne State University, Detroit, MI 48231, USA

Stephen M. Stahl Neuroscience Education Institute and Department of Psychiatry, University of California at San Diego, 9500 Gilman Drive, La Jolla, CA 92093-0603, USA

Werner Strik University Hospital of Clinical Psychiatry, Bollingenstrasse 111, Berne 60, 3000 Switzerland

Carol A. Tamminga Department of Psychiatry, University of Maryland, Maryland Psychiatric Research Center, Box 21247, Baltimore, MD 21228, USA

Thomas W. Uhde Department of Psychiatry and Behavioral Neurosciences, School of Medicine, Wayne State University, Detroit, MI 48231, USA

Contents

List of Contributors   v

Preface   ix

1. Genetic Research in Psychiatry   1
   Peter McGuffin

2. Molecular and Cellular Biology Research in Psychiatry   29
   Stephen M. Stahl and Alexander B. Niculescu III

3. Brain Imaging Research in Psychiatry   59
   Göran Sedvall and Stefan Pauli

4. Neuroendocrinological Research in Psychiatry   91
   Charles B. Nemeroff and David A. Gutman

5. Neurophysiological Research in Psychiatry   125
   John H. Gruzelier, Silvana Galderisi and Werner Strik

6. Neuropsychological Research in Psychiatry   181
   Karen Ritchie and Marcus Richards

7. Neurobiology of Schizophrenia   197
   Francine M. Benes and Carol A. Tamminga

8. Biological Research in Anxiety Disorders   237
   Thomas W. Uhde and Ravi Singareddy

9. Biological Research on Dementias   287
   Simon Lovestone

Index   323

Acknowledgements   331

Preface

Psychiatry has come on to good terms with the rest of neurosciences only very recently. Since then the achievements have been impressive and the opportunities unbelievable.

Modern psychiatry was born at the end of the eighteenth century, together with the rest of medical disciplines. This was when physicians abandoned old theories about diseases, many of them Galenic, and decided to describe what they saw, in accordance with the principles of modern science. Physicians learnt to see [1], and the site and causes of diseases were ascribed to organs. The title of Morgagni's seminal book, *On the site and causes of diseases, investigated by anatomical methods*, published in 1771, referred precisely to this.

The birth of psychiatry was more complex than that of the rest of medicine. It required three basic steps. The first was the delimitation of mental disorders from abnormal behaviours not accepted by society. It must be pointed out that the inmates in institutions such as the Hôpitaux Generaux in France or asylums in Great Britain or Germany included not only mentally ill individuals, but also others who were a nuisance to society. The clear-cut separation of these two populations is exemplified by the decision of the director of the Hôpital Charenton in Paris, in the first years of the French Revolution, to discharge the famous Marquis de Sade. The author of *Justine* had spent many years as an inmate as a consequence of an order of King Louis XVI. The director's reason for discharging him was literally: "He is not mad, his only madness is vice" [2].

The second step was quite straightforward: to ascribe what was left—that is, mental disease—to an organ, quite naturally the brain. Although it seems that Voltaire coined the expression "mental diseases are brain diseases", it was the French alienist Esquirol [3] who introduced this concept in medicine.

Immediately a third step was necessary, as psychiatry never fitted into a reductionistic medical model, and psychiatrists recognized among their patients some who seemed not to be suffering the consequences of brain disorders (on the contrary, their clinical manifestations seemed exaggerations of everyday behaviour). In 1777 Cullen defined neuroses as preternatural reactions [4], which could be translated as "statistically abnormal reactions". This introduced a dichotomy of mental disorders which has dominated up to very recent times, and is even present today.

From then on psychiatry developed in a dualistic way. Dualism is attributed to the French philosopher Descartes [5], who described two substances in human beings: one physical, which could be measured (*res extensa*), i.e. the body, and one characterized by thinking (*res cogitans*), i.e. the mind. It must be said that the trend to subdivide human nature is very ancient, and it is a powerful tool to explain the existence of evil, which according to Becker [6] is the main problem of the social sciences. This trend is present in gnostic philosophy and theology and in modern science. The German philosopher Dilthey [7] saw on the one side the sciences of nature (*Naturwissenschaften*), or natural sciences, ruled by the presence of causality, as in Newtonian physics. On the other side, however, he gave the status of sciences to other activities which today would be called "soft science", because they are unable to put forward causes and effects and experimental methods. History is the best example. Here research delves into motives which lead to consequences, and between the motives and the consequences there is a space of uncertainty, which is in contrast to the immediate relation between cause and effect. These sciences were called by Dilthey "sciences of the spirit" (*Geisteswissenschaften*); other names applied to them are cultural or humanistic sciences. Following this line, Jaspers [8] distinguished two methods of psychopathological research: explanation, which is the search for causes, and understanding, which is the search for motives.

This perspective shapes Kurt Schneider's [9] approach, which is at the core of current nosology, from DSM-III onwards. Schneider distinguished two kinds of mental disorders: the psychoses, which can be attributed to brain disorders, and the variations of the psychological way of being, essentially the neuroses and the psychopathic personalities. Looking closer and from the perspective of neuroscience, one of the branches of sciences of nature devoted to the nervous system, a series of problems appear.

The organic and symptomatic psychoses are straightforward. The medical scientific model rules with no difficulties. Brain malfunctions and clinical manifestations correlate smoothly.

Endogenous psychoses are different. They are characterized by manifestations that do not correspond to normal psychological phenomena, nor do they derive from them. They are, in the word of Jaspers, "incomprehensible", which means that there are no motives in them, and therefore they are not to be understood with the methods of humanistic sciences. Thus, they should have an explanation leading to the discovery of a cause following the principles of the sciences of nature. Well, yes and no.

Endogenous psychoses, schizophrenia and mood disorders, are the most characteristic of psychiatric disorders, and also the most enigmatic. For many clinicians they are the Delphic oracle of psychiatry [10]; for neuropathologists they were their graveyard. Schneider again clarifies the difficulties when he says that endogenous psychoses are only sets of manifestations accepted by convention (he says that when first-rank symptoms are present the diagnosis is *what I call schizophrenia*). Furthermore, the concept of "symptoms" does not apply properly to the clinical manifestations of endogenous psychoses. Tellenbach [11], for instance, refers to them as "phenomena". To summarize, according to Schneider, the realm of schizophrenia and mood disorders can never be fully explained from the perspective of natural neuroscience.

What about neurotic and personality disorders? Here Schneider lays stress on Griesinger's notion [12] that they are not brain diseases but variations of the mode of being. This has often been misunderstood as meaning that there is no biological basis for them. The point is that there is a biological background, as there is in every psychological manifestation of our life, but it is not different from the one lying under normal psychological phenomena.

Looking at the relationship between neuroscience and psychiatry from the other side, the problems have been also huge. First, there have been a series of paradigms, most of them too reductionist. Second, some methodological problems may never be solved. The fight between localizationists and their opponents still goes on today in the discussion as to whether modules or circuits are the basic structures to investigate and correlate with psychological activity. As to the methods, the lack of sufficient animal models leads to the search for new ways of research.

The different disciplines involved in the study of the nervous system have often developed in ignorance of the achievement of other disciplines. The concept of neuroscience as an integrated field of research is very young. Actually, it was born in 1969, when the Society for Neurosciences was created.

Science is better at explaining abnormal phenomena than normal ones. Physiology was born out of physiopathology and psychology out of psychopathology. The first neuroscientific disciplines delved into diseases, led by neuropathology. Normality is considered at a later stage. However, this is not enough as other aspects come into consideration, development being the first. Part of the success of Ramón y Cajal was to study how the nervous system grew in order to understand the role of its structure in adulthood.

During the last few decades the development of psychosocial sciences has reached a point where confluence with physiological and morphological sciences is a reachable target. Even Freud dared to write a highly speculative book on physiology for psychologists [13]. The founder of psychoanalysis was interested in developing an everyday scientific psychology and he did it from a physiological perspective. He was a physician, a pupil of Brücke, who was one of the four main disciples of Johannes Müller, the introducer

of physiopathology in Germany. It is highly significant that Freud's translators lost the everyday language which he used. For instance, where Freud
wrote *Seele* ("soul"), the French translators wrote *appareil psychique*, leading
to the notion that we have a "psychological organ" or "system", just as we
have a digestive or sexual one.

Today the situation is different from the one faced by Freud. There is
much to be done, if only to drop the plural "neurosciences" in favour of the
singular, a science integrating many different disciplines. This is the real
challenge. One of the important recent changes lies in the fact that neuroscientists are interested in how the brain functions while performing everyday
tasks such as recognizing faces or familiar environments. To investigate this,
it is necessary to analyse psychological and cognitive functions and to
identify their basic elements. For instance, seeing is split down into the
perceptions of lines, colour, inclination and so on—elements that have
different receptors at the retina, different pathways and cortical areas.
Further cortical areas are able to recompose the different kinds of stimuli,
and others, the secondary visual areas, to link them to other perceptions and
memories.

In this context, the question is not what can neuroscience do for psychiatry, the answer to which is obvious, but the opposite: what can psychiatry
do for neuroscience?

In my opinion, psychiatry can help to overcome the limitations of dualism. To do this, two approaches seem particularly important. The first is to
adopt a perspective beyond dualism. Following López-Ibor Sr. [14] and
others, we have tried to delve into the body experience, which is not the
experience of a body separated from a soul, but the unitary experience of a
corporality. Corporality is an incarnated mind, an animated body (using the
Latin meaning of *anima*, "soul").

The second approach is to define basic psychopathological disturbances
which relate to basic psychological functions that could be linked to basic
neurobiological activities. Here it is irrelevant whether these are cortical
modules or cortico-subcortical pathways. Zutt [15], a great German representative of the anthropological trends in psychiatry, gives us two good
examples of this perspective. The first is the Gerstmann syndrome, a well-
known neurological syndrome appearing with lesions of left parietal cortex.
The syndrome is characterized by finger agnosia, left-right agnosia and
acalculia. A strange combination indeed. No so much, Zutt points out, if
we take into account that the hands have an asymmetry which is the
reflection of the asymmetry of nature, for instance of the spins of electrons.
This is called "cheirality" (from the Greek word *cheiros*, "hand"). Therefore
there is a region of the brain which is able to recognize the hand and the
fingers. Damage at this level interferes with the recognition of hand and
fingers, and, simultaneously, with the other things we do with the internal-

ization of the perception of these parts of the body: namely, to distinguish right from left and to count. In other words, while differentiating right from left, we internally look for our hands, the right and the left one, and while doing mental calculations we make use of the internal image of our fingers—the same fingers we used in school to perform basic counting.

The second example of Zutt is also very basic. Why do patients with schizophrenia hear voices, and why is it not so common that they have visual hallucinations? To put it differently, is there an equivalent in the realm of seeing to the hearing of voices? The second formulation leads to the right answer: feeling watched. Therefore, the basic phenomenon of the schizophrenic experience is not having intruding hallucinations which interfere with normal perceptions. It is the fact of being overwhelmed by others: berated and spoken of in every aspect of life, be it visual, auditory or other.

The research on computerized models of the mind offered new possibilities for neuroscience. Gómez-Mont [16], in Mexico, has postulated the presence of a cortico-subcortical circuit involved in discriminating the relevance of perceptions. This circuit would be altered in patients with schizophrenia, for whom every single detail of perception is loaded with the certainty of a special meaning related to a delusion (the door opens, therefore the persecutors are coming in). Interestingly enough, this same circuit may be involved in obsessions, and indeed, neuroimaging techniques [17, 18] have shown a hyperactivity in an orbitofrontal–caudate–pallidus–thalamic circuit. One of the main characteristics of patients with obsessions is that they are unable to distinguish what is relevant from what is irrelevant, as Janet [19] described many decades ago. Therefore, the basic function of differentiating which new perception is relevant is linked to a specific circuit. This function is essential for survival, in order to detect possible threats or opportunities that require the activation of other functions and circuits. This basic function can be altered in several ways. For patients with schizophrenia, every new perception is relevant, is a threat, while those suffering from obsessions cannot reach a conclusion as to whether it is or not. Therefore, the circuit and the mind of the individual with obsessions turns on and on, until some external event interrupts it.

This approach to research is still speculative, but it opens new paths which are fascinating and go beyond dualism. Looking at Griesinger's views today we can say, first, that the brain is involved in every kind of mental disorder, be it an "organic" one or an "aberration of the intelligence" (an abnormal mode of being, in more modern words). Second, and even more important for psychiatry, we have to learn to see "the same order of facts" in healthy psychological functioning and in disease. The role of psychiatry as a neuroscience is to delve into the basic mechanisms underlying both normal and abnormal phenomena and, at the same time, to contribute to destigmatizing mental disorders so that they are not seen as something radically apart from the mental activity of everyday life, by understanding the adaptive mechanisms involved in them and the way these have gone astray.

Juan José López-Ibor

REFERENCES

1. Foucault M. (1963) *Naissance de la Clinique. Une Archéologie du Regard Médical*, Presses Universitaires de France, Paris.
2. Szasz T.S. (1970) *The Manufacture of Madness. A Comparative Study of the Inquisition and the Mental Health Movement*, Harper & Row, New York.
3. Esquirol J.E.D. (1816/1968) *Von den Geisteskrankheiten*, Huber, Bern.
4. Cullen W. (1777) *First Lines of the Practice of Physic*, London.
5. Descartes R. (1637/1963) *Discours de la Méthode*. In *Oeuvres Philosophiques*, Vol. 1, Garnier, Paris.
6. Becker E. (1980) *La Estructura del Mal. Un Ensayo sobre la Unificación de la Ciencia del Hombre*, Fondo de Cultura Económica, México.
7. Dilthey W. (1966) *Introducción a las Ciencias del Espíritu*, Revista de Occidente, Madrid.
8. Jaspers K. (1946) *Allgemeine Psychopathologie*, 4th ed., Springer, Berlin.
9. Schneider K. (1967) *Klinische Psychopathologie*, Thieme, Stuttgart.
10. Kolle K. (1957) *Der Wahnkranke im Lichte alter un Neuer Psychopathologie*, Thieme, Stuttgart.
11. Tellenbach H. (1976) *Melancholie*, Springer, Berlin.
12. Griesinger W. (1872/1968) *Gesammelte Abhandlungen*, Vol. 1, Bonset, Amsterdam.
13. Freud S. (1942) *Gesammelte Werke*, Imago Publishing, London.
14. López-Ibor J.J., López-Ibor Aliño J.J. (1974) *El Cuerpo y la Corporalidad*, Gredos, Madrid.
15. Zutt J. (1963) *Auf dem Wege zu einer anthropologischen Psychiatrie. Gesammelte Aufsätze*, Springer, Berlin.
16. Gómez-Mont F. (1993) Neuropsicología de la duda. *Salud Mental*, **16**: 9–16.
17. Baxter L.R., Schwartz J.M., Bergman K.S., Szuba M.P., Guze B.H., Mazziotta J.C., Alazraki A., Selin C.E., Ferng H.-K., Munford P. *et al.* (1992) Caudate glucose metabolic rate changes with both drug and behaviour therapy for obsessive-compulsive disorder. *Arch. Gen. Psychiatry*, **49**: 681–689.
18. López-Ibor A., Ortiz Alonso T., Encinas Mejías M., Fernández A., Maestú F., López-Ibor Aliño J.J. (2000) Avances en neuroimagen en el trastorno obsesivo-compulsivo. *Actas Español. Psiquiatría*, **28**: 304–310.
19. Janet P. (1903) *Les Obsessions et la Psychasthénie*, Alcan, Paris.

This volume is based in part on presentations delivered at the 11th World Congress of Psychiatry (Hamburg, Germany, August 6–11, 1999).

1

Genetic Research in Psychiatry

Peter McGuffin

Social, Genetic and Developmental Psychiatry Research Centre,
Institute of Psychiatry, De Crespigny Park,
Denmark Hill, London SE5 8AF, UK

INTRODUCTION

Psychiatric genetics and the application of molecular methods to studying psychiatric disorders is among the most rapidly expanding areas of research within neuroscience. In common with genetic approaches to other common and complex disorders, modern psychiatric genetics offers a compellingly attractive route to the understanding of aetiologies of conditions where the pathogenesis has until now been obscure. However, the prospect that genes may be involved in behaviour, both normal and abnormal, has often provoked controversy. For this reason I will begin by attempting to set modern psychiatric genetics within its historical context before going on to review what has been learned by the application of classic quantitative genetic approaches. New developments in both statistical and molecular genetics will then be surveyed and, finally, the clinical and broader implications for the whole field of psychiatry will be discussed.

A BRIEF HISTORY OF PSYCHIATRIC GENETICS

The idea that there is a hereditary component to mental illness is an ancient one, but psychiatric genetics, like genetics generally, only came into being as a branch of science at the beginning of the twentieth century. As far back as the 1820s, there was evidence that systematic attempts were being made to record the family histories of psychiatric patients. For example, patients' case records at the Bethlem Royal Hospital in London, England, showed that one of the routine questions that the admitting doctor was

Psychiatry as a Neuroscience. Edited by Juan José López-Ibor, Wolfgang Gaebel, Mario Maj and Norman Sartorius. © 2002 John Wiley & Sons Ltd.

required to answer about the illness of his patient was "whether heredi-tary?" [1].

The foundations of a scientific approach to the study of the inheritance of behaviour were laid by Francis Galton, an English polymath and largely self-taught scientist, in the second half of the nineteenth century. Stimulated by the theory of natural selection proposed by his cousin, Charles Darwin, Galton studied hereditary influence on behaviour, performed studies of families and was the first to propose that twin studies would be useful as a means of discriminating between *nature* and *nurture*. He also outlined the statistical techniques of correlation and regression in studying resemblance between relatives, and published the influential book *Hereditary Genius*, containing studies of men of high ability and their families, in 1869.

Although this was three years after Mendel's publication of his laws of inheritance, Galton, in common with most biologists of his day, appeared to be completely ignorant of Mendel's work. Mendel's writings and the veracity of his laws were "rediscovered" over 30 years later, in 1900, and thereafter recognized as fundamental to explaining patterns of inheritance. Nevertheless, Mendel studied dichotomous (present/absent) characteris-tics, whereas Galton's work emphasized the fact that human beings differ from each other mainly in terms of quantitative traits such as height, weight or intellectual ability. Consequently, many biologists questioned whether Mendelian laws had any general relevance and it was left to the statistician R.A. Fisher to demonstrate that the inheritance of continuous variation is readily explained by the combined affects of multiple genes, each of which is individually inherited in a Mendelian fashion [2].

Discovery of a theoretical basis for genetic inheritance, coinciding with the development of a workable system of classification of major psychiatric disorders largely resulting from the work of Emil Kraepelin in Heidelberg, paved the way for the beginnings of psychiatric genetics. Kraepelin moved to Munich in 1904 and soon established what was in effect the first research institute for psychiatry. Several of his senior staff began pioneering studies. They included Bruno Schultz and Ernst Rudin, who carried out the first sys-tematic family studies of schizophrenia, and Hans Luxemburger, who was the first to apply the twin method to schizophrenia and manic-depressive disorder in the 1920s. During the 1930s, the Munich Institute went from strength to strength and attracted visiting research fellows who included Erik Strömgren from Denmark and Eliot Slater from the UK. However, the situation became less favourable as the Nazis, who came to power in 1933, began to introduce laws based on their own interpretation of eugenics, which included first compulsory sterilization and later extermination of individuals believed to be suffering from hereditary disease. These included patients suffering from schizophrenia, manic-depressive disorder, Hunting-ton's disease and even alcoholism. Luxemburger and Schultz opposed such policies, on both moral and scientific grounds [2], and Luxemburger was banned from teaching at the University [3]. However, Rudin supported the Nazi policies and attained high eminence in German medicine under the Nazi regime. After the end of the Second World War, Rudin was tried by the Allies and found guilty of being a "fellow traveller" rather than a major perpetrator of war crimes. However, the depth of his involvement remains a subject of heated debate.

In the aftermath of the Second World War, psychiatric genetic research virtually ceased in Germany, its birthplace. However, it continued to progress, albeit on a small scale, elsewhere in Europe, particularly in Scandinavia and in the United Kingdom, where Slater set up a twin register at the Bethlem Royal and Maudsley Hospitals and developed a research group which eventually resulted in the setting up of a Medical Research Council (MRC) Psychiatric Genetics Unit in 1959.

Meanwhile, in the United States, psychiatric genetic research had continued: most notably, that carried out by Franz Kallmann, a German who had worked in Munich but who was half Jewish and had emigrated to the United States shortly after the Nazis came to power. Kallmann and others employed family and twin methods in research on a variety of traits and disorders, and twin research in particular was developed and refined both in the United States and in Europe.

By the later 1960s, the family and twin data on schizophrenia were beginning to make the case for a genetic component, with clear-cut results arising, for example, from Gottesman and Shields' [4] twin study in the London MRC Psychiatric Genetics Unit. However, schizophrenia at this stage was an ideological battleground in psychiatry, with "anti-psychiatrists" such as R.D. Laing arguing that schizophrenia was an understandable reaction to pathological family dynamics, and others, such as Thomas Szasz, arguing that schizophrenia was not an illness at all, but a "myth" created by doctors. For many mainstream psychiatrists, the vital pieces of evidence that clinched the argument in favour of genes having a role came from adoption studies. These were carried out first by Leonard Heston [5] and very soon after by Seymour Kety [6] and others in a landmark US–Danish collaboration. The results led Kety to make his famous remark that "if schizophrenia is a myth, it is a myth with a strong genetic component".

Despite the apparent triumph of these converging pieces of evidence from family, twin and adoption studies, psychiatric genetics remained unfashionable throughout the rest of the 1960s and 1970s. It was only really with the explosion of interest in biological psychiatry both in the United States and Europe that began in the later 1970s and continued into the 1980s, combined with the impact of the "new genetics" of recombinant DNA [7], that psychiatric genetics began again to find its place within the mainstream of research into mental illness. At the same time, the closing years of the twentieth century and the beginnings of the twenty-first have seen a dramatic increase in public interest in all things genetic or purportedly influenced by genes. Much of the media speculation has seen greatly overblown claims: not just of a genetic contribution to diseases, but reports that scientists have discovered the "gene for" such behaviours as aggression, intelligence, criminality, homosexuality and even feminine intuition [8]. Such reports often suggest a direct correspondence between carrying the gene and manifesting the trait or disorder, and only more rarely mention that complicated traits involving behaviour are likely to have a more complex genetic basis. In this chapter I will focus on the useful methods of research in quantitative and molecular studies of psychiatric disorders and attempt to clarify what they can really tell us about the aetiology of such conditions. I will then attempt to predict the likely impact of such knowledge on the development of psychiatry as a neuroscience in the twenty-first century.

FAMILIAL BEHAVIOUR

One of the fundamental pitfalls of studying the genetics of behaviour, or any other complex trait, is to assume that familial aggregation necessarily means that the trait is genetic, or that a strong clustering within families means that single gene effects are present. Although some disorders involving behaviour can be entirely explained by single genes, this is the exception rather than the rule. Alzheimer's disease (AD), for example, includes early-onset forms resulting from three different mutations in the genes called presenilin 1 on chromosome 14, presenilin 2 on chromosome 1 and the amyloid precursor protein gene on chromosome 21 [9]. However, these account for less than 1% of all cases of AD, whereas the vast majority of cases are of late onset and involve a combination of genetic and environment factors. Genes involved in later-onset AD have been identified, most notably the ε4 allele of the apolipoprotein E gene. However, carrying this allele is neither necessary nor sufficient to cause the disorder: that is, individuals who have the ε4 allele are at a higher risk of developing the disorder than those without, but the allele confers an increased risk, not a certainty, of getting AD, and many sufferers of the disease—more than half in some studies [10]—do not carry the ε4 allele at all.

By contrast, geneticists have long been aware that Mendelian inheritance can be simulated by other mechanisms [11]. For example, a study of the educational histories of the parents and siblings of medical students revealed that attending medical school was roughly 80 times more common in these family members than in the population at large. Segregation analysis showed that the trait "attending medical school" survived most of the statistical tests for autosomal recessive inheritance [12]. The point of the study was not to convince geneticists that they should embark on cloning the gene for attending medical school, but rather to show that an oversimple assumption about a complex trait can lead to highly misleading outcomes. On the other hand, there could well be *some* genetic contribution to attending medical school, for example, via the influence of genes on intellectual ability or on personality types associated with career choice.

The evidence that genes do in fact contribute to many types of behaviour comes from two types of natural experiments that, as we have already mentioned, have played an important part in the history of psychiatric genetics and continue to provide vital tools. Essentially, twin and adoption studies tell us whether traits running in families result from shared genes, shared environment or a combination of the two.

NATURAL EXPERIMENTS

Monozygotic (MZ) or identical twins have all of their genes in common and share a common environment. Dizygotic (DZ) or fraternal twins share, on average, half of their genes and again share a common environment. Assuming that common environmental effects are as influential in DZ as in MZ pairs, any greater similarity regarding a given trait in MZ pairs should reflect the influence of genes. Although this "equal environments" assumption has been criticized—because MZ twins may, for example, more often dress alike and share friends than DZ twins—various checks suggest that it is generally valid [1]. Twin studies have been important in demonstrating a genetic contribution to disorders such as schizophrenia [13], depression [14, 15] and manic-depressive disorder [16], as well as measures of normal behaviour such as cognitive ability as measured by IQ tests [17], and personality as measured by questionnaires [1]. Twin studies have also been important in locating a strong genetic contribution to childhood disorders such as attention deficit hyperactivity disorder (ADHD) [18] and autism [19], which in the comparatively recent past had been attributed largely to bad parenting. Some examples of twin study results are summarized in Figure 1.1, where resemblance is expressed as a correlation coefficient. The other commonly used statistic for summarizing resemblance in clinically ascertained samples is probandwise concordance, that is, the proportion of co-twins index cases (or probands) who are affected. Most of the syndromes shown in the figure show a clear MZ/DZ difference favouring a genetic contribution, whereas for others, such as bulimic behaviour and disabling fatigue in childhood, there is evidence of familiality, that is, there are positive correlations, but there are less clear genetic effects. In other words, there are only modest differences in the MZ and DZ correlations.

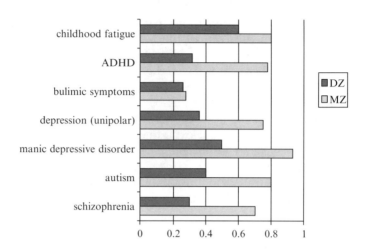

FIGURE 1.1 Monozygotic (MZ) and dizygotic (DZ) twin similarity expressed as correlations. Adapted from [8]

It is also worth noting that twin studies provide one of the most convincing pieces of evidence that environment influences behaviour. MZ twins who are "natural" clones of each other have only about a 70% correlation in liability for schizophrenia, and approximately the same is true if we take a normal trait such as IQ, where again the observed correlation in MZ twins is 70%, not 100% [17]. The effect of environment is perhaps even more striking if we consider discordance for particular disorders. For example, if one member of an MZ pair has a disorder such as schizophrenia [20] or depression [14], the risk of the other twin developing the same disorder is somewhat under 50%.

Another important approach to using twins to explore the effects of genes and environment on a complex trait is to focus on twins reared apart. In particular, identical twins who have been separated very early in life should, in theory, provide very clear evidence of the extent to which a trait is influenced by genes. In practice, the study of reared-apart identical (MZA) twins presents a number of problems. The most important is that MZA twins are rare, and it is not usually possible to ascertain a series of such twins in a systematic fashion. Thus, whereas twins reared together can be collected using hospital-based or population-based registers, most MZA series have depended on advertising for volunteer twins to come forward, which introduces the possible bias of those twins who are least dissimilar presenting for study. There is also the problem that if MZA twins are rare, those pairs where at least one individual has suffered from a particular disorder will be rarer still. Therefore, studies of reared-apart twins tended to focus on continuous characteristics within the normal range, such as IQ or personality, and here they have played an important role in confirming that there are substantial genetic effects [17].

ADOPTION STUDIES

For many, adoption studies offer a more convincing separation of the effects of genes and environment than do twin studies and, as we have already noted, adoption studies had an important role historically in turning the tide towards a more biological view of schizophrenia. However, because of the difficulties in carrying out adoption studies, they have been used much less than twin studies in investigating the genetics of behaviour. There are three principal designs, all of which have been used in studies of schizophrenia and which are summarized in Table 1.1.

Adoption studies have also had an important role in contributing to the evidence that genes play a part in antisocial behaviour, alcoholism and affective disorders. However, in the case of affective disorders, the pattern of findings has been less than clear-cut. Thus, in contrast to twin studies, all of which point to a genetic contribution, some of the adoption studies are inconclusive, and this seems at least in part a result of the fact that they have relied upon indirect sources of information rather than direct examination of the subject themselves [15].

MODELS OF INHERITANCE

One thing is clear from observing the patterns of inheritance of common psychiatric disorders and this is that usually we are not dealing with simple Mendelian traits. Although some neuropsychiatric diseases such as Huntington's disease and certain early-onset subtypes of familial AD show simple dominant inheritance, these are the rare exceptions rather than the rule. The patterns of segregation within families and the less than 100% concordance in MZ twins show that we are dealing with conditions that require more complex explanations of their inheritance than is allowed by classical Mendelian theory.

The most straightforward approach is to invoke the notion of incomplete penetrance. Penetrance can be defined as the probability of manifesting a phenotype given a particular genotype. Under Mendelian inheritance, penetrance is always either 0 or 1. Thus, in Table 1.2 we consider a disease (or more generally, a present/absent trait) where there is autosomal inheritance at a single locus with two alleles A_1 and A_2. There are therefore three genotypes, as shown in the table, and if A_1 is the normal or wild-type allele and A_2 is the disease or mutant allele, under a dominant model the heterozygotes

TABLE 1.1 The three main adoption study designs as exemplified by studies of schizophrenia

Study	Type of study	Diagnosis	Genetic relatives of a patient with schizophrenia	Not genetically related to a schizophrenic
Heston [5]	Adoptee	Schizophrenia	10.6% of 47 adoptees who had a schizophrenic biological mother	0% of 50 control adoptees
Rosenthal et al. [21]	Adoptee	Schizophrenia spectrum disorder	18.8% of 69 children of schizophrenics raised by normals	10.1% of 79 control adoptees
Tienari [22]	Adoptee	Any form of psychosis	9% of 138 adoptees who had a schizophrenic biological parent	1.2% of 171 control adoptees
Wender et al. [23]	Cross-fostering	Schizophrenia spectrum disorder	18.8% of 69 children of schizophrenics raised by normals	10.7% of 28 children of controls raised by future schizophrenics
Kety [6], Kety et al. [24]	Adoptee's family: national sample (47 chronic schizophrenic adoptees)	Chronic and latent (DSM-II) schizophrenics	15.8% of 279 biological relatives of adopted-away schizophrenics	1.8% of 228 adoptive relatives of schizophrenics and relatives of control adoptees

TABLE 1.2   Present/absent traits and the general single major locus model

Genotypes	A_1A_1	A_1A_2	A_2A_2
Penetrances			
Dominant	0	1	1
Recessive	0	0	1
General	$0 < f_1 < 1$	$0 < f_2 < 1$	$0 < f_3 < 1$
Frequency of genotype	$(1 - q)^2$	$2(1-q)q$	q^2
Population frequency of trait	$f_1(1 - q)^2$	$+f_2 2(1 - q)q$	$+f_3 q^2$

and the A_2A_2 homozygotes will show the disorder, whereas under a recessive model only the A_2A_2 homozygotes are affected. A more general model, called the two-allele single major locus (SML) model, allows the penetrances to have any value f_i that is between 0 and 1. In the table, the assumption is made that the frequency of the genotypes conforms to Hardy–Weinberg equilibrium [25]. Therefore, the frequency of the disorder in the population is simply the sum of the frequencies of each of the genotypes multiplied by their respective penetrances.

General SML models of this type have been explored in the past as possible explanations of the inheritance of schizophrenia [26, 27] and bipolar affective disorder [28]. However, the classic Slater–Cowie model of schizophrenia has been shown to give a very poor statistical fit to observed data [29], and the more recent studies strongly suggest that neither of these conditions show patterns of transmission that can be explained either by a single gene with incomplete penetrance, or by a collection of single genes each having incomplete penetrance [30, 31]. Nevertheless, the general SML model remains of both theoretical and practical importance, as the basis on which complex diseases are modelled in genetic linkage analysis, which will be discussed later.

By contrast, models assuming that there are combined effects of multiple genes tend to provide more satisfactory explanations of the available data [32]. It is assumed that *liability to a disease* is a (usually unobserved) continuous variable that is contributed to by multiple genes plus environmental effects. Liability would thus tend to be normally distributed in the population and only those individuals whose liability at some point in time exceeds a certain threshold manifest the disorder [33]. The relatives of affected individuals will have an increased liability compared with the general population, so that more of them will fall beyond the threshold for being affected. Knowing the proportion of affected individuals in the population, and the proportion among a certain class of relatives, allows the calculation of the correlation in liability [33, 34].

Knowing the correlations in liability for MZ and DZ twins allows model fitting to estimate how much genes and environment contribute to a trait. In the most straightforward, "ACE", model it is assumed that a trait is contributed to by additive genetic effects (A) resulting from several, perhaps many, genes at different loci, effects resulting from a common or shared environment (C) that increase the resemblance between members of a twin or sibling pair, and non-shared environment (E). Non-shared environment is specific to the individual and therefore tends to make twins or siblings differ from each other (in practice, estimates of this term also include measurement error and so E is sometimes also referred to as "residual environment"). The methods used to fit such models nowadays employ an approach called structural equation modelling [35]. Structural equation models can be used to explore the relationship between observed variables, i.e. phenotypes, in terms of underlying unobserved (or latent) variables including genotypes and shared or residual environment. This can be represented by a path diagram such as Figure 1.2. In classic path analysis [36], the expected values of the correlations between pairs of observed variables can be written down as the sum of the permitted paths connecting them. In Figure 1.2, the connecting paths between phenotypes 1 and 2 sum to give a correlation $r = \beta h^2 + c^2$. Where the individuals represented by phenotypes 1 and 2 are MZ twins, $\beta = 1$, and where they are DZ twins, $\beta = \frac{1}{2}$. Thus, where information is available on both types of twin, we would have two observations allowing a solution to the equations for the two unknowns h^2 and c^2.

In practice nowadays, when working with continuous data, it is more common to fit models using covariance matrices [35].

Figure 1.3 summarizes recent model fitting results for various traits and disorders. There are two striking findings. The first is that nearly all behaviours that have been studied showed moderate to high heritability [37]; the second is that although environment plays a role, this tends to be of the non-shared type. That is, environmental factors that make people different from

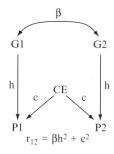

FIGURE 1.2 A simple univariate structural equation model

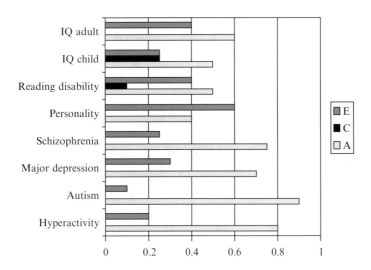

FIGURE 1.3   Estimates of genetic and environmental effects from recent twin studies. A is additive genetic variance, or heritability, C is variance explained by shared environment and E is variance resulting from non-shared environment and errors of measurement. Adapted from [8]

their relatives rather than similar to them (E) are more often involved in shaping behaviour than are shared environmental effects (C).

Although the polygenic/multifactorial model, as represented by the ACE model, appears for most psychiatric traits to be a better approximation to reality than single-gene models, there are further complications that need to be taken into account. One of these is shown in Figure 1.3 with respect to cognitive ability or IQ, where C, common environment, has a significant role in childhood, while in adult life, particularly in older adults, this appears not to be the case [17]. Thus, as we get older, our resemblance to our relatives with respect to IQ appears increasingly to result from the genes that we share with them rather than from the environments that we have in common. A similar pattern of increasing heritability and a decreasing role for common environment from childhood through to adolescent and adult life also appears to be the case for depressive symptoms [38] and antisocial behaviour [39].

Another complication is that, although standard classification schemes such as ICD-10 and DSM-IV attempt to define discrete and mutually exclusive categories, in real life there is a tendency for patients to have the symptoms of more than one disorder or even fulfil the diagnostic criteria for two or more disorders. An example of disorders that frequently occur together are anxiety and depression. Model-fitting approaches using bivariate analysis, i.e. investigating the co-occurrence of two disorders in twins rather than analysing one disorder at a time, suggest that the genes contributing to anxiety and depression are mainly the same [38, 40] and that the different phenotypic manifestations are strongly influenced by the environment.

There is also evidence that, in certain behavioural traits, genes and environment may be correlated. One mechanism is that certain genotypes predispose the individual to seek out certain environments. For example, those with the better innate abilities in, say, sport, music or general academic skills may be more likely to choose environments in which their talents can flourish [1]. There may also be gene–environment interactions that differ from simple gene plus environment co-action. One example of this is antisocial behaviour. It has been shown that adoptees with a biological parent who exhibited antisocial behaviour tended themselves to show antisocial behaviour when raised in adverse environments. In contrast, in those adoptees who did not have an antisocial biological parent, the frequency of antisocial personality did not differ between those raised in favourable and those raised in unfavourable social circumstances [41].

A more complicated example, where so far it has been difficult to tease out gene–environment correlation and gene–environment interaction completely, concerns the relationship between genes, life events and depression. A study by McGuffin *et al.* [42] produced the initially surprising finding that the relatives of depressed index cases not only had an increased risk of depression but also had higher rates of life events than the general population. Subsequent twin studies confirmed the familiality of life events [14, 43, 44]. Although part of the familiality of life events can be explained by the same life event impinging on more than one member of the family [45], this does not offer a complete explanation for all categories of events, and in particular those events that have variously been classified as "dependent" or "controllable" seem to be partly influenced by genetic factors [14, 43]. There is even some evidence that part of the overlap between depressive symptoms and life events can be explained by the fact that the ways that subjects report both are partly influenced by the same genes [46]. This is an area where more work is required, but where the data so far tell us that the interplay between genes and environment is much more complex than it appears at first sight.

Finally, gene–gene interactions present a further complication beyond simple additive models. The most familiar interaction is between two alternative genes or alleles at the same locus—the phenomenon of dominance—but in addition there may be interaction between genes at different loci—the phenomenon called "epistasis". Whereas purely additive polygenic models predict that the similarity or correlation between relatives is in direct proportion to the number of genes that they share, epistasis will tend to exaggerate the similarity between relatives who share a high proportion of genes. For example, the pattern seen in schizophrenia, where MZ twins show around 50% concordance, DZ twins or first-degree relatives show around 10–15% concordance, and the rate in second-degree or more distant relatives falls to 3 or 4%, may reflect the epistatic interactions of several loci [47]. A statistical study of the familial aggregation of autism has also suggested epistasis [48], and the phenomenon could be widespread in polygenic systems that influence behaviour.

MOLECULAR GENETIC APPROACHES

The implication of the finding that genes play a substantial, albeit complicated, role in common psychiatric disorders, and most normal behaviours, is that it should be possible to find and identify such genes. The dramatic advances over the past three decades in using genetic markers to chart the human genome—23 pairs of chromosomes on which our genetic material is carried—are summarized in Box 1.1. The first draft sequence of the entire human genome was published in 2000, and a more detailed initial sequencing and analysis of the human genome [49] shows that there are about 32 000–40 000 protein-coding genes in the human genome. Although this is half as many as was once thought and only about twice as many as in worms or flies, it remains an enormous task to search through them and find the genes involved in psychiatric disorders.

Broadly, there are two conventional approaches to identifying the genes involved in complex traits. These are candidate gene studies and positional cloning. "Candidate genes" are those that encode for proteins that might be involved in a trait or disorder. Since at least half of all genes are expressed in the brain, the potential number of candidates is overwhelming and has to be narrowed down by informed guesswork. In psychiatric disorders, useful leads may be provided by the mode of action of drugs. For example, all the standard drug treatments used in schizophrenia (e.g. chlorpromazine or

---

Box 1.1   Progress in gene mapping

1970s: "Classical" markers (6% coverage of genome)
1980: The "New Genetics" and restriction fragment length polymorphisms (RFLPs)
1987: (Nearly) complete linkage map (95%)
1990: Microsatellites
1996: Comprehensive map (100%)
1999: Single nucleotide polymorphism (SNP) consortium set up
2000: > 200 000 SNPs on map
2001: 1.42 million SNPs

haloperidol) are known to block dopamine D2 receptors, while the newer "atypical" antipsychotics, such as clozapine or olanzapine, block both dopamine receptors and serotonin receptors, particularly 5HT2A. There have now been numerous studies comparing the frequency of polymorphisms (variants) in the 5HT2A receptor gene in schizophrenic and control subjects. Although not all results are clear-cut, a meta-analysis suggests a small but significant effect in conferring susceptibility to schizophrenia of allele 2 of a bi-allelic polymorphism (T102C) found in the first exon or coding region of the gene. Although T102C is in an exon, it appears to be a "silent" polymorphism, i.e. it does not result in an amino acid change in the protein. It is therefore likely that the effect of the variant on susceptibility to schizophrenia results from another polymorphism that is nearby. For example, it is has been shown that there is a polymorphism in the promoter region of the gene, where the same allele is always found in combination with the 5HT2A T102C allele 2 [50], a phenomenon called linkage disequilibrium.

Among dopamine receptor genes studied in relation to schizophrenia, there has been greatest interest in the DRD3, one of the D2-like family. Although, again, results are somewhat conflicting, a matter analysis overall shows a significant association with being homozygotic for a polymorphism in the first exon of DRD3 [51]. Neither DRD3 or 5HT2A variance on their own is sufficient to cause schizophrenia, but it seems likely that both are part of the set of polygenes that contribute to liability to the disorders.

Similarly, the most effective medication in ADHD, methylphenidate, is known to increase the availability of dopamine in the brain, and a polymorphism in a different dopamine receptor, DRD4, has been shown in several studies to be associated with the disorder [45, 52].

The above examples using candidate gene approaches have all used an allelic association design. In its simplest form, an allelic association study just compares the frequency of a particular marker allele or a haplotype (two or more alleles at closely adjacent loci carried on the same chromosome) in a sample of cases with the frequency in a sample of control subjects. Until recently, association studies were essentially confined to candidate genes. More systematic genome searching depended (and to a large extent still does depend) on detection of a related but slightly different phenomenon, genetic linkage. Linkage detection provides the starting point for positional cloning. This approach to identifying genes makes use of the fact that there are now excellent marker maps available, with polymorphisms providing thousands of approximately equally spaced reference points spread throughout the 23 pairs of chromosomes. The classic starting point for positional cloning is to collect a set of families containing multiple members affected by a disorder and to detect genetic linkage. Linkage occurs when a pair of gene loci are close together on the same chromosome and fail to follow Mendel's law of independent disorder. That is, within families, the same alleles are found together more than would be expected by chance (although it may be different alleles in different families). In gene mapping studies, the genome is measured in units called centimorgans (cM). One cM corresponds to a pair of loci showing crossing over, or recombination, one meiosis in a hundred. Loci that are on different chromosomes or that are far apart on the same chromosome show crossing over half of the time; that is, they obey Mendel's law and assort at a frequency no higher than chance. Loci that are close together tend to depart from chance assortment and, within certain limits, the frequency of recombination between loci is proportional to the physical distance between them. The whole genome, averaged across the sexes, is about 3500 cM long, with 1 cM roughly corresponding to just under a megabase of DNA (or a million base pairs).

Linkage can be detected over relatively long distances—10 cM or more—so it is possible to mount a whole genome search using just a few hundred evenly spaced markers. The disadvantage of linkage is that it is capable only of detecting large effects. Linkage analysis is therefore straightforward in simple Mendelian disorders, such as Huntington's disease or early-onset AD (Table 1.3). However, in the case of complex traits, such as schizophrenia, it is more of a challenge [53]. Despite this, a number of regions of interest have been identified by more than one study. Furthermore, for another complex trait, reading disability, there appears to be a fairly high degree of consistency across linkage studies. In particular, there have been notable successes in the detection of loci on chromosomes 6 [54–56] and 15 [57]. There is also reasonable consistency in linkage studies on childhood autism. In particular, several groups have reported evidence of a locus on chromosome 7 [58].

One of the difficulties that has beset attempts to detect linkage in psychiatric disorders and other common diseases is that the mode of transmission is unknown. That is, the disease does not follow a simple Mendelian pattern of segregation in families. The standard statistical approach to detecting linkage and to estimating recombination is to calculate LOD (log of the odds) scores [59]. A LOD scores the common log of the ratio of the probability that the recombination fraction has a certain value, $\theta < 0.5$, to the probability that $\theta = 5$. The LOD scores are calculated for a range of values of θ from 0 to 5 and the value that gives the maximum LOD is taken as the most likely value of θ. By convention, a LOD of 3 or more is accepted as providing sufficient support for linkage and a LOD of -2 or less excludes linkage. Unfortunately, LOD scores were originally intended for use with simple traits. Using the general SML approach described earlier, it is possible to adapt the LOD method to traits that do not show simple Mendelian patterns, but this requires correct specification of the parameters defining the model, the penetrances and the gene frequency (Table 1.1) for the particular disease. Otherwise, at best the estimation of recombination will be incorrect, and at worst linkage will not be detected even when it is present [60].

TABLE 1.3 Some behavioural disorders and traits, their pattern of inheritance and the status of gene mapping studies. Adapted from [8]

Behavioural trait	Pattern of inheritance	Gene mapping
Huntington's disease	Rare autosomal dominant dynamic mutation	Gene identified (huntingtin) with unstable trinucleotide repeat.
Early-onset (familial) Alzheimer's disease	Rare autosomal dominant	Three distinct genes identified (presenilins 1 and 2, and amyloid precursor protein).
Fragile X mental retardation	Non-standard X-linked dynamic mutation	Two genes identified (FMR1 and 2), both with unstable trinucleotide repeats.
Late-onset Alzheimer's disease	Common complex	Increased risk with apolipoprotein ε4 allele firmly established.
Attention deficit hyperactivity disorder	Common complex	Three contributory loci in the dopamine system, DRD4, DAT1 and DRD5; DRD4 best replicated, others less certain.
Dyslexia	Common complex	Two contributory loci suggested on chromosomes 6 and 15; findings replicated.
Schizophrenia	Common complex	Numerous reported linkages including chromosomes 1, 5, 6, 10, 13, 15 and 22 but no consensus; a few promising candidate genes include 5-HT2A and CHRNA7.
Aggression	Common complex	Mutation reported in X-linked MAO-A gene in one family; no evidence of broader relevance.
Male homosexuality	Common complex	Association reported at X-linked marker locus in sib pairs; not replicated.

Other problems include possible genetic heterogeneity in common disorders and lack of precision in defining who is affected or unaffected (not a problem with clear-cut cases or clearly healthy family members, but a difficulty with relatives who have "spectrum" disorders). The most straightforward way of dealing with these problems has been to concentrate on extended multiplex pedigrees, i.e. families with many affected members, to make an informed guess at the mode of transmission and to assume that, even if there is heterogeneity in the disorder as a whole, there is homogeneity within each family. These simplifying assumptions have worked well with some common diseases. Most notable among psychiatric successes has been AD (Table 1.3). However, in other disorders, such as schizophrenia, concentration on large multiplex families has produced less clear results and there has been a move toward alternative approaches, such as focusing on affected sib pairs [51]. Affected sib pairs may be more representative of a common disorder generally than subjects from multiplex pedigrees and they lend themselves to "model-free" methods of analysis. This depends on the fact that at any given locus the probabilities of a pair of siblings inheriting zero, one or two alleles identical by descent from their parents are respectively ¼, ½ and ¼. Greater allele sharing than would be expected by chance in pairs of sibs who are both affected by the disease suggests that the locus is close to a gene conferring susceptibility to the disease.

A disadvantage of sib pair methods is that the price paid for simplicity and robustness is a comparative lack of power. Whatever the method used, both practical experience and simulation studies [61] suggest that, unless the sample sizes are extremely large, linkage is difficult to detect with genes that confer a relative risk of a disorder of much less than about 3 or account for less than around 10% of the variation in liability. Genes with effects that are that large may be rare in common diseases. For example, a genome scan for linkage in schizophrenia in almost 200 families effectively excluded a gene having a relative risk of 3 from most of the genome [51].

The need to detect genes having only small effects has brought about a renewed interest in allelic association in a more systematic fashion, that is, not just focusing on potential candidate genes. As noted, association is the phenomenon whereby a particular allele at a marker locus is found together with a trait or disorder more than would be expected by chance. In contrast with linkage, the same allele is found across the population (rather than just within particular families). The simplest study design is just to compare allelic frequency between affected cases and controls. It has long been known that association can detect genes that account for as little as 1% of the variance in a trait [62]. However, association only occurs either if the marker itself confers liability to a disorder or the marker and the disease susceptibility locus are so close together that there is linkage disequilibrium (LD), that is, association is undisturbed over many generations of recombination.

One of the hazards of association studies is recent admixtures of populations, which can result in a phenomenon called stratification. This occurs when two ethnic groups have different frequencies of the disease or trait being studied and also have different frequencies of marker alleles. Consequently, in mixed populations from these groups there may be a spurious association unless cases and controls are carefully matched for ethnicity. To overcome the need to carry out case–control matching, which may be very difficult in some highly admixed populations where there has been much recent immigration, one can use family-based methods with "internal" controls. For example, the transmission disequilibrium test (TDT) [63] depends on at least one parent of each affected subject being heterozygous at the marker locus and compares the frequency of affected offspring to whom a particular allele is transmitted with the frequency of those who do not receive that allele.

Another issue to do with control selection if family-based methods are not used is whether to rigorously exclude affected individuals (or those with a family history of the disorder) from the control sample. Doing careful screening of controls obviously increases the time and costs of association studies. It turns out that for comparatively uncommon disorders—those with a population frequency of 1% or less—power is not much reduced by failing to screen out affected individuals from the control group, whereas for common disorders, with a frequency of 10% or more, it pays in terms of maximizing power to carefully screen controls for the disorder [64].

In most populations LD can only be detected over very short distances: hence thousands not hundreds of markers are needed to carry out the genome scan for LD. There is considerable current debate over the approximate number of markers that would be required to perform a thorough genome scan by LD. One controversial suggestion based on simulations is that it might be as many as 500 000 [65]. However, some empirical studies have shown that LD can readily be detected in moderately outbred populations over a distance up to 1 cM [66]. Although LD is not evenly distributed across the genome, this would mean that a few thousand markers would suffice for a first trawl. Even so, until recently a genome search using this number of markers was not feasible (and hence, as we have noted, association studies were restricted to candidate genes). However, now maps based on thousands of polymorphisms of a type called short sequence repeats are already available, and a map based upon hundreds of thousands of single nucleotide polymorphisms (SNPs) is rapidly being developed. Linkage and association are compared in Table 1.4 and are best regarded as complementary rather than competing strategies in complex diseases [67].

The implication of carrying out a genome search using LD is that very large amounts of genotyping must be carried out. New methods of high-throughput genotyping are being developed that can accomplish this based on a variety of methods to detect SNPs on microarrays, using mass spectrometry, or other methods such as denaturing high-performance liquid chromatography (dHPLC) [68]. Another approach is to use DNA pooling, where the first stage involves combined analysis of the pooled DNA of all of the cases and compares the results with findings on the pooled DNA of all of the controls. Any differences are then checked out by individual

TABLE 1.4   A comparison of linkage and association

Linkage	Association
Uses families	Uses cases and controls or families with "internal controls"
Detectable over large distances, >10 cM	Detectable only over very small distances, 1 cM or much less
Can usually only detect fairly large effects, e.g. a relative risk >2 or >10% of variance	Capable of detecting small effects, e.g. odds ratios <2 or as little as 1% of variance

genotyping [69]. The first "top-to-bottom" searches of whole chromosomes using DNA pooling had been published as a part of a search for genes involved in cognitive ability [56, 70]. With such technical advances, the problems of genome-wide searches using LD are beginning to appear tractable.

The classic approach to positional cloning, once a region of interest has been identified, involves a combination of molecular techniques, including physically cutting the DNA from the region into smaller, more manageable pieces. These are then cloned into a vector such as yeast or bacteria. Now, because of advances resulting from the human genome project, much of the hard work of positional cloning has been replaced by cloning by computer ("cloning *in silica*"). Thus, genome sequence, gene sequence or even identification of polymorphisms can be achieved by searching appropriate databases.

Ultimately, the combination of ever more complete information on the genome sequence, the genes and the control elements contained therein, together with ready accessibility via computers attached to the Internet,

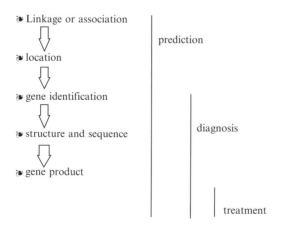

FIGURE 1.4   A schematic representation of positional cloning

means that the genes involved in psychiatric disorders and even those involved in normal behaviours will be tracked down and identified. The systematic genome search approach and candidate gene strategies will, in effect, converge very rapidly once all genes have been definitely identified and characterized. This will occur because all genes that are expressed in the brain can be considered as candidates, and SNPs, including those in coding regions (cSNPs), together with SNPs in promoter regions, will become the obvious targets for association studies. Even if the number of these is large, as is likely to be the case, high-throughput genotyping methods will make such studies practicable. The only obstacle, therefore, to detecting and identifying genes of even small effect will be having samples of DNA from well-characterized populations. This means that assembling large-scale collections of cases, controls and families containing affected individuals and making this material available to the research community is likely to entail a massive combined effort from multiple centres. The outcome of such research is likely to have a very profound implication for the scientific and clinical development of psychiatry in the twenty-first century.

IMPACT OF GENETICS ON PSYCHIATRY IN THE TWENTY-FIRST CENTURY

The first area that is likely to receive an important impact from what we can now call "behavioural genomics" [8] is an improved understanding of the neurobiology of disease. Currently, not only do we have a draft of the human genome, but there are also complete genome sequences available on databases of over 60 species [71]. Comparing genomes across species and noting differences in those genes that have been conserved will show the major variations between species and offer an understanding of the basis for a biological evolution. Knowing the structure and function of all human genes has been compared with discovering a "periodic table of life" [71]. It paves the way for a series of paradigm shifts where the emphasis moves from the structure of the genome to a functional genomics and to proteomics, the study of proteins at a functional level. A striking example of how one complex aspect of human behaviour, circadian rhythms, can be dissected and its basis understood at a molecular level is given by the recent discovery of new "clock" genes simply by analysis of the draft sequence of the human genome, searching for genes with a high similarity to known clock genes originally discovered in mice or fruit flies [72].

Even before the publication of the draft sequence of the human genome, discoveries arrived at by positional cloning in AD had begun to provide important new understandings of neuropathological mechanisms, as described in Chapter 9 of this volume. Although AD has a characteristic neuropathology that was described at the beginning of the twentieth century, the problem of uncovering its pathogenesis did not appear to have a tractable solution until the discovery of the role of mutations in amyloid precursor protein and the presenilin genes. Interestingly, although presenilin 1 on chromosome 14 was identified by positional cloning, presenilin 2 was discovered essentially by its homology with presenilin 1 and subsequently demonstrated to have an aetiological role by linkage analysis. As with the discovery of new clock genes, we can expect the discovery of families of genes involved in abnormal and normal behaviours to become more commonplace.

Identification of the genes and gene products involved in psychiatric disorders should have very important implications for pharmacotherapy in two ways. The first of these is in directing drug discovery [73]. At present the drugs used in the treatment of psychiatric or other central nervous system diseases have their actions at a limited number of target sites that include cell surface receptors, nuclear receptors, ion channels and enzymes. It is likely that detecting the genes involved in the pathogenesis of psychiatric disorders will identify new targets, some of which fall within these categories, but will include others that have thus far not been included as target sites of drug action. In addition to targeting of treatments, advances in genomics will allow tailoring of treatments. There is already some evidence that response to atypical antipsychotics such as clozapine is influenced by the individual's 5HT2A genotype [74]. It is also well established that the rate at which most psychoactive drugs are metabolized is influenced by genetic factors, in particular genes in the cytochrome P450 system, of which variants in the CYP2D6 gene have particular importance. This may be relevant to the development of side effects as well as to treatment response [75]. This whole area of pharmacogenetics is still comparatively novel, but holds enormous potential for individual tailoring of treatments that will be a major advance on current trial and error approaches.

There has been a degree of public concern that the current pace of advance will tend to "geneticize" common diseases and encourage deterministic attitudes. In particular, worries have been expressed that insurance companies may wish to force DNA testing on individuals thought to be at high genetic risk of disorder. While prediction with a high degree of accuracy is already possible for rare early-onset dementia such as Huntington's disease or the single-gene forms of AD, this is not possible for complex disorders. For example, the apolipoprotein ε4 allele, despite the confirmed association with risk of late-onset AD in the general population, is of limited value as a predictor at an individual level [10]. The situation is likely to prove even more complicated with disorders such as schizophrenia. At best, DNA-based tests may be used to modify the predicted risk in individuals who are already at high risk because of having a schizophrenic close relative. However, it is unlikely that risk prediction will ever be better than about 50% accurate, since genetically identical individuals, MZ twins, are discordant for schizophrenia 50% of the time. This means that DNA-based population screening for complex psychiatric disorders (including AD of late onset) will never become a reality, but the option of offering screening to high-risk individuals probably will, with the caveat that such testing will refine risk prediction but not give clear yes/no answers. Given that most common diseases, and not just psychiatric ones, will depend upon the combined action of multiple common gene variations together with environmental risk factors, batteries of genetic tests will be of limited usefulness to insurance companies and are not likely to be widely employed.

Finally, the other potentially worrying aspect of psychiatric disorders becoming "geneticized" is, it has been suggested, an increase in stigma. Of course, just the opposite could be the case, so that increasing knowledge about the causation of disorders may serve to demystify them and therefore make them, in the public eye, something that is more tangible and accept-able. Part of post-genomic psychiatry's impact on disorders such as schizo-phrenia, bipolar affective disorder and depression might therefore be to legitimize them as "real" diseases rather than, as is all too often the case, being seen as phenomena that result from personal failing or weakness. AD might be taken as a good example of how public perceptions clearly have changed. "Becoming senile" in old age was once seen by many as somehow morally reprehensible, whereas it is now acceptable for the families of a past President of the United States or a famous novelist such Iris Murdoch to "come out" and admit that they suffer from AD. In the present author's view, this could turn out to be a general effect. Therefore, rather than an increasing stigma, it is quite possible that the ultimate effect of genetic research on the public image of psychiatric diseases will be wholly positive.

CONCLUSIONS

Psychiatric genetics is a field of research that has expanded rapidly in recent years, but it has a history almost as long as that of the field of genetics as a whole. Indeed, the recognition that mental illness runs in families probably dates back to ancient times. Despite this, genetic studies of psychiatric disorders have often been the subject of controversy and debate, largely arising from a misplaced notion that the involvement of genes in a disorder necessarily means that the causes are predetermined and that once the disorder develops it will be fixed and immutable. On the contrary genetic studies such as those on twins provide probably the most compelling evidence available that most psychiatric disorders have a substantial contribution from environmental factors. With the exception of some comparatively rare Mendelian disorders, the disorders that present in psychiatric clinics involve the effects of multiple genes that, together with environmental factors, confer a liability to disease rather than a certainty of illness. For most disorders which have been thoroughly researched, these environmental effects appear to be largely or totally of the non-shared (or non-familial) type. That is, the familial aggregation of most disorders is explained by shared genes and very little, if any, by shared environment.

Attempts to locate and identify genes involved in common psychiatric disorders are impeded by the multifactorial nature of the conditions and by the fact that most of the genes involved, by themselves, only have small effects. Nevertheless, technical advances in gene mapping and sequencing of the human genome, leading to the eventual identification of all common variants in all genes, makes it a virtual certainty that the genes involved in all common disorders will be identified. This will have important implications for our understanding of the neurobiological underpinnings of psychiatric disorders, for the discovery of new drug treatments, and the replacement of current trial-and-error presciption of medication with individually tailored treatments. There are also important implications for the general public perception of psychiatric disorders, which are more difficult to predict, but in my view these will turn out to be beneficial.

REFERENCES

1. Plomin R., DeFries J., McClearn G., McGuffin P. (2001) *Behavioral Genetics*, 4th ed., Freeman, San Francisco.
2. Cardno A., McGuffin P. (1999) Psychiatric genetics. In *A Century of Psychiatry*, Vol. 2 (Ed. H. Freeman), pp. 343–347, Mosby-Wolfe Medical Communications, London.
3. Farmer A.E., McGuffin P. (1999) Ethics and psychiatric genetics. *Psychiatric Ethics*, 3rd ed. (Ed. S. Bloch), pp. 479–493, Oxford University Press, New York.
4. Shields J., Gottesman I.I. (1971) *Man, Mind and Heredity: Selected Papers of Eliot Slater on Psychiatry and Genetics*, Johns Hopkins Press, Baltimore.
5. Heston L.L. (1966) Psychiatric disorders in foster home reared children of schizophrenic mothers. *Br. J. Psychiatry*, 112: 819–825.
6. Kety S.S. (1983) Mental illness in the biological and adoptive relatives of schizophrenic adoptees, findings relevant to genetic and environmental factors in etiology. *Am. J. Psychiatry*, 140: 720–727.
7. Weatherall D.J. (1984) DNA in medicine. Implications for medical practice and human biology. *Lancet*, 2: 1440–1444.
8. McGuffin P., Riley B., Plomin R. (2001) Toward behavioral genomics. *Science*, 291: 1232–1233.
9. Masters C.L., Beyreuther K. (2000) Genetic basis of resistance to Alzheimer's disease and related neurodegenerative diseases. In *Genes and Resistance to Disease* (Eds V. Boulyjenkov, K. Berg, Y. Chrisen), pp. 121–131, Foundation IPSEN, Paris.

10. Liddell M.B., Lovestone S., Owen M.J. (2001) Genetic risk of Alzheimer's disease: advising relatives. *Br. J. Psychiatry*, **178**: 7–11.
11. Edwards J.H. (1960) The simulation of Mendelism. *Acta Genet.*, **10**: 63–70.
12. McGuffin P., Huckle P. (1990) Simulation of Mendelism revisited: the recessive gene for attending medical school. *Am. J. Hum. Genet.*, **46**: 994–999.
13. McGuffin P., Owen M.J., Farmer A.E. (1995) The genetic basis of schizophrenia. *Lancet*, **346**: 678–682.
14. McGuffin P., Katz R., Rutherford J., Watkins S. (1996) A hospital based twin register of the heritability of DSM-IV unipolar depression. *Arch. Gen. Psychiatry*, **53**: 129–136.
15. Sullivan P.F., Neale M., Kendler K.S. (2000) Genetic epidemiology of major depression: review and meta-analysis. *Am. J. Psychiatry*, **157**: 1552–1562.
16. Craddock N., Jones I. (1999) Genetics of bipolar disorder. *J. Med. Genet.*, **36**: 585–594.
17. Bouchard T.J. (1998) Genetic and environmental influences on adult intelligence and special mental abilities. *Hum. Biol.*, **70**: 257–280.
18. Thapar A., Harrington R., Ross K., McGuffin P. (2000) Does the definition of ADHD affect heritability? *J. Am. Acad. Child Adolesc. Psychiatry*, **39**: 1528–1536.
19. Bailey A., Phillips W., Rutter M. (1996) Autism: towards an integration of clinical, genetic, neuropsychological, and neurobiological perspectives. *J. Child Psychol. Psychiatry*, **37**: 89–126.
20. Cardno A.G., Gottesman I.I. (2000) Twin studies of schizophrenia: from bow-and-arrow concordances to star wars mx and functional genomics. *Am. J. Med. Genet.*, **97**: 12–17.
21. Rosenthal D., Wender P.H., Kety S.S., Schulsinger F., Welner J., Østergaard L. (1968) Schizophrenics' offspring reared in adoptive homes. In *The Transmission of Schizophrenia* (Eds D. Rosenthal, S.S. Kety), pp. 377–391, Pergamon Press, Oxford.
22. Tienari F. (1991) Gene–environment interaction in adoptive families. In *Search for the Causes of Schizophrenia*, Vol. 2 (Eds H. Hafner and W.F. Gattaz), pp. 126–143, Springer, Berlin.
23. Wender P.H., Rosenthal D., Kety S.S., Schulsinger F., Welner J. (1974) Cross-fostering. A research strategy for clarifying the role of genetic and experimental factors in the etiology of schizophrenia. *Arch. Gen. Psychiatry*, **30**: 121–128.
24. Kety S.S., Wender P.H., Jacobsen B., Ingraham L.J., Jansson L., Faber B., Kinney D.K. (1994) Mental illness in the biological and adoptive relatives of schizophrenic adoptees: replication of the Copenhagen study in the rest of Denmark. *Arch. Gen. Psychiatry*, **51**: 442–455.
25. Falconer D.S., Mackay F.C. (1996) *Introduction to Quantitative Genetics*, Longman, Essex.
26. Slater E., Cowie V. (1971) *The Genetics of Mental Disorder*, Oxford University Press, London.
27. Elston R.C., Campbell M.A. (1970) Schizophrenia: evidence for the major gene hypothesis. *Behav. Genet.*, **1**: 101–106.
28. O'Rourke D., McGuffin P., Reich T. (1983) Genetic analysis of manic depressive illness. *Am. J. Phys. Anthropol.*, **62**: 51–59.
29. McGuffin P. (1990) Models of the heritability and genetic transmission. In *Search for the Causes of Schizophrenia*, Vol. 2 (Eds H. Hafner, W.F. Gattaz), pp. 109–125, Springer, Berlin.
30. O'Rourke D.H., Gottesman I.I., Al E. (1982) Refutation of the general single-locus model for the etiology of schizophrenia. *Am. J. Hum. Genet.*, **34**: 630–649.

31. Craddock N., Khodel V., Van Eerdewegh P., Reich T. (1995) Mathematical limits of multilocus models: the genetic transmission of bipolar disorder. *Am. J. Hum. Genet.*, **57**: 690–702.
32. Mcgue M., Bouchard T.J., Lykken D.T, Feuer D. (1984) Information-processing abilities in twins reared apart. *Intelligence*, **8**: 239–258.
33. Falconer D.S. (1965) The inheritance of liability to certain diseases, estimated from the incidence among relatives. *Ann. Hum. Genet.*, **29**: 51–76.
34. Reich T., James J.W., Morris C.A. (1972) The use of multiple thresholds in determining the mode of transmission of semi-continuous traits. *Ann. Hum. Genet.*, **36**: 163–184.
35. Neale M.C., Cardon L.R. (1990) *Methodology for Genetic Studies of Twins and Families*, Kluwer, Dordrecht.
36. Li C.C. (1975) *Path Analysis—A Primer*, Boxwood Press, California.
37. Plomin R., McClearn G.E., Gora-Maslak G. (1991) Use of recombinant inbred strains to detect quantitative trait loci associated with behavior. *Behav. Genet.*, **21**: 99–116.
38. Thapar A., McGuffin P. (1995) Are anxiety symptoms in childhood heritable? *J. Child Psychol. Psychiatry*, **36**: 439–447.
39. Lyons M.J., True W.R., Eisen A., Goldberg J., Meyer J.M., Faraone S.V., Eaves L.J., Tsuang M.T. (1995) Differential heritability of adult and juvenile antisocial traits. *Arch. Gen. Psychiatry*, **52**: 906–915.
40. Kendler K.S., Heath A.C., Martin N.G., Eaves L.J. (1987) Symptoms of anxiety and symptoms of depression. *Arch. Surg.*, **122**: 451–457.
41. Cadoret, R.J., Yates W.R., Troughton E., Woodworth G., Stewart M.A. (1995) Genetic-environmental interaction in the genesis of aggressivity and conduct disorders. *Arch. Gen. Psychiatry*, **52**: 916–924.
42. McGuffin P. (1988) Genetics of schizophrenia. In *Schizophrenia: The Major Issues*, (Eds P. Bebbington, P. McGuffin), pp. 107–126, Heinemann Medical, London.
43. Kendler K.S, Neale M., Kessler R., Heath A., Eaves L. (1993) A twin study of recent life events and difficulties. *Arch. Gen. Psychiatry*, **50**: 789–796.
44. Plomin R., Litchenstein P., Pedersen N.L., McClearn G.E., Nesselroade J.R. (1990) Genetic influences on life events during the last half of the life span. *Psychol. Aging*, **5**: 25–30.
45. Farmer A., Harris T., Redman K., Sadler S., Mahmood A., McGuffin P. (2000) The Cardiff Depression Study—a sib pair study of life events and familiality in major depression. *Br. J. Psychiatry*, **176**: 150–155.
46. Thapar A., Harold G., McGuffin P. (1998) Life events and depressive symptoms in childhood—shared genes or shared adversity? A research note. *J. Child Psychol. Psychiatry*, **39**: 1153–1158.
47. Risch N. (1990) Linkage strategies for genetically complex traits. III: The effect of marker polymorphism analysis on affected relative pairs. *Am. J. Hum. Genet.*, **46**: 242–253.
48. Pickles A., Bolton P., Macdonald H., Bailey A., Le Couteur A., Jordan H., Sim C.H., Rutter M. (1995) Latent class analysis of recurrence risks for complex phenotypes with selection and measurement error: a twin and family history study of autism. *Am. J. Hum. Genet.*, **57**: 717–726.
49. Anonymous (2000) Help in accessing human genome information. The International Human Genome Sequencing Consortium. *Science*, 289: 1471.
50. Spurlock G., Heils A., Holmans P., Williams J., D'Souz U.M., Cazdno A., Murphy K.C., Jones L., Buckland P.R., McGuffin P. *et al.* (1998) A family based association study of T102C polymorphism in 5HT2A and schizophrenia

plus identification of new polymorphisms in the promoter. *Mol. Psychiatry*, **3**: 42–49.

51. Williams J.T., Begleiter H., Porjesz B., Edenberg H.J., Foroud T., Reich T., Goate A., Eerdewegh P.V., Almasy L., Blangero J. (1999) Joint multipoint linkage analysis of multivariate qualitative and quantitative traits. II. Alcoholism and event-related potentials. *Am. J. Hum. Genet.*, **65**: 1148–1160.

52. Faraone S.V., Biederman J., Monuteaux M.C. (2000) Toward guidelines for pedigree selection in genetic studies of attention deficit hyperactivity disorder. *Genet. Epidemiol.*, **18**: 1–16.

53. Riley B.P., McGuffin P. (2000) Linkage and associated studies of schizophrenia. *Am. J. Med. Genet.*, **97**: 23–44.

54. Cardon L.R., Smith S.D., Fulker, D.W., Kimberling W.J., Pennington B.F., De Fries J.C. (1994) Quantitative trait locus for reading disability on chromosome 6. *Science*, **265**: 276–279.

55. Grigorenko E.L., Wood F.B., Meyer M.S., Hart L.A., Speed W.C., Shuster A., Pauls D.L. (1997) Susceptibility loci for distinct components for developmental dyslexia on chromosomes 6 and 15. *Am. J. Hum. Genet.*, **60**: 27–39.

56. Fisher P.J., Turic D., McGuffin P., Asherson P., Ball D., Craig I., Eley T., Hill L., Chorney K., Chorney M.J. *et al.* (1999) DNA pooling identifies QTLs for general cognitive ability in children on chromosome 4. *Hum. Mol. Genet.*, **8**: 915–922.

57. Schulte-Korne G., Grimm T., Nothen M.M., Muller-Myhsok B., Cichon S., Vogt I.R., Propping P., Remschmidt H. (1998) Evidence for linkage of spelling disability to chromosome 15. *Am. J. Hum. Genet.*, **63**: 279–282.

58. Rutter M., Silberg J., O'Connor T., Simonoff, E. (1999) Genetics and child psychiatry: I. Advances in quantitative and molecular genetics. *J. Child Psychol. Psychiatry*, **40**: 3–18.

59. Morton N.E. (1955) Sequential tests for the detection of linkage. *Am. J. Hum. Genet.*, **7**: 277–318.

60. Clerget-Darpoux F., Babron M.C., Bonaiti-Pellie C. (1990) Assessing the effect of multiple linkage tests in complex diseases. *Genet. Epidemiol.*, **7**: 245–253.

61. Risch N., Merikangas K. (1996) The future of genetic studies of complex human diseases. *Science*, **273**: 1516–1517.

62. Edwards T.H. (1965) The meaning of the associations between blood groups and disease. *Ann. Hum. Genet.*, **29**: 77–83.

63. Spielman R.S., Ewens W.J. (1996) The TDT and other family-based tests for linkage disequilibrium and association. *Am. J. Hum. Genet.*, **59**: 983–989.

64. Owen M.J., Holmans P., McGuffin P. (1997) Association studies in psychiatric genetics. *Mol. Psychiatry*, **2**: 270–273.

65. Kruglyak L. (1999) Prospects for whole-genome linkage disequilibrium mapping of common disease genes. *Nature Genet.*, **22**: 139–144.

66. Kendler K.S., MacLean C.J., Ma Y., O'Neill F.A., Walsh D., Straub R.E (1999) Marker-to-marker linkage disequilibrium on chromosomes 5q, 6p, and 8p in Irish high-density schizophrenia pedigrees. *Am. J. Med. Genet.*, **88**: 29–33.

67. Owen M.J., McGuffin P. (1993) Association and linkage: complementary strategies for complex disorders. *J. Med. Genet.*, **30**: 638–639.

68. O'Donovan M.C., Oefner P.J., Roberts S.C., Austin J., Hoogendoorn B., Guy C., Speight G., Upadhyaya M., Sommer S.S., McGuffin P. (1998) Blind analysis of denaturing high-performance liquid chromatography as a tool for mutation detection. *Genomics*, **52**: 44–49.

69. Daniels J., Holmans P., McGuffin P., Plomin R., Owen M.J. (1998) A simple method for analysing microsatellite allele image patterns generated from DNA

pools and its application to allelic association studies. *Am. J. Hum. Genet.*, **62**: 1189–1197.

70. Hill L., Asherson P., Ball D., Thalia E., Ninomiya T., Craig I.W., Fisher P.J., Turic D., McGuffin P., Owen M.J. *et al.* (1999) DNA pooling and dense marker maps: a systematic search for genes for cognitive ability. *Neuroreport*, **10**: 843–848.

71. Peltonen L., McKusick V.A. (2001) Genomics and medicine—dissecting human disease in the postgenomic era. *Science*, **291**: 1224.

72. Clayton J.D., Kyriacou C.D., Reppert S.M. (2001) Keeping time with the human genome. *Nature*, **409**: 829–831.

73. Roses A.D. (2000) Pharmacogenetics and future drug development and delivery. *Lancet*, **355**: 1358–1361.

74. Arranz M.J., Pons J., Gutierrez B., Mulcrone J., Cairns N., Makoff A., Kerwin R. (2000) Investigation of 5–HT2A differential expression and imprinting in schizophrenia. *Am. J. Med. Genet.*, **96**: 391.

75. Wolf R., Smith G., Smith R.L. (2000) Pharmacogenetics. *Br. Med. J.*, **320**: 987–990.

2

Molecular and Cellular Biology Research in Psychiatry

Stephen M. Stahl and Alexander B. Niculescu III

Neuroscience Education Institute and Department of Psychiatry, University of California at San Diego, 9500 Gilman Drive, La Jolla, CA 92093-0603, USA

INTRODUCTION

Paradigm shifts and new technologies are revolutionizing psychiatry at the dawn of the new millennium. Psychiatry, much beholden to Freud in the past, is finding a new patron saint in Darwin. Freud himself, if his early career as a neurologist and scientist is any indication, might very well have chosen to be a molecular neurobiologist were he alive and active today. We will attempt in this chapter to provide a highly selective view of current and future trends, rather than an exhaustive overview of the data accumulated so far, and integrate it into the larger clinical picture, in the hope that this will provide the reader with a useful framework for understanding the rapid evolution in the field.

Paradigm Shifts

Clinical Comorbidity Underlined by Overlapping Biological Mechanisms

The growing understanding and appreciation of shared genes and overlapping molecular and cellular mechanisms on the one hand, and of the global impact of psychiatric syndromes on the brain on the other hand, provide a potential biological explanation for clinical comorbidity as the rule rather than the exception. It may also provide a basis for future more precise, mechanism-based classifications of psychiatric illnesses, rather than the current descriptive complexity of the DSM-IV.

Psychiatry as a Neuroscience. Edited by Juan José López-Ibor, Wolfgang Gaebel, Mario Maj and Norman Sartorius. © 2002 John Wiley & Sons Ltd.

Tissue Remodelling

The brain is being increasingly viewed as just another organ, only more complex. The structural and functional plasticity of the brain, not unlike that of a muscle, is beginning to be appreciated [1]. The molecular and cellular changes in neural function that are produced as adaptations to chronic administration of addictive drugs, such as psychostimulants, and therapeutic drugs, such as antidepressants, have been proposed as a basis for their long-term effects on the brain, and for the latency of their therapeutic actions [2]. Moreover, the role of cell proliferation and cell death in psychiatric disorders is coming into focus [3, 4], prompting analogies with, and benefiting from concepts and techniques from, cancer biology [5, 6].

Glial cells, long thought to play mainly a supportive role to neurons, are increasingly identified as active players [7]. Post-mortem studies in mood disorders indicate altered numbers of neurons and glial cells [8]. Glial cells but not neurons were reported to be reduced in the subgenual prefrontal cortex in mood disorders [9].

A new concept that may inform psychiatry in the coming years is that of cumulative end-organ damage, in this case of (different regions of) the brain. The analogy to make is with diabetes, where cumulative glycosylation of artery walls and other tissues leads to retinal, kidney, neuropathic and other damage. This paradigm may explain why, for example, a medication tried earlier in the course of the illness may not work as well or at all when tried again later.

Endocrinology and Psychiatry

The brain, just like any other organ, is constantly exposed to and regulated by the hormones in the internal milieu, as a way of integrating its activity with the rest of the organism. The powerful influence of hormones on neuronal activity is an area that has received and will continue to receive increasing scrutiny, and the wealth of clinical observations from classical endocrinology regarding changes in mood and cognition in endocrinological disorders is now being revisited at a molecular and cellular level. Furthermore, not only the extremes of endocrinological pathology but also the physiological variations in hormonal levels are emerging as being of importance in modulating psychiatric syndromes.

Peripheral Molecular Markers

At present, diagnosis in psychiatry relies mainly on descriptive behavioural and symptomatic information. Measurable peripheral molecular markers are being actively pursued, and may enable simpler, more rapid, more objective and more accurate diagnosis and monitoring.

Infectious Aetiologies for Psychiatric Disorders

This interesting emerging area of research holds promise in identifying endogenous retroviruses, integrated in the genome and hereditarily transmitted, as important in the pathogenesis of a subset of psychiatric disorders [10]. Another avenue being followed is that of infectious agents as "second hits" that may lead to overt disease development in individuals with an inherited genetic susceptibility [11, 12]. The parallels with cancer biology are intriguing and may be methodologically fruitful.

Concerted Approaches to a Problem

It is beginning to be appreciated that a successful way to understand mental disorders is to use and integrate different approaches concurrently: phenotypical assessment, pharmacological studies, animal models, molecular and cellular biology, genetics and brain imaging [5, 13]. At the same time, strenuous efforts are being made in the field to perfect each approach as much as possible.

METHODOLOGY

Overview

Rapid progress was made during the past decade in several important areas relevant to cellular and molecular research in psychiatry. They include a better understanding of the neural circuitry involved in mental disorders, the cloning of complementary DNAs encoding important molecular targets of drugs, including the whole extended family of dopamine and serotonin receptors [14], and progress in understanding the molecular basis of long-term adaptive processes and their role in illness progression.

New methodologies that are revolutionizing psychiatry, as they are other fields of medicine, are molecular biology, genomic research, and combinatorial chemistry coupled to rational drug design.

Molecular biology has led to the development of powerful techniques such as the polymerase chain reaction (PCR) and DNA microarrays, like the so-called GeneChips (Affymetrix Inc., USA). It has also led to the possibility of engineering gene deletions or insertions in experimental animals, the most notable example being transgenic mice. The human genome project has been identifying the sequence of the complete set of genes, estimated to be over 30 000, variants of which are associated in different individuals with different illnesses. The number of proteins is estimated to be ten times as high, about 300 000, since a gene can encode for multiple proteins by its subsequent "tailoring" and processing.

Combinatorial chemistry has increased the pool of compounds that can be generated and tested against a specific protein target, and rational drug design based on structural imaging and modelling of proteins speeds up the drug discovery process by providing specific key-in-lock parameters for lead compounds.

Further on the horizon, neuronal stem cells may lead to transplant approaches for those mental disorders where cell loss is involved, as is currently attempted in neurology for Parkinson's disease, for example. Also on the horizon is the possibility of gene therapy, mostly for now in an early development stage and used as a research tool in animal models [15], but currently moving towards clinical applications in humans in at least one area, Alzheimer's disease (AD) [16, 17].

Gene Expression and Microarrays

The ability to simultaneously assess the expression of thousands of genes with microarray technology is opening new vistas in basic neurobiological research in both animal models and human post-mortem tissue samples [5, 18–20]. While gene expression is just part of the story of what is mechanistically happening in specific brain regions, it is an important first step in terms of identifying targets for more detailed studies, as well as for pharmaceutical drug development. More recent approaches have added the same massive parallel approach to protein assays [21] in the emerging field of proteomics [22]. The ultimate goal is the physiome, where molecular changes are integrated at a whole-organ or system level [23].

Animal Models

Obvious technical and ethical limitations dictate that studies on molecular changes in mental disorders cannot be performed on live human beings. Animal models of neuropsychiatric disorders are being developed in species as diverse as monkeys [16], rats and mice. While careful attention to animal welfare and minimizing pain and distress is a must, and ethical discussions of conducting research on animals are warranted, one should bear in mind that the ultimate goal is a worthy one, at least from our species' viewpoint—understanding and curing illness.

Monkeys are closer to humans, but more difficult and expensive to breed and conduct research on. Rats and mice are less expensive to breed and have faster generation times. Rats have bigger brains than mice, but less work has been done on creating transgenic rats. While mice have smaller brains, they are extensively used in genetic research due to their amenability to transgenic manipulation of their genome. Useful models of human psychiatric illnesses have been generated in this way [24].

Functional Imaging

Functional imaging is more developed in humans, due to a diagnostic medical impetus from fields like neurology and neurosurgery, although studies in psychiatry have yet to take full advantage of the spectrum of technologies currently available [25]. Imaging of primates and even rodents (rats, mice) is gradually being developed and standardized and may benefit basic research significantly, especially in concert with molecular genetics in well-defined animal models of disease.

Convergent Functional Genomics

The intersection of multiple lines of evidence upon a gene or biological mechanism for a particular disorder—what we would term *convergent functional genomics*—can be a powerful discovery engine. It may also reduce the uncertainty inherent in individual methodologies or lines of evidence. An approach to bridge insights from animal models and human genetic and brain imaging models has been described [5]. The basic idea is to use data from brain imaging studies to select brain regions of interest in a specific mental disorder and analyse gene expression patterns in those regions in post-mortem human brains or a germane animal model. The next step is to integrate human genetic linkage data with the gene expression data. This is done by seeing whether the genes that show a changed pattern of expression in the animal model or post-mortem human brains (compared to controls) map to linkage hotspots from human family tree genetic studies. This approach, which combines imaging, animal models and molecular genetics, is arguably quite useful in terms of identifying specific candidate genes involved in a particular mental disorder. Those genes are then the targets of extensive investigation, and the protein encoded by them becomes a potential target for pharmacological drug development.

Pharmacological Studies

Drug development in psychiatry is progressing at a particularly rapid pace, especially in view of the relative paucity of the pharmacological armamentarium available to psychiatrists until recently, compared with other fields of medicine. This can make even a recent psychopharmacology textbook an out-of-date tome gathering dust on a shelf. We will outline some of the interesting current insights from pharmacological studies, with a clear feeling that this may be one of the more rapidly obsolescing parts of this chapter.

For at least two reasons, one has to be careful in extrapolating the results of clinical trials, with their very particular enrolled patient populations, to patients at large seen in primary psychiatric practice [26]. First, patients enrolled in clinical trials may have a more severe and refractory form of the illness. Second, due to the exclusion criteria, patients may lack the comorbidities that are the rule rather than the exception in the general patient population.

Matching a drug to a given patient in psychiatry has been and still is largely a trial-and-error process, with broadly acting drugs being administered to a large range of patients with a broadly descriptive disorder. Determining whether a given patient will respond to a given drug, or whether a given patient will tolerate a given drug, cannot be done in advance of an empirical trial. In the future, pharmacogenomic profiles are expected to predict particularly those patients who are unlikely to tolerate a given drug, and may even be able to define in advance those most likely to respond successfully to a given drug. Thus, future drugs may be indicated not for broadly descriptive mental disorders defined in the DSM-IV, but for behavioural syndromes associated with a given genotype.

Drugs serve not only therapeutic purposes, but also as probes unravelling pathophysiology, due to our still incomplete knowledge of brain function and somewhat empirical black-box approach to psychopharmacology. While the information garnered this way is no doubt useful, this chapter, and in fact the whole volume, outlines approaches that will make psychopharmaceutical research less of a hit-and-miss proposition.

SCHIZOPHRENIA AND OTHER COGNITIVE DISORDERS

Clinical Comorbidity Underlined by Overlapping Biological Mechanisms

Disorders of cognition have traditionally been classified into psychoses and dementias. Other disorders of cognition include delirium and amnestic disorders. Psychoses were deemed to occur at an earlier age, to be biochemical/genetic in nature and to be at least partially reversible pharmacologically. Dementias were deemed to occur at a more advanced age, be degenerative in nature and to be mostly irreversible. The prototypical examples of psychoses were the schizophrenias, and the prototype dementia was AD. These distinctions are becoming strained and blurred as we learn more about the underlying pathophysiology, nowhere more so than in geropsychiatry. It is now being increasingly recognized that degenerative changes underlined by cell loss occur in schizophrenias, and that partially correctable biochemical neurotransmitter abnormalities occur in dementias. Moreover, other mental disorders such as mood and anxiety disorders, in addition to neurological disorders such as Parkinson's disease and Lewy body dementia, have an impact on cognition, with psychotic or pseudo-dementia-like end results.

Tissue Remodelling

The occurrence of macroscopic and microscopic end-organ brain damage in dementia as well as in schizophrenia has been appreciated for some time, more so than for other psychiatric syndromes. There is increasing evidence that the schizophrenic disease process begins before psychotic symptoms become overt [27]. These findings may also explain the limited functional recovery produced by even state-of-the-art psychopharmacological treatment, and suggest that early intervention, perhaps with agents that prevent cell death or promote cell growth, may be a valid strategy in the future.

An interesting line of work in the realm of brain plasticity has been the exploration at a molecular level in experimental animals of the effects of nurturing maternal behaviour [28]. The authors report that variations in maternal care in the rat promote hippocampal synaptogenesis and spatial learning and memory through systems known to mediate experience-dependent neural development. Thus, the offspring of mothers that show high levels of pup licking, grooming and arched-back nursing showed increased expression of N-methyl-D-aspartate (NMDA) receptor subunit and brain-derived neurotrophic factor (BDNF) mRNA, increased cholinergic innervation of the hippocampus and enhanced spatial learning and memory. A cross-fostering arm of the study, in which pups from neglectful mothers were raised by high-nurturing mothers, provided evidence for a direct relationship between maternal behaviour and hippocampal development. Interestingly, not all neonates were equally sensitive to variations in maternal care, illustrating the permanent intricate interrelationship between genes and environment.

Tissue changes in AD are well established. However, early diagnosis and detection of AD has been a challenging problem. Post-mortem studies had revealed that patients with AD have neurofibrillary tangles in the olfactory epithelium and entorhinal–hippocampal–subicular regions. Based on this, a study was conducted to assess whether olfactory impairment in individuals with mild cognitive impairment may predict subsequent AD [29]. In this study, tests of olfaction and olfaction-related anosognosia were both sensitive and specific in predicting subsequent illness. Interestingly, one of the candidate genes for psychosis identified through a convergent functional genomics approach, G-protein-coupled receptor kinase 3 (GRK3) [5], is highly expressed in olfactory cortex, where it plays a role in odorant receptor desensitization [30]. This opens the interesting possibility that direct or indirect alterations in this gene's activity could lead to early, detectable phenotypical changes in a subset of psychotic disorders.

Mutations in the amyloid precursor protein (APP) and presenilin-1 and -2 genes (PS-1, PS-2) cause AD. Transgenic mice engineered to carry both mutant genes (PS/APP) develop AD-like deposits composed of β-amyloid (Aβ) at an early age. A study using these mice showed an inflammatory response occurring in response to the amyloidosis [31]. Both fibrillar and nonfibrillar Aβ (diffuse) deposits were visible in the frontal cortex by 3 months, and the amyloid load increased dramatically with age. The number of fibrillar Aβ deposits increased up to the oldest age studied (2.5 years old), whereas there were less marked changes in the number of diffuse deposits in mice over 1 year old. Activated microglia and astrocytes increased synchronously with amyloid burden and were, in general, closely associated with deposits. Cyclooxygenase-2, an inflammatory response molecule involved in the prostaglandin pathway, was up-regulated in astrocytes associated with some fibrillar deposits. Complement component 1q, an immune response component, strongly co-localized with fibrillar Aβ, but was also up-regulated in some plaque-associated microglia. These results, showing that cyclooxygenase-2 and complement component 1q levels increase in response to the formation of fibrillar Aβ in a transgenic model of AD, are of interest in view of human clinical epidemiological data suggesting that the use of nonsteroidal anti-inflammatory drugs (NSAIDs), among other things, down-regulates cyclooxygenase-2, delaying the onset and progression of the illness [32].

Peripheral Molecular Markers

Because, at present, the diagnosis of schizophrenia relies principally on descriptive behavioural and symptomatic information, the identification of a peripheral measurable marker might enable simpler, more rapid and more accurate diagnosis and monitoring. Human peripheral blood lymphocytes have been found to express several dopamine receptors (D3, D4 and D5) by molecular biology techniques and binding assays. It has been speculated that these dopamine receptors found on lymphocytes may reflect receptors found in the brain. The D3 dopamine receptor on lymphocytes has been demonstrated to correlate with schizophrenia [33]. In that study there was a significant elevation (at least two-fold) in the mRNA level of the D3 but not of the D4 dopamine receptor in schizophrenic patients. This increase was not affected by different antipsychotic drug treatments (typical or atypical). Patients not receiving medication exhibited the same pattern, indicating that this change is not a result of medical treatment. The authors propose that the D3 receptor mRNA in blood lymphocytes could constitute a trait marker for identification and follow-up of schizophrenia.

A similar study from another group confirmed findings of changes of dopamine receptor mRNA levels in schizophrenic patients [34]. Forty-four schizophrenics who had been receiving drug medication for more than 3 years, 28 schizophrenics who had been drug-free for more than 3 months, 15 drug-naive schizophrenic patients, and 31 healthy persons were enrolled. Quantitative PCR of the mRNA was used to investigate the expression of D3 and D5 dopamine receptors in peripheral lymphocytes. The gene expression of dopamine receptors was compared in each group. In drug-free and drug-naive patients, the dopamine receptors of peripheral lymphocytes were sequentially studied in the second and eighth weeks after administration of antipsychotic medication. In the drug-free schizophrenic group, the D3 dopamine receptor mRNA expression of peripheral lymphocytes was significantly increased compared to that in controls and the drug-medicated schizophrenics, and D5 dopamine receptor mRNA expression was increased compared to that in the drug-medicated schizophrenics. Interestingly, the group of patients with increased dopamine receptor expression had more severe psychiatric symptoms. These results seem to suggest that the molecular biologically determined dopamine receptors of peripheral lymphocytes are reactive in response to antipsychotic treatment, and that increased expression of dopamine receptors in peripheral lymphocytes has possible clinical significance for subgrouping of schizophrenic patients.

Heterotrimeric G proteins play a pivotal role in post-receptor information transduction in cells and have been implicated in the pathophysiology and treatment of mood disorders. Changes have also been detected in G protein levels in post-mortem brains of patients with schizophrenia, where they could reflect an underlying abnormality or be an effect of antipsychotic treatment. A study aiming to eliminate this confound looked at receptor-coupled G proteins in mononuclear leukocytes obtained from 23 untreated patients with schizophrenia and 30 healthy controls [35]. Dopamine-enhanced guanine nucleotide binding capacity to G_s protein through D1/D5 receptors in mononuclear leukocytes of untreated patients with schizophrenia was significantly increased in comparison with that in healthy subjects, and positively correlated with both the total Positive and Negative Syndrome Scale (PANSS) score and the positive subscale. β-adrenergic and muscarinic receptor-coupled G protein functions, as well as $G_{s\alpha}$, $G_{i\alpha}$ and G_β immunoreactivities, were similar to those in healthy subjects. The lack of relationship to drug treatment makes these findings of elevated dopamine receptor-coupled G_s protein measures in mononuclear leukocytes of patients with schizophrenia useful as potential trait diagnostic markers.

GRK3, a candidate gene for mania and psychosis identified through a convergent functional approach [5], has been implicated in dampening signal transduction from G-protein-coupled receptors in neuronal and other tissues, and is present in human lymphocytes. There are some preliminary data indicating alterations of its levels in lymphocytes from patients with bipolar disorders [5], and it may deserve further scrutiny in subtypes of schizophrenia also, as a possible peripheral marker.

Advances and Insights from Convergent Functional Genomic Studies

A recently published study [18] looked at gene expression changes in the prefrontal cortex (PFC), an area implicated in schizophrenia by imaging studies in post-mortem brains of matched pairs of schizophrenics and control subjects. It identified a number of genes involved in presynaptic function as being abnormally decreased, the most strongly implicated being N-ethylmaleamide sensitive factor and synapsin II. The data suggest that subjects with schizophrenia may share a common abnormality in presynaptic function.

Advances and Insights from Pharmacological Studies

An interesting emerging direction is the study of the use of potential neuroprotective agents. Damage from free radicals and oxidative stress has been proposed as a cause of tardive dyskinesia. A recent study in rats [36] investigated whether neuroleptic medications may affect the motor system through the creation of free radicals, and whether structural brain changes related to oxidative damage may disrupt normal striatal function. The study showed that rats treated chronically with fluphenazine had significantly lower striatal cholinergic neuron densities than those that did not receive antioxidants. Rats exposed to a diet consisting of antioxidants had significantly higher neuron densities in each of the three regions tested than did those that did not receive antioxidants. Clinical trials of the antioxidant vitamin E for reducing the severity of symptoms of tardive dyskinesia have had mixed results [37], but it may be that irreversible neuronal loss had already occurred and that antioxidant supplementation should be instituted very early on during neuroleptic and other treatments that may lead to oxidative damage, in order to have an impact.

Lithium has recently been added to the list of potential neuroprotective agents. Rodent studies have shown that lithium exerts neurotrophic or neuroprotective effects [6]. An imaging study in patients [38] used three-dimensional magnetic resonance imaging and brain segmentation to study grey-matter volume with chronic lithium use in patients with bipolar mood disorder. Grey-matter volume increased after 4 weeks of treatment, probably because of neurotrophic effects. This has led the authors to propose that low-dose lithium may have a potential use as a prophylactic agent for age-related neuronal loss and dementia [39].

The role of nicotine in improving cognition [40] may explain the high incidence of smoking in schizophrenics as a form of self-medication. Pharmacological, clinical and epidemiological data also support a role for nicotine in delaying the onset and perhaps slowing down the progression of AD. Interestingly, nicotine produces a long-lasting elevation of nerve growth factor (NGF) production when administered experimentally directly to the hippocampus of rats. In the central nervous system (CNS), NGF has powerful effects on the cholinergic system. It promotes cholinergic neuron survival after experimental injury as well as maintaining and regulating the phenotype of uninjured cholinergic neurons. In addition to these neurotrophic effects mediated by gene expression, NGF has a rapid neurotransmitter-like action to regulate cholinergic neurotransmission and neuronal excitability. Consistent with its actions on the cholinergic system, NGF can enhance function in animals with cholinergic lesions and has been suggested as being to be useful in humans with AD [16, 17]. However, the problems of CNS delivery, and of potential side effects such as pain, limit the clinical efficacy of NGF. Drug treatment strategies to enhance production of NGF in the CNS may be useful in the treatment of AD. Nicotine may be one such agent [41].

MOOD DISORDERS

Clinical Comorbidity Underlined by Overlapping Biological Mechanisms

We will consider in this section bipolar disorders and depression. Anxiety disorders, often closely related and comorbid, will be considered in the next section. Three emerging themes in the biology of mood disorders are:

1. Mood disorders, even what was considered unipolar depression, involve cycling and can broadly be viewed as part of a bipolar spectrum, or spectra [42].
2. There is extensive comorbidity with other mental disorders; it is the rule rather than the exception.
3. There is a longitudinal organic progression in the lifetime history of mood disorder, with progressive end-organ changes and damage.

Tissue Remodelling

Increasing evidence suggests that mood disorders are associated with a reduction in regional CNS volume and neuronal and glial cell atrophy or loss. Catecholamines have been recently implicated in both neurotoxic and neuroprotective phenomena [43, 44], and lithium has been demonstrated to increase robustly the levels of the cytoprotective, anti-apoptotic B-cell lymphoma protein-2 (bcl-2) in both cultured cells and areas of rodent brain [6]. Therefore, tissue remodelling may be relevant as a mechanistic substrate underlying the behavioural phenotypes and long-term effects of drugs, as well as the progressive nature of mood disorders, which may best be understood as an end-organ damage paradigm.

The influence of stress and glucocorticoids on neuronal pathology has been demonstrated in animal and clinical studies. It has been proposed that stress-induced changes in the hippocampus may be central to the development of depression in genetically vulnerable individuals. A study investigating the effect of antidepressants on hippocampal neurogenesis in the adult rat [45] used the thymidine analogue bromodeoxyuridine (BrdU) as a marker for dividing cells. The study demonstrated that chronic antidepressant treatment significantly increased the number of BrdU-labelled cells in the dentate gyrus and hilus of the hippocampus. Administration of several different classes of antidepressant, but not non-antidepressant, agents was found to increase BrdU-labelled cell number, indicating that this was a common and selective action of antidepressants. In addition, up-regulation of the number of BrdU-labelled cells was observed after chronic, but not acute, treatment, consistent with the time course for the therapeutic action of antidepressants. Additional studies demonstrated that antidepressant treatment increased the proliferation of hippocampal cells and that these new cells matured and become neurons, as determined by triple labelling for BrdU and neuronal- or glial-specific markers. These findings raise the interesting possibility that increased cell proliferation and increased neuronal number may be a mechanism by which antidepressant treatment overcomes the stress-induced atrophy and loss of hippocampal neurons and may contribute to the therapeutic actions of antidepressant treatment. Their likely trophic actions on other areas of the brain merit further exploration.

Additional evidence implicates the PFC in addition to the hippocampus as a site of neuropathology in depression. The PFC may be involved in stress-mediated neurotoxicity because stress alters PFC functions and glucocorticoid receptors, the PFC is directly interconnected with the hippocampus, and metabolic alterations are present in the PFC in depressed patients. Post-mortem studies in major depression and bipolar disorders provide evidence for specific neuronal and glial histopathology in mood disorders [8]. Three patterns of morphometric cellular changes were observed in that study: cell loss (subgenual PFC), cell atrophy (dorsolateral PFC and orbito-frontal cortex) and increased numbers of cells (hypothalamus, dorsal raphe nucleus). The study suggests that cellular changes in mood disorders may be due to stress and prolonged PFC remodelling, with a role played by neurotrophic/neuroprotective factors. Furthermore, the precise anatomic localization of dysfunctional neurons and glia in mood disorders may lead to specific cortical targets at molecular and cellular level for the development of novel antidepressants and mood stabilizers.

Physical activity may also impact mood through neurotrophic effects on the brain. In mice, running was shown to increase neurogenesis in the dentate gyrus of the hippocampus, a brain structure that is important for memory function [46]. Additionally, in that study, spatial learning and long-term potentiation (LTP) were tested in groups of mice housed either with a running wheel (runners) or under standard conditions (controls). Mice were injected with BrdU to label dividing cells and trained in the Morris water maze. LTP was studied in the dentate gyrus and area CA1 in hippocampal slices from these mice. Running improved water maze performance, increased BrdU-positive cell numbers, and selectively enhanced dentate gyrus LTP. The results suggest that physical activity can regulate neurogenesis, synaptic plasticity and learning.

There are clinical observations that are possible correlates for these effects. Several reports indicate that physical activity can reduce the severity of symptoms in depressed patients. Some data suggest that even a single exercise bout may result in a substantial mood improvement. A study evaluating the short-term effects of a 10-day training programme on patients with moderate to severe major depression [47] found clinically relevant and statistically significant reduction in depression scores, suggesting that aerobic exercise can produce substantial improvement in mood in patients with major depressive disorders in a short time. Another study compared physical exercise with standard drug treatment for depression [48]. The study assessed the status of 156 adult volunteers with major depressive disorder (MDD) 6 months after completion of a study in which they were randomly assigned to a 4-month course of aerobic exercise, sertraline therapy, or a combination of exercise and sertraline. After 4 months, patients in all three groups exhibited significant improvement; the proportion of participants with remission was comparable across the three treatment conditions. After 10 months, however, subjects in remission in the exercise group had significantly lower relapse rates ($p < 0.01$) than subjects in the medication group. Exercising on one's own during the follow-up period was associated with a reduced probability of depression diagnosis at the end of that period. Obviously, exercise has a variety of physiological and endocrinological effects on the body, but an intriguing possibility exists that neurotrophic effects may underlie some of the positive effects of exercise on mood.

Endocrinological Aspects

Several studies have underlined the high prevalence of psychiatric symptoms and disorders in endocrine diseases. More recently, the role of sex hormones in the differential spectrum of mood disorders in women versus men
[42] and the role of hormone replacement therapy as an adjuvant treatment in
mood disorders [49–51] are receiving increasing recognition and attention.
The underlying biology may be related to the integration and cross-talk of
signal-processing cascades from membrane-bound neurotransmitter receptors with those from nuclear ligand-activated transcription factors such as
hormone receptors for oestrogen, progesterone and testosterone.

Estradiol is known to affect a number of neurotransmitter systems in the
brain. Stress and corticotropin-releasing hormone inhibit the reproductive
axis. A study examining whether reproductive axis hormone secretion is
inhibited in women with depression, similar to what has been observed to
be caused by stress in numerous species, found that the blood levels of
reproductive hormones were mostly normal in women with depression, but
the blood level of estradiol was significantly lower [52].

Decreased *growth hormone* (GH) response to pharmacological stimulation
has been found in children and adolescents during an episode of major
depressive disorder and after recovery. GH secretion is similarly altered in
children and adolescents who had never experienced depression but were
at high risk of developing depression [53]. These results suggest that the
decreased GH response found in high-risk subjects may represent a trait
marker for depression in children and adolescents. It is interesting to note
that one of the candidate psychogenes identified by our work using convergent functional genomics [5] described below is insulin-like growth factor
1 (IGF1), a downstream effector in the GH pathway.

Thyroid disorders also strongly affect mood. A study to evaluate the prevalence of mental disorders in 93 inpatients affected by different thyroid diseases
during their lifetimes, by means of standardized instruments, showed higher
rates of panic disorder, simple phobia, obsessive-compulsive disorder, MDD,
bipolar disorder and cyclothymia in thyroid patients than in the general
population [54]. These findings may suggest either that thyroid abnormalities
effect secondary mood changes, or that the co-occurrence of mental and
thyroid diseases may be the result of common biochemical abnormalities.

Lithium is known to interact with the thyroid axis and causes hypothyroidism in a subgroup of patients, which compromises its mood-stabilizing effects.
Lithium was reported to alter thyroid hormone metabolism in the rat brain,
and a study investigating whether these effects were mediated through regulation of thyroid hormone receptor (THR) gene expression found that chronic
lithium treatment appeared to regulate THR gene expression in a subtype-
(isoform) and region-specific manner in the rat brain [55]. This study raises the

possibility that the observed effects of lithium on THR gene expression may be related to its therapeutic efficacy in the treatment of bipolar disorders.

Advances and Insights from Convergent Functional Genomic Studies

The initial description and application of the concept of convergent functional genomics was in identifying genes involved in mania and psychotic mania [5]. Methamphetamine treatment of rats as an animal model for psychotic mania was used. Specific brain regions—PFC, amygdala—were analysed comprehensively for changes in gene expression using oligonucleotide GeneChip microarrays. These regions had been implicated in mood and psychotic disorders by previous studies in animal models and imaging studies in humans. The data were cross-matched against human genomic loci associated with either bipolar disorder or schizophrenia, which had been previously identified by human genetic linkage studies. Using this convergent approach, we have identified several novel possible candidate genes that may be involved in the pathogenesis of mood disorders and psychosis—signal transduction molecules like GRK3, transcription factors like the clock gene D-box binding protein (DBP), growth factors such as IGF1, metabolic enzymes like farnesyl-diphosphate farnesyltransferase 1 (FDFT1) involved in cholesterol biosynthesis and sulfotransferase 1A1 (SULT1A1) involved in dopamine metabolism, and others. Furthermore, for one of these genes, GRK3, preliminary experiments by Western blot analysis found evidence for decreased protein levels in a subset of patient lymphoblastoid cell lines that correlated with disease severity.

We also proposed a novel paradigm for classification of these and other candidate genes involved in mental disorders, by analogy to cancer biology, into two prototypical categories, psychogenes and psychosis-suppressor genes. Genes whose activity promotes processes that lead to mania or psychosis could be called "psychogenes", by analogy to oncogenes. Conversely, genes whose activity suppresses processes that lead to these mental disorders could be called "psychosis-suppressor genes". This classification, while probably oversimplistic, may have heuristic value for psychiatry as it has had for cancer biology, by providing a framework for understanding the roles of putative disease genes in pathophysiology and as targets for developing treatment strategies. Using this paradigm, and on the basis of their biology, DBP, IGF1 and FDFT1 were classified as candidate psychogenes, and GRK3 and SULT1A1 were classified as candidate psychosis-suppressor genes [5].

Furthermore, it is possible that genes that show concomitant changes in expression levels in such studies may be interacting pathophysiologically, and warrant further analysis as co-acting gene groups. The concept that "genes that change together act together" provides a straightforward testable model for unravelling complex polygenic diseases like bipolar disorders, schizophrenia and others, including non-mental disorders.

Advances and Insights from Pharmacological Studies

An interesting study supporting the concept of progressive end-organ changes was reported recently [56]. The authors investigated the relationship between the number of lifetime episodes of affective disorder and the antimanic response to lithium, divalproex or placebo. An apparent transition in the relationship between number of previous episodes and response to antimanic medication occurred at about 10 previous episodes. For patients who had experienced more episodes than this, the response to lithium resembled the response to placebo but was worse than the response to divalproex. For patients who had experienced fewer episodes, however, the responses to lithium and divalproex did not differ and were better than the response to placebo. This differential response pattern was not related to rapid cycling or mixed states. The authors conclude that a history of many previous episodes was associated with poor response to lithium or placebo but not to divalproex.

Medications have potential side effects, which may reduce patient compliance. Some patients also have a psychological resistance to being on psychotropic medications long-term, hence their seeking other approaches, including "alternative medicine". One such approach for which there are actually good epidemiological, clinical and biological data is using supplementation with omega-3 fatty acids, which are long-chain, polyunsaturated fatty acids that are a normal component of cell membranes. They are found in the diet in enriched form in plant and marine sources, such as fish oil. Unlike saturated fats, which may have negative health consequences, omega-3 fatty acids have been associated with health benefits in cardiovascular disorders and arthritis.

Omega-3 fatty acids have been proposed to be potentially efficacious in a number of mental disorders [57–59]. Diminished levels of omega-3 fatty acids have been reported in mood disorders like depression. An epidemiological study looking at fish consumption and depressive symptoms in the general population in Finland found that the likelihood of having depressive symptoms was significantly higher among infrequent fish consumers than among frequent fish consumers, even after adjusting for potential confounders [60]. One double-blind placebo-controlled trial reported favourable results using omega-3 fatty acids as an adjunctive treatment in bipolar disorder [61]. Their molecular mechanism of action is still being elucidated, but, like the case in mood stabilizers, it seems to have to do with impacting on cell membrane function and signal transduction from the membrane to the nucleus through protein kinase signalling [62].

ANXIETY DISORDERS

Clinical Comorbidity Underlined by Overlapping Biological Mechanisms

From an evolutionary standpoint, anxiety is probably a signal of alarm to the organism in uncertain and potentially dangerous situations. While pure, or, more precisely, *mainly* anxiety disorders may exist, there is an emerging recognition that there are significant interactions and impact with both mood and cognition. In terms of interactions with mood, anxiety and low mood may translate as fear, whereas anxiety and high mood may translate as irritability and anger. In terms of interactions with cognition, high anxiety may be a component of paranoid ideation, and lack of anxiety a component of antisocial psychotic acts.

Tissue Remodelling

Preclinical studies demonstrate that early anxiety and stress can alter the development of the hypothalamic–pituitary–adrenal (HPA) axis, hypothalamic and extrahypothalamic corticotropin-releasing hormone (CRH), mono-aminergic and γ-aminobutyric acid/benzodiazepine systems. Stress has also been shown to promote structural and functional alterations in brain regions similar to those seen in adults with chronic anxiety and depression [63].

As mentioned, stress has been shown to lead over time to cell death in the hippocampus. Elevated glucocorticoid levels produce hippocampal dysfunction and correlate with individual deficits in spatial learning in aged rats. Aged humans with significant prolonged cortisol elevations showed reduced hippocampal volume and deficits in hippocampus-dependent memory tasks compared to normal-cortisol controls [64]. Moreover, the degree of hippocampal atrophy correlated strongly with both the degree of cortisol elevation over time and current basal cortisol levels in the studied population. Therefore, basal cortisol elevation may cause hippocampal damage and impair hippocampus-dependent learning and memory in humans.

Endocrinological Aspects

CRH is a critical coordinator of the HPA axis. In response to stress, CRH released from the paraventricular nucleus (PVN) of the hypothalamus activates CRH receptors on anterior pituitary corticotropes, resulting in release of adrenocorticotropic hormone (ACTH) into the bloodstream. ACTH in turn activates ACTH receptors in the adrenal cortex to increase synthesis and release of glucocorticoids. The receptors for CRH, CRHr1 and CRHr2 are found throughout the CNS and periphery. Mice engineered by a gene knockout approach to be deficient for CRHr2 display anxiety-like behaviour and are hypersensitive to stress [65].

Circulating corticosterone and insulin are involved in regulation of the hypothalamic neuropeptide Y system, which in turn is involved in regulation of the HPA axis. The HPA axis and stress responsivity is altered in diseases such as anxiety and depression. A study in rats found a differential regulation of neuropeptide Y mRNA expression in the hypothalamic arcuate nucleus and the brainstem locus coeruleus by stress and antidepressants [66], and provided further evidence for the importance of circulating insulin in the regulation of the arcuate nucleus neuropeptide Y system. The GH/IGF1 pathway has been implicated in studies of mood disorders, as described in the section on mood disorders above. Insulin and insulin-like growth factors are emerging as interesting players in mood and anxiety disorders.

Advances and Insights from Convergent Functional Genomic Studies

GRK3, a protein implicated in mood disorders by a convergent functional genomic approach [5], was shown to mediate homologous desensitization of corticotropin-releasing factor (CRF) type 1 (CRF1) receptors in a human brain-derived cell line [67]. CRF is an important mediator of stress and anxiety responses. These data speak to the overlap at a molecular level between what we currently define clinically as mood and anxiety disorders.

Advances and Insights from Pharmacological Studies

CRF is a major mediator of adaptive responsiveness to stress. The development of CRF inhibitors is a very active area of interest pharmacologically.

A preclinical pharmacological study measured changes in extracellular concentrations of catecholamines and indoleamines in the hippocampus or the PFC in rats in response to administration of the CRF1 antagonist CP-154, 526 by using in vivo microdialysis [68], and found that this CRH1 receptor antagonist suppresses the release of norepinephrine and serotonin in the hippocampus, which may be of relevance to understanding and treating anxiety and mood disorders.

Another reported study evaluated the effects of the lipophilic non-peptide CRH1 receptor antagonist antalarmin, developed at the National Institutes of Health, on the behavioural, neuroendocrine and autonomic components of the stress response in adult male rhesus macaques [69]. The study was carried in a double-blind, placebo-controlled fashion in monkeys exposed to an intense social stressor: namely, placement of two unfamiliar males in adjacent cages separated only by a transparent Plexiglas screen. Antalarmin significantly inhibited a repertoire of behaviours associated with anxiety and fear such as body tremors, grimacing, teeth gnashing, urination and defecation. In contrast, antalarmin increased exploratory and sexual behaviours that are normally suppressed during stress. Moreover, antalarmin significantly diminished the increases in cerebrospinal fluid CRH as well as the pituitary–adrenal, sympathetic and adrenal medullary responses to stress. Use of this pharmacological tool revealed that CRH plays a broad role in the physiological responses to psychological stress in primates. Furthermore, it is possible that a CRH1 receptor antagonist may be of therapeutic value in human psychiatric, reproductive and cardiovascular disorders associated with CRH system hyperactivity.

SUBSTANCE ABUSE AND EATING DISORDERS

Clinical Comorbidity Underlined by Overlapping Biological Mechanisms

Drug addiction is defined as the compulsive seeking and taking of a drug despite adverse consequences. Multiple psychological and social factors come into play, but at its core it represents a biological process underlined by the effects of repeated drug exposure on a vulnerable brain [70]. A dysregulation and resetting of the threshold for reward mechanisms in the brain, termed allostasis, is proposed to occur with long-term drug use and to underlie addiction [71].

One emerging theme in the field of substance addiction is the intricate relationship at a molecular level with other mental disorders. Substances of abuse modulate some of the same biochemical pathways and circuits involved in mood and anxiety disorders. It is also increasingly being appreciated that there is a strong interplay with cognitive disorders. Eating disorders can also be viewed from the perspective of a substance abuse disorder, both in aetiology and treatment. Active areas of research include: substance abuse propensity and affective disorders, substance abuse as a way of self-treating affective disorders, and substance abuse and cognitive disorders. This ongoing work may have strong practical implications in terms of treatment strategies.

Dopaminergic neurotransmission plays a central role in cognition, mood and substance abuse. A study in mice looking at the effects of targeted disruption in mice of dopamine and adenosine $3',5'$-monophosphate-regulated phosphoprotein (32 kDa) (DARPP-32), a gene regulating the efficacy of dopaminergic neurotransmission, illustrates this point [72]. Dopaminergic neurons exert a major modulatory effect on the forebrain. DARPP-32, which is enriched in all neurons that receive a dopaminergic input, is converted in response to dopamine into a potent protein phosphatase inhibitor. Mice generated to contain a targeted disruption of the DARPP-32 gene showed profound deficits in their molecular, electrophysiological and behavioural responses to dopamine, drugs of abuse and antipsychotic medication.

Further illustrating the intimate interplay between cognition and addiction, dopamine mediated mechanisms of addiction are also likely to involve some of the molecular mechanisms of memory formation [73].

Tissue Remodelling

Another emerging theme is that of progressive brain changes and end-organ damage resulting from sustained abuse of drugs. Behavioural abnormalities associated with addiction are very long-lived. It is being increasingly appreciated that chronic drug exposure causes stable changes in the brain at the molecular and cellular levels that underlie these behavioural abnormalities [74].

A recent study with methamphetamine users illustrates this point. While illicit stimulants are often used to enhance attention and alertness and generally speed up the thought process, chronic users had a dose-dependent decrease of performance in neuropsychological tests that assess recall, ability to manipulate information, ability to ignore irrelevant information, and abstract thinking [75]. A positron tomography study in methamphetamine abusers revealed an association of dopamine transporter reduction with psychomotor impairment [76]. A parallel study from the same group of investigators found higher cortical and lower subcortical metabolism in detoxified methamphetamine abusers [77]. These results suggest that, in humans, methamphetamine abuse results in lasting changes in the function of dopamine- and non-dopamine-innervated brain regions.

One such molecular switch underlying long-term neural plasticity is DeltaFosB, a transcription factor that has been implicated in drug addiction and movement disorders [78].

Advances and Insights from Convergent Functional Genomic Studies

Acute methamphetamine administration in rats has been used as an animal model of mania [5]. The candidate genes identified in that study through a convergent functional genomics approach, as discussed in the section on mood disorders, may also represent players involved in stimulant addiction and provide a mechanistic basis for comorbidity between bipolar disorders and stimulant abuse and addiction.

Cocaine enhances dopamine-mediated neurotransmission by blocking dopamine re-uptake at axon terminals. The striatum is one such site of action. Chronic exposure to cocaine up-regulates several transcription factors that alter gene expression and which could mediate the long-term neural and behavioural changes induced by the drug. One such transcription factor is DeltaFosB, a protein that persists in striatum long after the end of cocaine exposure. Using DNA microarray analysis of striatal tissue from both inducible transgenic mice engineered to overexpress DeltaFosB and mice treated with cocaine, cyclin-dependent kinase 5 (Cdk5) was identified as a downstream target gene of DeltaFosB [79]. Overexpression of DeltaFosB, or chronic cocaine administration, raised levels of Cdk5 messenger RNA, protein and activity in the striatum. Interestingly, injection of Cdk5 inhibitors into the striatum potentiated behavioural effects of repeated cocaine administration. This elegant study implicates the neuronal protein Cdk5 as a regulator of the effects of chronic exposure to cocaine, and identifies a novel cellular pathway as a potential target for pharmaceutical drug development.

Changes in brain gene expression are thought to be responsible for the tolerance, dependence and neurotoxicity produced by chronic alcohol abuse. DNA microarrays have been used recently with some success in studies of alcoholism [20]. RNA was extracted from post-mortem samples of superior frontal cortex of alcoholics and non-alcoholics. Relative levels of RNA were determined by array techniques. Expression levels were determined for over 4000 genes, and 163 of these were found to differ by 40% or more between alcoholics and non-alcoholics. Analysis of these changes revealed a selective reprogramming of gene expression in this brain region, particularly for myelin-related genes, which were down-regulated in the alcoholic samples. In addition, cell cycle genes and several neuronal genes were changed in expression. The investigators conclude that the observed gene expression changes suggest a mechanism for the loss of cerebral white matter in alcoholics as well as alterations that may lead to the neurotoxic actions of ethanol.

A recent study comprehensively catalogued gene expression changes in rat brains following acute and chronic exposure to δ-9-tetrahydrocannabinol (THC), the active ingredient in marijuana, using microarray technology profiling a total of 24456 cDNAs [80]. Of these, only 49 different genes showed specific changes in expression compared to control animals, including some signal transduction molecules (prostaglandin D synthase, calmodulin), and structural molecules [neural cell adhesion molecule (NCAM), myelin basic protein].

The sequencing of the human and other mammalian genomes is a watershed event that will help us to understand the biology of addiction by enabling us to identify genes that contribute to individual risk for addiction and those through which drugs cause addiction. A preliminary search of a draft sequence of the human genome for genes related to desensitization of receptors that mediate the actions of drugs of abuse on the nervous system yielded multiple potential candidates and illustrates the impact this methodology can make in speeding up the discovery process [70].

Advances and Insights from Pharmacological Studies

Ondansetron, an anti-nausea drug best known for its use in cancer chemotherapy, has been reported to be effective in reducing drinking, especially in patients with early-onset alcoholism (before age 25) [81]. In their discussion, the authors speculate that ondansetron changes the balance of activity among the neurotransmitters dopamine and serotonin. In particular, it reduces the activity at one of the serotonin receptors, 5-HT3; in previous animal studies, blocking this receptor had been found to reduce the consumption of alcohol. It is hypothesized that early-onset alcoholics may carry a genetic variant of the receptor that makes them more vulnerable to the addictive effects of alcohol. Interestingly, the blood test used to measure alcohol use in this study is a new one: it measures carbohydrate-deficient transferrin (CDT), which accumulates in the blood with sustained heavy drinking, as haemoglobin A_{1c} does in diabetes, and persists at elevated levels for weeks after drinking stops. The test was recently approved by the US Food and Drug Administration for use in alcohol treatment centres and may soon become widespread.

SLEEP DISORDERS

Clinical Comorbidity Underlined by Overlapping Biological Mechanisms

Sleep is altered in a variety of mental disorders, both as a consequence of the illness and secondary to pharmacological treatment. Mania and anxiety disorders can lead to sleep decrease, whereas anergic depression and negative-symptoms schizophrenia can lead to increases in the duration of sleep. As one of the few objective parameters to be investigated during a psychiatric interview, sleep may be viewed as the "temperature" of the psychiatric clinical exam. The extreme phenotype of narcolepsy has led to the identification of a family of brain peptides called hypocretins as involved in sleep regulation. Another promising line of research is represented by clock genes. Clock genes regulate circadian rhythms, are highly conserved from plants to man [82] and may be molecular substrates mediating the interface of sleep and psychiatric syndromes.

Tissue Remodelling

Narcolepsy is a disorder characterized by sleep attacks, cataplexy, disrupted sleep patterns and hypnogogic hallucinations. Neurons containing the neuropeptide hypocretin (orexin), identified using a combination of animal models and genetics as described below, are located exclusively in the lateral hypothalamus and send axons to numerous regions throughout the CNS, including the major nuclei implicated in sleep regulation. In a post-mortem study of human brains [83], investigators have found that narcoleptics had 85–95% fewer hypocretin-expressing neurons in their hypothalamus than did matched controls. This suggests that a neurodegenerative process may have affected the hypocretin neurons.

Advances and Insights from Convergent Functional Genomic Studies

Two animal models of narcolepsy that have been instrumental in understanding the pathophysiology of the disease are the canarc-1 mutant dogs, which have a spontaneous mutation, and the orexin knockout mice, where hypocretin/orexin was deleted by a purposeful experimental transgenic approach.

Positional cloning was used to identify an autosomal recessive mutation responsible for narcolepsy in the canine model [84]. The study determined that canine narcolepsy is caused by disruption of the hypocretin (orexin) receptor 2 gene (Hcrtr2).

Assessed using behavioural and electroencephalographic criteria, orexin knockout mice [85] exhibit a phenotype strikingly similar to that of human narcolepsy patients, as well as to canarc-1 mutant dogs, the only known monogenic model of narcolepsy. Modafinil, an anti-narcoleptic drug with ill-defined mechanisms of action, was observed in those mice to activate orexin-containing neurons.

These results identify hypocretins as major sleep-modulating neurotransmitters and open novel potential therapeutic approaches for narcoleptic patients.

Familial advanced sleep phase syndrome (FASPS) is an autosomal dominant circadian rhythm variant; affected individuals are "morning larks" with a 4-hour advance of the sleep, temperature and melatonin rhythms. Human genetic linkage studies localized the FASPS gene near the telomere of chromosome 2q. A strong candidate gene (hPER2), a human homologue of the period gene in *Drosophila*, maps to the same locus. Affected individuals were shown to have a serine-to-glycine mutation within the casein kinase Iε (CKIε) binding region of hPER2, which causes hypophosphorylation by CKIε in vitro [86]. A stable alteration in human sleep behaviour can thus be attributed to a missense mutation in a clock component, hPER2, which alters the circadian period.

Another clock gene, D-box binding protein (DBP), was identified as a candidate for being involved in mood and psychotic disorders by a convergent functional genomics approach [5], as described earlier in this chapter. DBP is a transcriptional activator that shows a robust circadian rhythm. DBP knockout mice show a reduced amplitude of circadian modulation of sleep time, a reduction in the consolidation of sleep episodes and reduced locomotor activity, a picture that is not unlike depression [87]. Clock genes have been shown to be important for the development of behavioural sensitization to repeated stimulant exposure [88]. Taken together, the converging lines of evidence about connections between clock genes, stimulant sensitization, circadian rhythmicity, sleep and mood disorders make DBP an interesting target for further studies of the bidirectional interface between disorders of sleep and other psychiatric disorders.

Advances and Insights from Pharmacological Studies

The interplay between sleep disturbances and mood disorder is underlined, for example, by the use of stimulants to augment antidepressant treatment in patients who have had only a partial response to first-line therapy. Modafinil is a novel psychostimulant that has shown efficacy in, and is marketed for, treating excessive daytime sleepiness associated with narcolepsy. The mechanism of action of modafinil is unknown, but, unlike other stimulants, the drug is highly selective for the CNS, has little effect on dopaminergic activity in the striatum, and appears to have a lower abuse potential. In a retrospective case series of seven patients with DSM-IV depression (four with major depression and three with bipolar depression) in whom modafinil was used to augment a partial or non-response to an antidepressant, all patients achieved full or partial remission within 1–2 weeks [89]. These preliminary results suggest that modafinil may be of use as an augmenter of antidepressants, especially in patients with residual tiredness or fatigue. It may also be an interesting choice in treating negative symptoms associated with schizophrenia, although rigorous controlled studies need to be carried out.

CONCLUSIONS AND FUTURE DIRECTIONS

Increasing Confluence of Psychiatry and Neurology

As psychiatry better understands the underlying structural and molecular changes associated with mental disorders, and as neurology explores further the behavioural, cognitive and affective aspects of neurological disorders of the brain, there is increasing overlap between the two specialties that may lead down the road to a unified specialty, brainology [13].

Blurring of the Separation Between Axis I and Axis II

The constantly increasing psychopharmacological armamentarium at our disposal is significantly impacting axis II disorders, and has revealed the separation between axis I and axis II to be somewhat artificial. An example of this is that personality disorder scores improve with effective pharmacotherapy of depression [90]. Molecular genetic research will also benefit from viewing axis I and axis II as lying on a continuum-of-severity spectrum, together with even softer forms that are currently classified as temperaments. Illustrating this trend is a recent study identifying the association between a polymorphism in the promoter region of the human dopamine receptor D4 (DRD4) gene and novelty-seeking personality traits [91].

Better Phenotypical Definitions

Psychiatry needs better, more precise quantitative descriptions of mental phenomena and the phenotypes of different disorders in order to improve patient care and speed up the convergent functional genomics and pharmacological discovery processes. This has not kept pace with the contemporary progress in molecular genetics and brain imaging, and may provide a rate-limiting step for future progress [42]. Our expectation is that the constant interplay between molecular and cellular biology, imaging and clinical research will avoid this roadblock.

REFERENCES

1. Gage F.H. (2000) Structural plasticity: cause, result, or correlate of depression. *Biol. Psychiatry*, **48**: 713–714.
2. Hyman S.E., Nestler E.J. (1996) Initiation and adaptation: a paradigm for understanding psychotropic drug action. *Am. J. Psychiatry*, **153**: 151–162.
3. Jacobs B.L., Praag H., Gage F.H. (2000) Adult brain neurogenesis and psychiatry: a novel theory of depression. *Mol. Psychiatry*, **5**: 262–269.
4. Duman R.S., Malberg J., Nakagawa S., D'Sa C. (2000) Neuronal plasticity and survival in mood disorders. *Biol. Psychiatry*, **48**: 713–714.
5. Niculescu A.B., Segal D., Kuczenski R., Barrett T., Hauger R., Kelsoe J.R. (2000) Identifying a series of candidate genes for mania and psychosis: a convergent functional genomics approach. *Physiol. Genomics*, **4**: 83–91.

6. Chen G., Rajkowska G., Du F., Seraji-Bozorgzad N., Manji H.K. (2000) Enhancement of hippocampal neurogenesis by lithium. *J. Neurochem.*, **75**: 1729–1734.
7. Coyle J.T., Schwarcz R. (2000) Mind glue: implications of glial cell biology for psychiatry. *Arch. Gen. Psychiatry*, **57**: 90–93.
8. Rajkowska G. (2000) Postmortem studies in mood disorders indicate altered numbers of neurons and glial cells. *Biol. Psychiatry*, **48**: 766–777.
9. Ongur D., Drevets W.C., Price J.L. (1998) Glial reduction in the subgenual prefrontal cortex in mood disorders. *Proc. Natl. Acad. Sci USA*, **95**: 13 290–13 295.
10. Yolken R.H., Karlsson H., Yee F., Johnston-Wilson N.L., Torrey E.F. (2000) Endogenous retroviruses and schizophrenia. *Brain Res. Brain Res. Rev.*, **31**: 193–199.
11. Torrey E.F., Yolken R.H. (2000) Familial and genetic mechanisms in schizophrenia. *Brain Res. Brain Res. Rev.*, **31**: 113–117.
12. Yolken R.H., Bachmann S., Rouslanova I.I., Lillehoj E., Ford G., Torrey E.F., Schroder J. (2001) Antibodies to Toxoplasma gondii in individuals with first-episode schizophrenia. *Clin. Infect. Dis.*, **32**: 842–844.
13. Niculescu A.B. (1999) Brainology. *MedGenMed.*, Aug 4; **E21**.
14. Cravchik A., Goldman D. (2000) Neurochemical individuality: genetic diversity among human dopamine and serotonin receptors and transporters. *Arch. Gen. Psychiatry*, **57**: 1105–1114.
15. Carlezon W.A. Jr., Nestler E.J., Neve R.L. (2000) Herpes simplex virus-mediated gene transfer as a tool for neuropsychiatric research. *Crit. Rev. Neurobiol.*, **14**: 47–67.
16. Smith D.E., Roberts J., Gage F.H., Tuszynski M.H. (1999) Age-associated neuronal atrophy occurs in the primate brain and is reversible by growth factor gene therapy. *Proc. Natl. Acad. Sci. USA*, **96**: 10 893–10 898.
17. Tuszynski M.H. (2000) Intraparenchymal NGF infusions rescue degenerating cholinergic neurons. *Cell Transplant.*, **9**: 629–636.
18. Mirnics K., Middleton F.A., Marquez A., Lewis D.A., Levitt P. (2000) Molecular characterization of schizophrenia viewed by microarray analysis of gene expression in prefrontal cortex. *Neuron*, **28**: 53–67.
19. Watson S.J., Meng F., Thompson R.C., Akil H. (2000) The "chip" as a specific genetic tool. *Biol. Psychiatry*, **48**: 1147–1156.
20. Lewohl J.M., Dodd P.R., Mayfield R.D., Harris R.A. (2001) Application of DNA microarrays to study human alcoholism. *J. Biomed. Sci.*, **8**: 28–36.
21. MacBeath G., Schreiber S.L. (2000) Printing proteins as microarrays for high-throughput function determination. *Science*, **289**: 1760–1763.
22. Stahl S.M. (2000) New drug discovery in the postgenomic era: from genomics to proteomics. *J. Clin. Psychiatry*, **61**: 894–895.
23. Bassingthwaighte J.B. (2000) Strategies for the physiome project. *Ann. Biomed. Eng.*, **28**: 1043–1058.
24. Gainetdinov R.R., Caron M.G. (2001) Genetics of childhood disorders: 24. ADHD, part 8: hyperdopaminergic mice as an animal model of ADHD. *J. Am. Acad. Child Adolesc. Psychiatry*, **40**: 380–382.
25. Stoll A.L., Renshaw P.F., Yurgelun-Todd D.A., Cohen B.M. (2000) Neuroimaging in bipolar disorders: what have we learned? *Biol. Psychiatry*, **48**: 505–517.
26. Stahl S.M. (2001) Does evidence from clinical trials in psychopharmacology apply in clinical practice? *J. Clin. Psychiatry*, **62**: 6–7.
27. Cosway R., Byrne M., Clafferty R., Hodges A., Grant E., Abukmeil S.S., Lawrie S.M., Miller P., Johnstone E.C. (2000) Neuropsychological change in young people at high risk for schizophrenia: results of the first two neuropsychological assessments of the Edinburgh High Risk Study. *Psychol. Med.*, **30**: 1111–1121.

28. Liu D., Diorio J., Day J.C., Francis D.D., Meaney M.J. (2000) Maternal care, hippocampal synaptogenesis and cognitive development in rats. *Nature Neurosci.*, **3**: 799–806.
29. Devanand D.P., Michaels-Marston K.S., Liu X., Pelton G.H., Padilla M., Marder K., Bell K., Stern Y., Mayeux R. (2000) Olfactory deficits in patients with mild cognitive impairment predict Alzheimer's disease at follow-up. *Am. J. Psychiatry*, **157**: 1399–1405.
30. Peppel K., Boekhoff I., McDonald P., Breer H., Caron M.G., Lefkowitz R.J. (1997) G protein-coupled receptor kinase 3 (GRK3) gene disruption leads to loss of odorant receptor desensitization. *J. Biol. Chem.*, **272**: 25 425–25 428.
31. Matsuoka Y., Picciano M., Malester B., LaFrancois J., Zehr C., Daeschner J.M., Olschowka J.A., Fonseca M.I., O'Banion M.K., Tenner A.J. *et al.* (2001) Inflammatory responses to amyloidosis in a transgenic mouse model of Alzheimer's disease. *Am. J. Pathol.*, **158**: 1345–1354.
32. Hull M., Lieb K., Fiebich B.L. (2000) Anti-inflammatory drugs: a hope for Alzheimer's disease? *Expert Opin. Investig. Drugs*, **9**: 671–683.
33. Ilani T., Ben-Shachar D., Strous R.D., Mazor M., Sheinkman A., Kotler M., Fuchs S. (2001) A peripheral marker for schizophrenia: increased levels of D3 dopamine receptor mRNA in blood lymphocytes. *Proc. Natl. Acad. Sci. USA*, **98**: 625–628.
34. Kwak Y.T., Koo M.S., Choi C.H., Sunwoo I. (2001) Change of dopamine receptor mRNA expression in lymphocyte of schizophrenic patients. *BMC Med. Genet.*, **2**: 3.
35. Avissar S., Barki-Harrington L., Nechamkin Y., Roitman G., Schreiber G. (2001) Elevated dopamine receptor-coupled G(s) protein measures in mononuclear leukocytes of patients with schizophrenia. *Schizophr. Res.*, **47**: 37–47.
36. Lohr J.B., Caligiuri M.P., Manley M.S., Browning J.A. (2000) Neuroleptic-induced striatal damage in rats: a study of antioxidant treatment using accelerometric and immunocytochemical methods. *Psychopharmacology*, **148**: 171–179.
37. Lohr J.B., Caligiuri M.P. (1996) A double-blind placebo-controlled study of vitamin E treatment of tardive dyskinesia. *J. Clin. Psychiatry*, **57**: 167–173.
38. Moore G.J., Bebchuk J.M., Wilds I.B., Chen G., Manji H.K. (2000) Lithium-induced increase in human brain gray matter. *Lancet*, **356**: 1241–1242.
39. Manji H.K., Moore G.J., Rajkowska G., Chen G. (2000) Neuroplasticity and cellular resilience in mood disorders. *Mol. Psychiatry*, **5**: 578–593.
40. Rezvani A.H., Levin E.D. (2001) Cognitive effects of nicotine. *Biol. Psychiatry*, **49**: 258–267.
41. Rattray M. (2001) Is there nicotinic modulation of nerve growth factor? Implications for cholinergic therapies in Alzheimer's disease. *Biol. Psychiatry*, **49**: 185–193.
42. Niculescu A.B., Akiskal H.S. (2001) Putative endophenotypes of dysthymia: evolutionary, clinical and pharmacogenomic considerations. *Mol. Psychiatry* (in press).
43. Noh J.S., Kim E.Y., Kang J.S., Kim H.R., Oh Y.J., Gwag B.J. (1999) Neurotoxic and neuroprotective actions of catecholamines in cortical neurons. *Exp. Neurol.*, **159**: 217–224.
44. Bozzi Y., Vallone D., Borrelli E. (2000) Neuroprotective role of dopamine against hippocampal cell death. *J. Neurosci.*, **20**: 8643–8649.
45. Malberg J.E., Eisch A.J., Nestler E.J., Duman R.S. (2000) Chronic antidepressant treatment increases neurogenesis in adult rat hippocampus. *J. Neurosci.*, **20**: 9104–9110.

46. van Praag H., Christie B.R., Sejnowski T.J., Gage F.H. (1999) Running enhances neurogenesis, learning, and long-term potentiation in mice. *Proc. Natl. Acad. Sci. USA*, **96**: 13 427–13 431.

47. Dimeo F., Bauer M., Varahram I., Proest G., Halter U. (2001) Benefits from aerobic exercise in patients with major depression: a pilot study. *Br. J. Sports Med.*, **35**: 114–117.

48. Babyak M., Blumenthal J.A., Herman S., Khatri P., Doraiswamy M., Moore K., Craighead W.E., Baldewicz T.T., Krishnan K.R. (2000) Exercise treatment for major depression: maintenance of therapeutic benefit at 10 months. *Psychosom. Med.*, **62**: 633–638.

49. Stahl S.M. (1998) Basic psychopharmacology of antidepressants, part 2: Estrogen as an adjunct to antidepressant treatment. *J. Clin. Psychiatry*, **59**: 15–24.

50. Stahl S.M. (2001) Sex and psychopharmacology: is natural estrogen a psychotropic drug in women? *Arch. Gen. Psychiatry* (in press).

51. Daly R.C., Su T.P., Schmidt P.J., Pickar D., Murphy D.L., Rubinow D.R. (2000) Cerebrospinal fluid and behavioral changes after methyltestosterone administration: preliminary findings. *Arch. Gen. Psychiatry*, **58**: 172–177.

52. Young E.A., Midgley A.R., Carlson N.E., Brown M.B. (2000) Alteration in the hypothalamic–pituitary–ovarian axis in depressed women. *Arch. Gen. Psychiatry*, **57**: 1157–1162.

53. Birmaher B., Dahl R.E., Williamson D.E., Perel J.M., Brent D.A., Axelson D.A., Kaufman J., Dorn L.D., Stull S., Rao U. *et al.* (2000) Growth hormone secretion in children and adolescents at high risk for major depressive disorder. *Arch. Gen. Psychiatry*, **57**: 867–872.

54. Placidi G.P., Boldrini M., Patronelli A., Fiore E., Chiovato L., Perugi G., Marazziti D. (1998) Prevalence of psychiatric disorders in thyroid diseased patients. *Neuropsychobiology*, **38**: 222–225.

55. Hahn C.G., Pawlyk A.C., Whybrow P.C., Gyulai L., Tejani-Butt S.M. (1999) Lithium administration affects gene expression of thyroid hormone receptors in rat brain. *Life Sci.*, **64**: 1793–1802.

56. Swann A.C., Bowden C.L., Calabrese J.R., Dilsaver S.C., Morris D.D. (1999) Differential effect of number of previous episodes of affective disorder on response to lithium or divalproex in acute mania. *Am. J. Psychiatry*, **156**: 1264–1266.

57. Fenton W.S., Hibbeln J., Knable M. (2000) Essential fatty acids, lipid membrane abnormalities, and the diagnosis and treatment of schizophrenia. *Biol. Psychiatry*, **47**: 8–21.

58. Freeman M.P. (2000) Omega-3 fatty acids in psychiatry: a review. *Ann. Clin. Psychiatry*, **12**: 159–165.

59. Maidment I.D. (2000) Are fish oils an effective therapy in mental illness?—An analysis of the data. *Acta Psychiatr. Scand.*, **102**: 3–11.

60. Tanskanen A., Hibbeln J., Tuomilehto J., Uutela A., Haukkala A., Viinamaki H., Lehtonen J., Vartiainen E. (2001) Fish consumption and depressive symptoms in the general population in Finland. *Psychiatr. Serv.*, **52**: 529–531.

61. Stoll A.L., Severus W.E., Freeman M.P., Rueter S., Zboyan H.A., Diamond E., Cress K.K., Marangell L.B. (1999) Omega-3 fatty acids in bipolar disorder: a preliminary double-blind, placebo controlled trial. *Arch. Gen. Psychiatry*, **56**: 407–412.

62. Mirnikjoo B., Brown S.E., Seung Kim H.F., Marangell L.B., Sweatt J.D., Weeber E.J. (2001) Protein kinase inhibition by omega-3 fatty acids. *J. Biol. Chem.* (in press).

63. Kaufman J., Plotsky P.M., Nemeroff C.B., Charney D.S. (2000) Effects of early adverse experiences on brain structure and function: clinical implications. *Biol. Psychiatry*, **48**: 778–790.

64. Lupien S.J., de Leon M., de Santi S., Convit A., Tarshish C., Nair N.P., Thakur M., McEwen B.S., Hauger R.L., Meaney M.J. (1998) Cortisol levels during human aging predict hippocampal atrophy and memory deficits. *Nature Neurosci.*, **1**: 69–73.

65. Bale T.L., Contarino A., Smith G.W., Chan R., Gold L.H., Sawchenko P.E., Koob G.F., Vale W.W., Lee K.F. (2000) Mice deficient for corticotropin-releasing hormone receptor-2 display anxiety-like behaviour and are hypersensitive to stress. *Nature Genet.*, **24**: 410–414.

66. Makino S., Baker R.A., Smith M.A., Gold P.W. (2000) Differential regulation of neuropeptide Y mRNA expression in the arcuate nucleus and locus coeruleus by stress and antidepressants. *J. Neuroendocrinol.*, **12**: 387–395.

67. Dautzenberg F.M., Braun S., Hauger R.L. (2001) GRK3 mediates desensitization of CRF(1) receptors: a potential mechanism regulating stress adaptation. *Am. J. Physiol. Regul. Integr. Comp. Physiol.*, **280**: R935–R946.

68. Isogawa K., Akiyoshi J., Hikichi T., Yamamoto Y., Tsutsumi T., Nagayama H. (2000) Effect of corticotropin releasing factor receptor 1 antagonist on extracellular norepinephrine, dopamine and serotonin in hippocampus and prefrontal cortex of rats in vivo. *Neuropeptides*, **34**: 234–239.

69. Habib K.E., Weld K.P., Rice K.C., Pushkas J., Champoux M., Listwak S., Webster E.L., Atkinson A.J., Schulkin J., Contoreggi C. *et al.* (2000) Oral administration of a corticotropin-releasing hormone receptor antagonist significantly attenuates behavioral, neuroendocrine, and autonomic responses to stress in primates. *Proc. Natl. Acad. Sci. USA*, **97**: 6079–6084.

70. Nestler E.J., Landsman D. (2001) Learning about addiction from the genome. *Nature*, **409**: 834–835.

71. Koob G.F., Le Moal M. (2001) Drug addiction, dysregulation of reward, and allostasis. *Neuropsychopharmacology*, **24**: 97–129.

72. Fienberg A.A., Hiroi N., Mermelstein P.G., Song W., Snyder G.L., Nishi A., Cheramy A., O'Callaghan J.P., Miller D.B., Cole D.G. *et al.* (1998) DARPP-32: regulator of the efficacy of dopaminergic neurotransmission. *Science*, **281**: 838–42.

73. Berke J.D., Hyman S.E. (2000) Addiction, dopamine, and the molecular mechanisms of memory. *Neuron*, **25**: 515–532.

74. Nestler E.J. (2001) Molecular basis of long-term plasticity underlying addiction. *Nature Rev. Neurosci.*, **2**: 119–128.

75. Simon S.L., Domier C., Carnell J., Brethen P., Rawson R., Ling W. (2000) Cognitive impairment in individuals currently using metamphetamine. *Am. J. Addict.*, **9**: 223–231.

76. Volkow N.D., Chang L., Wang G.J., Fowler J.S., Leonido-Yee M., Franceschi D., Sedler M.J., Gatley S.J., Hitzemann R., Ding Y.S. *et al.* (2001) Association of dopamine transporter reduction with psychomotor impairment in metamphetamine abusers. *Am. J. Psychiatry*, **158**: 377–382.

77. Volkow N.D., Chang L., Wang G.J., Fowler J.S., Franceschi D., Sedler M.J., Gatley S.J., Hitzemann R., Ding Y.S., Wong C. *et al.* (2001) Higher cortical and lower subcortical metabolism in detoxified methamphetamine abusers. *Am. J. Psychiatry*, **158**: 383–389.

78. Kelz M.B., Nestler E.J. (2000) DeltaFosB: a molecular switch underlying long-term neural plasticity. *Curr. Opin. Neurol.*, **13**: 715–720.

79. Bibb J.A., Chen J., Taylor J.R., Svenningsson P., Nishi A., Snyder G.L., Yan Z., Sagawa Z.K., Ouimet C.C., Nairn A.C. *et al.* (2001) Effects of chronic exposure to cocaine are regulated by the neuronal protein Cdk5. *Nature*, **410**: 376–380.

80. Kittler J.T., Grigorenko E.V., Clayton C., Zhuang S.Y., Bundey S.C., Trower M.M., Wallace D., Hampson R., Deadwyler S. (2000) Large-scale analysis of gene expression changes during acute and chronic exposure to delta 9-THC in rats. *Physiol. Genomics*, **3**: 175–185.

81. Johnson B.A., Roache J.D., Javors M.A., DiClemente C.C., Cloninger C.R., Prihoda T.J., Bordnick P.S., Ait-Daoud N., Hensler J. (2000) Ondansetron for reduction of drinking among biologically predisposed alcoholic patients: a randomized controlled trial. *JAMA*, **284**: 963–971.

82. Wager-Smith K., Kay S.A. (2000) Circadian rhythm genetics: from flies to mice to humans. *Nat. Genet.*, **26**: 23–27.

83. Thannickal T.C., Moore R.Y., Nienhuis R., Ramanathan L., Gulyani S., Aldrich M., Cornford M., Siegel J.M. (2000) Reduced numbers of hypocretin neurons in human narcolepsy. *Neuron*, **17**: 469–474.

84. Lin L., Faraco J., Li R., Kadotani H., Rogers W., Lin X., Qiu X., de Jong P.J., Nishino S., Mignot E. (1999) The sleep disorder canine narcolepsy is caused by a mutation in the hypocretin (orexin) receptor 2 gene. *Cell*, **98**: 365–376.

85. Chemelli R.M., Willie J.T., Sinton C.M., Elmquist J.K., Scammell T., Lee C., Richardson J.A., Williams S.C., Xiong Y., Kisanuki Y. *et al.* (1999) Narcolepsy in orexin knockout mice: molecular genetics of sleep regulation. *Cell*, **98**: 437–451.

86. Toh K.L., Jones C.R., He Y., Eide E.J., Hinz W.A., Virshup D.M., Ptacek L.J., Fu Y.H. (2000) An hPer2 phosphorylation site mutation in familial advanced sleep phase syndrome. *Science*, **291**: 1040–1043.

87. Franken P., Lopez-Molina L., Marcacci L., Schibler U., Tafti M. (2000) The transcription factor DBP affects circadian sleep consolidation and rhythmic EEG activity. *J. Neurosci.*, **20**: 617–625.

88. Andretic R., Chaney S., Hirsh J. (1999) Requirement of circadian genes for cocaine sensitization in Drosophila. *Science*, **285**: 1066–1068.

89. Menza M.A., Kaufman K.R., Castellanos A. (2000) Modafinil augmentation of antidepressant treatment in depression. *J. Clin. Psychiatry*, **61**: 378–381.

90. Black K.J., Sheline Y.I. (1997) Personality disorder scores improve with effective pharmacotherapy of depression. *J. Affect. Disord.*, **43**: 11–18.

91. Okuyama Y., Ishiguro H., Nankai M., Shibuya H., Watanabe A., Arinami T. (2000) Identification of a polymorphism in the promoter region of DRD4 associated with the human novelty seeking personality trait. *Mol. Psychiatry*, **5**: 64–69.

3

Brain Imaging Research in Psychiatry

Göran Sedvall and Stefan Pauli

*Department of Clinical Neuroscience, Hubin Project, Karolinska Institute and Hospital,
SE-171 76 Stockholm, Sweden*

INTRODUCTION

The evolution of the brain constitutes the basis for the emergence of all the psychological functions of the human mind. Animal and clinical work during the past 200 years has clearly demonstrated that consciousness, memories, language, concepts, feelings and emotions are dependent on activity in more or less well-defined neuronal networks in the brain. Diagnostic work in psychiatry has until recent years been exclusively based upon psychological interaction and careful observation of the patient's behaviour. Needless to say, more direct information about the integrity of the structure and function of the brain in individual patients would be of great value as a complement to conventional psychiatric skills and methods. Recent developments make it likely that the objective analyses of anatomical and functional brain correlates of mental phenomena will be indispensable for major progress in psychiatric diagnostic and therapeutic work.

This dream for many psychiatrists started to materialize at the end of the 1970s. Developments in the natural sciences including computer technology made it possible to apply physical principles discovered during the previous phase of the twentieth century to obtain images of the living human brain. In the early 1970s, advances in applied physics and computer science laid down the background for the development of instruments that permitted, for the first time, detailed visualization and analysis of the anatomy and function of the brain within the skull of living patients. These technical achievements include computed tomography (CT), magnetic resonance imaging (MRI) and the emission tomographic methods, single photon emission tomography (SPECT), and positron emission tomography (PET). These methods of brain imaging have since been the subject of intense technical development and are currently having a marked impact on clinical

Psychiatry as a Neuroscience. Edited by Juan José López-Ibor, Wolfgang Gaebel, Mario Maj and Norman Sartorius. © 2002 John Wiley & Sons Ltd.

psychiatric research, and to some extent also on clinical practice. In the present chapter the history and physical principles of each of these methods will be described and their application in psychiatric research projects outlined.

SPECIFIC BRAIN IMAGING METHODS

Computed Tomography

History and Physical Principles

X-rays were discovered by Wilhelm Conrad Röntgen in 1899. For this he was awarded the Nobel Prize in 1901. The high energy of X-rays makes them penetrate most biological tissues as a function of the electron density or the chemical composition of the tissue. Some tissues with a high calcium content (e.g. bone) have a high X-ray absorbing capacity (attenuation); soft tissues (e.g. brain) produce little attenuation. Accordingly, the conventional skull X-ray gives a distinct image of the bone structure surrounding the brain but is virtually useless with regard to information concerning brain structure. In 1918, Dandy developed the principle that X-rays are absorbed by air to a much lower extent than brain tissue. He injected air into the ventricular system and partly filled the cerebrospinal fluid (CSF) space with air, which allowed visualization of the ventricular system [1]. This principle, called pneumoencephalography, was used for several decades to examine brain structure in neurology. It was also used to describe ventricular enlargements in many patients with schizophrenia [2]. The painful side effects of this procedure precluded its use when other methods became available.

In commercial X-ray procedures, the X-ray tube and the detector (or film) are fixed in position and a single shot of X-rays is allowed to pass through the structure to be imaged. In 1973, Allan McCormac and Godfrey Hounsfield developed methods based upon mathematical linear integrals developed by Radon in 1919 for calculation of projections (transforms) and used the information from a number of X-ray exposures of the tissue from different angles [3]. They developed algorithms to reconstruct the tomographic distribution of the X-ray absorbtion in cross-sectional planes throughout the brain. The term "tomography" comes from *tomos*, the Greek word for cut. McCormac and Hounsfield were awarded the Nobel Prize in Physiology or Medicine in 1979 for developing the principle of computerized axial tomography (now called computed tomography, CT).

The CT technique is accordingly based on the principle of X-ray absorbtion (attenuation) in tissues. The information from a number of X-ray exposures of the brain from different angles is used to reconstruct tomographic image planes through the brain (Figure 3.1). This is accomplished by moving the X-ray tube and the detector in a circular or spiral process around the head. In every position the attenuation profile of the patient's brain is measured. This profile is called a projection. For each turn around the head, thousands of projections are measured. Each projection is transferred to the computer for image reconstruction. This procedure markedly increases the sensitivity at low absorption or attenuation levels. Recent CT cameras use scintillation crystals that produce light when hit by an X-ray and semiconductor technique. The light signal is converted to an electric signal which is fed into the computer. Modern X-ray cameras have several hundred detector elements to record the projection. Using this technique, the absorption in many brain sections can be recorded. Various soft tissues in the brain can be imaged with reasonably good contrast. In CT scan images, various shades of grey, black or white can then be assigned to a density number corresponding to each volume element (voxel). Thus, CSF, which has a low attenuation similar to that of water, appears almost black, whereas bone appears white. As shown in Figure 3.2, the best available CT scanners produce images of brain sections where details of the tissue structures can be visualized. The outline of the ventricular system is easily distinguished from the brain tissue proper. Although it is difficult to distinguish grey from white matter, several brain nuclei such as the basal ganglia and the thalamus can often be outlined. Using various contrast media that absorb X-rays, blood flow distribution can also be visualized (Figure 3.2).

Currently available CT scanners have a resolution of approximately 1 mm. The recent elaboration of computer techniques allows the imaging of the brain of living patients through several geometrical planes. Conventional high-resolution CT scanners show morphological features of about 2 to 5-mm thick sections throughout the brain.

A major advantage of CT is that it is quite patient-friendly in comparison with MRI and PET. It takes only 5–10 minutes to make a brain investigation. It is also quite cost-effective; for routine use the cost is in the order of US$ 500. It is also available in most medical institutions.

The major disadvantage is the radiation exposure, which is of the same order as that of an ordinary skull or chest X-ray. This precludes carrying out many repeated investigations. Another disadvantage is that it can only be used to examine structural features of the brain. Compared to MRI it gives rather low resolution and poor tissue differentiation, e.g. with regard to grey and white matter.

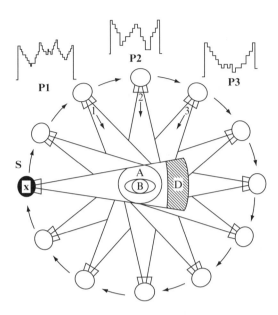

FIGURE 3.1 Computed tomography (CT) acquisition of data. The X-ray tube (X) and the detector (D) rotate stepwise (S) around the patient. In each position of the detector system (1, 2, etc.), the attenuation profile of the patient's head is measured. The profile is called a projection (P1, P2, etc.). For each turn thousands of projections can be created. Each projection is sent to the computer for image reconstruction

Modified after Siemens-Elema AB. Copyright Per-Åke Påhlstorp

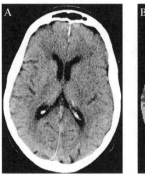
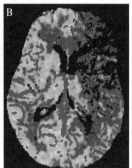

Precontrast CT   Flow Image

FIGURE 3.2 CT images of the brain of a 75-year-old woman with acute ischaemic stroke. **A** Precontrast CT (note visualization of the ventricular system and bone structure; note also poor contrast between grey and white matter). **B** CT image after injection of X-ray absorbing contrast medium reflecting blood flow. See colour plates

Modified after Siemens-Elema AB. Copyright Per-Åke Påhlstorp

Research Findings

The first systematic application of the CT technique in psychiatric research was made by Johnstone *et al.* [4]. These authors demonstrated unequivocally the occurrence of wide ventricles, wide cortical sulci and reduced size of cortical gyri in patients with schizophrenia as compared to healthy control subjects. Since then many studies have replicated these findings, and recent meta-analyses of studies in schizophrenic patients demonstrate a high consistency in this regard [5]. Alterations of the attenuation property of brain tissue and a reduced volume of specific neocortical and cerebellar regions in schizophrenia have also been reported in studies using the CT technique [6–9]. However, similar changes are often observed in pre-senile and senile dementia as well as in many cases of affective disorders, chronic alcoholism and drug abuse. Brain morphology as examined by CT also varies considerably with regard to the age of the patient and other individual factors. For this reason, all CT scanning measures in all studies have demonstrated a considerable overlap of data between psychiatrically specific diagnostic groups and control subjects. There is also evidence from several studies that subjects with apparently normal mental activity may have signs of marked cerebral changes on a CT scan. Thus, the specificity of changes reported from CT studies in various psychiatric diagnostic groups as well as their functional significance are still matters for further analysis and exploration.

CT scanning as hitherto applied by psychiatric research cannot be of diagnostic value as a single technique in psychiatry, even in dementia. In the future more refined analyses of brain morphology and the establishment of standardized quantitative reference values for various brain structures will be necessary before brain morphological dimensions as measured by CT can be introduced in psychiatric diagnostics. For this to be accomplished, the development of standardized databases for various features of human brain morphology will have to be developed. Comprehensive methods of assessing routine CT scans have recently been developed, allowing the pooling of data obtained by different research groups [10].

During recent years, developments in MRI and PET technology have to a large extent led to their gaining over the use of the CT technique in psychiatric research, because of the radiation hazards. However, it is evident that CT was the first brain imaging technique successfully used to examine biological changes in psychiatric disorders. Before the development of CT scanning, the occurrence of morphological brain alterations in such disorders besides dementias was generally not accepted by the scientific community.

Magnetic Resonance Imaging

History and Physical Principles

The word magnetism comes from the name of the city Magnesia in Turkey, where many naturally occurring magnets can be found. The first physical principles for magnetism were formulated by Karl Friedrich Gauss in the eighteenth century. James Clerk Maxwell discovered the fundamental laws of electromagnetism in the following century. Felix Bloch [11] and Edward Mills Purcell *et al.* [12] independently discovered the nuclear magnetic resonance (NMR) phenomenon and were jointly awarded the Nobel Prize for Physics in 1952.

The NMR phenomenon was first used to examine magnetic resonance spectroscopic (MS) properties of compounds in solution. In the 1960s, superconducting magnets and more efficient computers were developed. When they were combined with the image reconstruction techniques developed by Godfrey Hounsfield for X-ray tomography, the first in vivo magnetic resonance images could be reconstructed, which took place in the early 1970s [13]. Several kinds of MRI data can be acquired without exposing subjects to ionizing radiation or radioactive isotopes. Initially MRI was mainly used for visualizing the structure of the brain. In the early 1990s, functional magnetic resonance imaging (fMRI) was developed for the recording of rapid changes in local cerebral blood flow. The term "functional" MRI is related to neurovascular coupling, a phenomenon first reported by Roy Sherrington in 1894, who reported that local variations of functional neuronal activity are followed by local changes in blood flow. fMRI has been extensively used for mapping the functional anatomy of the human brain in living subjects. The first successful application of fMRI was when it was used to describe the functional activation of the occipital cortex by visual stimulation and the motor cortex by finger movements [14, 15]. A third modality using the NMR phenomenon is NMR spectroscopy (MRS). Although this method has not yet reached the status of an imaging technique, topographically covering widespread areas of the brain, it can currently be used to examine concentrations of some specific organic compounds and metabolites in blocks of brain tissue of living subjects.

Compared to the other imaging techniques mentioned in this chapter, the physical principles of MRI are more complex. The brain is largely composed of water, and each water molecule contains atoms of hydrogen and oxygen. The hydrogen nucleus is a positively charged proton that has an impulse momentum such that the charges within the nucleus can be regarded as rotating around an axis, i.e. the nucleus is said to have spin. When placed in a powerful magnetic field, nuclei show a precessional motion about the field direction (precession is similar to the wobbling of a spinning top). The precessional frequency increases as the field strength increases. Protons aligned with a static magnetic field precess at very high frequency around the axis of the external field. The precession frequency (Larmor frequency) is constant for a given type of atomic nucleus and the external field strength. All the hydrogen nuclei in the brain precess at the same frequency in the same field; however, they precess with different phases. Thus, at a given moment different nuclei have reached different points in their rotation around the axis of the external field. Bloch and Purcell showed that if radiofrequency stimuli were supplied to the atoms at the right angle to the magnetic field, the nuclei absorbed energy and precessed at a wider and wider angle from the magnetic field. When the radiofrequency stimulus was discontinued, the precessing nuclei emitted a brief radiofrequency signal (i.e. magnetic resonance signal) at the same frequency as the precession frequency. If a pulse of radiofrequency energy is applied at the Larmor frequency to a brain located in a magnetic field, the protons within the brain will absorb the energy and resonate. When the radiofrequency pulse has ceased, the resonating nuclei gradually relax back to the state of random precession. There are two components of this relaxation process, character-ized by so-called relaxation times. T_1 reflects the longitudinal and T_2 the transverse relaxation in relation to the magnetic field [11, 12].

The first relaxation time (T_1) is the time taken for the strength of longitu-dinal magnetization (parallel to the magnetic field) to return to 63% of its value before the end of the radiofrequency stimulation. T_1 is determined by interaction between protons and their long-range molecular environment.

The second relaxation time (T_2) describes the time it takes for the nuclei to stop marching in step around (perpendicular to) the axis of the magnetic field. When the radiofrequency pulse stops, the dephasing begins, but its rate is determined by the immediate atomic environment of the protons. When the protons relax, they emit energy absorbed from the radiofrequency pulse in the form of a weak radiofrequency signal which decreases at a rate normally determined by T_2. The character of these emitted signals consti-tutes the data from which magnetic resonance images are constructed.

MRI is the current method of choice for anatomical examination of the brain, because it is possible to produce marked image contrast between grey matter, white matter and CSF. Tissue contrast in MRI images is related to proton density. The physical and chemical environment of the protons also influences relaxation times. The location of the radiofrequency emitted is encoded in the three spatial dimensions by slice-selective radiofrequency pulses (Z-dimension) combined with the use of frequency- and phase-encoding magnetic field gradients for the XY dimensions.

The fast spin echo sequence represents a further refinement. Instead of eliciting a single echo after the pulse, fast spin echo imaging elicits several pulses (an echo train). Earlier echoes generate a proton-density-weighted image, and the latter can be used to form a T_2-weighted image. A fast spin echo sequence provides further tissue contrast with about the same scan time.

Diffusion-weighted imaging is another development of the MRI technique. Protons move by random brownian motion or diffusion within solutions. The rate of diffusion is greatest for protons in the CSF and less for protons limited by physical barriers such as myelinated axons. The diffusion rate affects the relaxation times. It is also possible to use diffusion-weighted imaging to show how compactly organized the white matter is and to estimate the orientation of fibre tracts. To obtain images weighted for diffusion, two extra magnetic gradients are applied during a spin echo sequence.

An MR system consists of the following components: a main magnet, magnetic gradient coils, a radiofrequency emitter and receiver, a computer and a patient data retrieval system. The key to a good MR magnet is its homogeneity. Currently superconducting magnets cooled by liquid helium are used. Most current machines have magnets with up to 1.5 Tesla (T) field strengths. However, magnets up to about 4 T are also available and are used for animal experimentation, but they are presumed to represent the limit of health hazards for human subjects. The gradient coils are used to generate magnetic field gradients in three dimensions for spatial localization. The gradient coils are placed between the patient and the main magnet. There is great demand on the current generators for the coils, since currents in the order of 50 A and voltages of 80 V with very rapid (>1 ms) alternations of current direction are required. The switching of the gradient coils produces the loud bumping sound (magnetostriction) one can hear when an MR machine is used. The radiofrequency coil has a two-fold function, to transmit the radiofrequency pulses for the imaging sequences and to receive the emitted signal. Head coils with a three-dimensional "bird cage" design are often used with good sensitivity throughout the volume they enclose.

Practically all general hospitals in the Western world have active MRI units. The within-plane resolution with 1.5 T magnets is of the order of 0.5–2 mm, with a slice thickness down to about 2 mm. With higher magnetic field strengths, higher resolution can be obtained. Currently some 3 T MRI scanners are used for neuropsychiatric research.

Visual inspection of MRI images allows the qualitative estimation of gross anatomical changes that are relatively often found in psychiatric patients. For more detailed analysis, quantitative methods have to be used. The previously most widely used method of measuring volumes of brain structures from MRI was based upon manual drawing of a line around the region of interest (ROI) on the image and determining the number of volume elements (voxels) in the image enclosed by the line. Measurements of several manually drawn ROIs through several sections were combined to produce three-dimensional volumes of different structures. Manual ROI morphometry is conceptually simple but very time-consuming. In recent years procedures have been developed that use automatic techniques for classification or segmentation of brain tissue. In one method based on discriminant analysis, the operator selects subsets of voxels in the image that are representative of each tissue class, i.e. white matter, grey matter and CSF [16]. These training data are then used to make a probabilistic assignment of each voxel in the image to one of the three classes (Figure 3.3). Before, or when the brain image has been divided into its tissue classes by segmentation, the image can be registered in a standard anatomical space, using mathematical transformation minimizing the difference between image and a template image in standard space. This procedure allows comparison of brain structure and volume between individuals. The parameters used for the transformation to line the image with a template can in turn be used as measures of brain structure [17].

The main advantage of nuclear magnetic imaging is the lack of radiation exposure. MRI with current technology also has a higher resolution than CT, SPECT and PET imaging. It is the only technique that allows reproducible differentiation of grey matter, white matter and CSF. Intra- and interrater

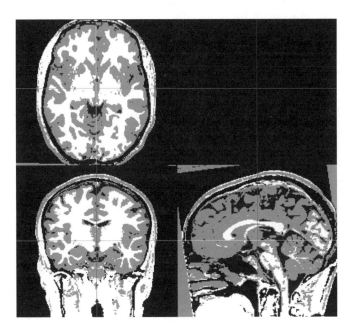

FIGURE 3.3 Tissue classification by magnetic resonance imaging (MRI). MRI of a 32-year-old healthy man. Discrete (categorical) classification of cerebrospinal fluid (black), grey matter (grey) and white matter (white)

By courtesy of Ingrid Agartz

reliability of measurements with structural MRI is usually better than 0.9 even for relatively small structures [18]. The investigation takes about 30 minutes and is relatively expensive, costing about US$ 750. The major disadvantage of MRI is that it is stressful for the subject (both the placement within the magnetic tunnel, which is critical for claustrophobic subjects, and also the relative noisiness of the investigation due to the bumping of the gradient coils). Currently there are no known health hazards with a magnetic field strength below 4 T. Other limitations of MRI are that it is quite sensitive to motion artefacts and the presence of metals.

Research Findings with Structural MRI

Schizophrenia. A large number of MRI studies performed during the past decade have confirmed previous findings with CT demonstrating expansion of lateral and third ventricles and other CSF spaces, as well as reduction of gyral size and widened sulci in the brain of many schizophrenic patients. Reduced volumes of total brain, dorsolateral prefrontal cortex, hippocampus and parts of the cerebellar vermis have also been demonstrated [19]. Although there is significant variability in all these studies and a considerable overlap in data between patients and control subjects, a number of studies have found significant volume reductions of specific brain regions in groups of schizophrenic patients. The studies appear to be most consistent with regard to reductions in prefrontal, temporal and specific lobules of the vermis in groups of patients with schizophrenia [18]. Several studies also indicate a clear tendency to lower intracranial cavities in patients with schizophrenia [20]. This is particularly evident for patients with childhood-onset schizophrenia [21]. MRI analysis of the volume of grey matter in a number of brain regions also tends to indicate that there are reductions in prefrontal brain regions, particularly the medial temporal cortex [22, 23]. Several studies examined lateralization of volume changes in schizophrenia; some investigators found more reduction on the left side in prefrontal and medial temporal cortex, but other groups were unable to verify such a lateralization [24–26].

In order to examine possible relationships between etiological factors for schizophrenia and brain morphological changes, several studies examined the brain morphology with MRI in patients with versus without a family history of the disorder. In this respect, too, results were not consistent. Some investigators found fewer morphological deviations in patients with a family history of the disorder, whereas most investigators found no marked differences in brain morphological features between schizophrenic patients with and without family history of the disorder. Studies in monozygotic twins discordant for the disorder demonstrated wider ventricles in the sick co-twin, indicating that expansion of CSF volume in schizophrenic patients is related to environmental rather than genetic factors [20, 27]. Interestingly, analysis of birth complications in monozygotic twins discordant for the disorder also indicated that the ill twin had suffered more perinatal complications and also had wider ventricles than the healthy twin [28].

Over the last few years several diffusion tensor imaging studies have indicated alterations in water diffusion parameters in several white matter tracts in patients with schizophrenia. However, here, too, results were divergent with regard to the region in the brain where such alterations could be demonstrated [29, 30]. Steel *et al.* [31] were unable to detect such differences between schizophrenic patients and controls.

Affective disorders. Comparisons of brain MRI data generally find more morphological deviations in schizophrenic patients than in those with affective disorders or alcohol abuse [32, 33]. The most consistent structural change in depressive patients is the observation of deep subcortical hyperintensities in patients with severe and old-age depression [34, 35]. In some studies, expansion of the ventricular system and reduction of prefrontal lobe volumes have also been observed [36]. Although authors of the latter study found reduced volumes of the left hippocampus in depressed patients, such a change has been questioned by other authors [37]. In a structural brain MRI study of depressed children, Steingard *et al.* [38] found a significantly lower frontal lobe volume in the depressive patients with early onset. The incidence of cavum septum pellucidum, which has often been regarded as a neurodevelopmental anomaly, has been found to be higher in patients with schizophrenia. Shioiri *et al.* [39] found that the frequency of this anomaly in patients with bipolar disorder was significantly higher than in control subjects, but slightly lower than in schizophrenic patients.

Functional Magnetic Resonance Imaging

History and Physical Principles

During the past decade, another important application of MRI has emerged, functional magnetic resonance imaging (fMRI). This technique has been applied to a number of important questions with regard to brain function. Two independent phenomena have made the development of fMRI possible. The first is the principle of neurovascular coupling, i.e. the fact that when neuronal activity is increased in a brain region, it is followed by a local increase in blood flow through the region. When the neurons in a local region of the neocortex are activated, e.g. by sensory stimulation, the local blood supply to the activated cortical area increases a few seconds after the onset of stimulation. The blood flow is elevated to a greater extent than the oxygen uptake in the region, causing a local increase in the ratio of oxygenated to deoxygenated haemoglobin [40]. This change in the ratio of oxyhaemoglobin to deoxyhaemoglobin affects the MRI signal, since deoxyhaemoglobin is more paramagnetic than oxyhaemoglobin (Figure 3.4). This will lead to prolongation of T_2 times in the area in relation to increased blood flow and functional activation. This haemodynamic effect can be recorded by a T_2-weighted signal which is *b*lood *o*xygen *l*evel-*d*ependent (BOLD) [42].

To optimize the signal for fMRI, special radiofrequency sequences paired with very rapid data acquisition are required. The advantage of this so-called *gradient echo imaging* is that both time for excitation and time between consecutive excitations can be markedly reduced, giving a reduction in scanning time. In less than three seconds, slices a few millimetres thick can be acquired covering the entire cortex. The technology required for this rapid gradient echo sequence has become available in most MR centres during the last few years, allowing the recording of functional changes with high temporal resolution over the entire brain.

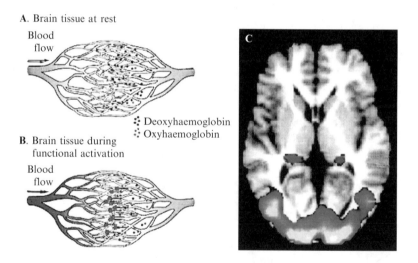

FIGURE 3.4 Functional magnetic resonance imaging (fMRI): blood oxygen level-dependent (BOLD) phenomenon reflecting blood flow. **A** Brain tissue at rest, containing a relatively low proportion of deoxyhaemoglobin in relation to oxyhaemoglobin. **B** After activation the proportion of deoxyhaemoglobin increases, giving a stronger signal from the tissue. **C** Image showing the increased signal in the visual cortex generated from a comparison of the cortex at rest and the activated cortex after visual stimulation. See color plates

Modified after [41]

The most common experimental design for psychiatric studies is to alter the subject's experience or behaviour in a reproducible way that is likely to produce a specific neuronal and neurovascular response. The most common is the blocked periodic design, useful for a range of investigations. It involves alternately presenting an activation condition and a baseline condition to the subject. During each condition several stimuli are presented. The cycle of alternation between the two conditions is repeated a number of times during the course of the experiment. Functional MRI data in the form of T_2-weighted signals are acquired repeatedly throughout the experiment.

Research Findings

The great potential of fMRI is to visualize brain regions involved in specific neuropsychological and neurophysiological processes. During the relatively few years since the development of this technique, it has been applied in a number of studies of considerable importance for neuropsychiatric research. Initial demonstrations that functional activations take place in primary cortical regions in relation to specific sensory stimulation verified the previously known localizations of brain visual, auditory and motor cortices. Of particular interest are studies of memory and cognition. Such studies have demonstrated relationships between activation in a number of brain regions, probably reflecting distributed neuronal networks in relation to memory acquisition and retrieval, with short- and long-term memory showing different activation patterns [43–45]. Specific cognitive tasks in relation to fMRI studies have since been elaborated in order to examine possible alterations in specific psychiatric patient groups.

Schizophrenia. Weinberger and his group examined activation of the dorsal prefrontal cortex in relation to complicated cognitive tasks, using the Wisconsin Card Sorting Test (WCST). Schizophrenic patients exhibited reduced activation of the prefrontal cortex and the medial temporal cortex compared to control subjects in this test [46]. Menon *et al.* [47], using fMRI, found evidence for disrupted basal ganglia function in schizophrenia. Woodruff *et al.* [48] found that auditory hallucinatory states in schizophrenic patients were associated with reduced activation in temporal cortical regions that normally express activity during external speech. These studies were performed in relatively small subject groups and showed considerable variability between subjects with regard to the magnitude of changes in relation to activation and also with regard to location of regions activated. For this reason, the effects observed in fMRI studies performed so far have to be replicated in substantially greater patient groups with standardization of research test paradigms before definitive conclusions can be drawn. The problem with fMRI is that activation patterns are relative and semiquantitative and can only be poorly recorded in subcortical brain regions, which complicates the interpretation of the location of primary perturbations in mental disorders as schizophrenia.

Affective disorders. To date little fMRI research has been done in psychiatric disorders besides schizophrenia. In order to examine the neuroanatomy of major depression, Beauregard *et al.* [49] performed an fMRI study using an emotion-activation paradigm. Subjects were exposed to an emotionally laden film aimed at inducing a transient state of sadness. Patients with unipolar depression as well as normal subjects had significant activation in the medial and inferior prefrontal cortices, the middle temporal cortex, the cerebellum and the caudate. The depressed patients exhibited significantly greater activation in the left medial prefrontal cortex and in the right cingulate gyrus compared with controls, indicating alterations in these regions in the pathophysiology of depressive states.

Anxiety disorders. A few fMRI studies have so far been performed in phobic states. Birbaumer *et al.* [50] found excessive activation of the amygdala in human social phobics. In the same category of patients, Schneider *et al.* [51] found that conditioned stimuli with negative odour led to signal increase, whereas an opposite decrease in the same regions was obtained in normal subjects.

Single Photon Emission Tomography and Positron Emission Tomography

Another principle employed to obtain information about events within the living brain is to introduce specific compounds labelled with radioactive isotopes into the brain. The signals emitted from these radioactively labelled compounds reflect the dynamic distribution of the compounds in the brain. This is the principle of emission tomography. By selecting compounds that participate in brain functions without fundamentally altering them, kinetic information about the fate of the compound may be used as an index of such functions in brain regions.

Gamma radiation easily penetrates the skull and brain tissue. When gamma-ray-emitting isotopes are used to label compounds that interact with brain metabolism or constituents thereof, their location in brain tissue can be externally determined by crystal detectors that emit photons, or light, when hit by gamma rays. Using systems of such scintillation detectors positioned around the head, it is possible to follow dynamic metabolic or molecular events by measuring radioactivity in regions of the brain over time. Currently, there are two types of emission tomography: single photon emission computed tomography (SPECT) and positron emission tomography (PET).

History and Physical Principles

SPECT and PET are based upon radiotracer principles. Several types of radioactive isotopes are used to label specific compounds as markers for different physiological and biochemical pathways. The radiotracers are usually administered intravenously and the emission resulting from the decaying radioactive isotope is recorded externally by sensitive detectors.

In 1961, Lassen and Ingvar introduced the first method for determination of regional cerebral blood flow (rCBF), using arterial administration of inert radioactive gases such as krypton-85 (^{85}Kr), or xenon-133 (^{133}Xe) [52]. They recorded the gamma radiation emitted from these isotopes using several scintillation detectors and measured the clearance of these isotopes from cortical regions of the brain. This method allowed them to describe a hypofrontal rCBF distribution pattern in chronic schizophrenic patients [53]. The introduction of SPECT in ^{133}Xe rCBF measurements by Stokeley *et al.* [54] enabled three-dimensional studies of rCBF using rotating detector systems and reconstruction of images reflecting the isotope distribution in the brain.

Recent developments in multidetector systems have made the SPECT technique highly sensitive and given it high resolution. The SPECT camera is less expensive than PET cameras and less technically demanding, which has made it more readily available in many hospitals and research units. The random occurrence of gamma radiation in nature creates a relatively high noise level for the detectors used in SPECT. The most common radioisotopes used for SPECT are technetium-99 (^{99m}Tc) and iodine-123 (^{123}I). These isotopes have half-lives of about 6 and 13 hours respectively. SPECT radiotracers useful for measurement of blood flow, dopamine, serotonin and benzodiazepine receptors, and monoamine transporters are presented in Table 3.1.

SPECT cameras currently have a resolution of the order of about 5 mm in all three dimensions. Using the appropriate radiotracer, selective relative measurements of blood flow and receptor or transporter molecules related to the monoamine and γ-aminobutyric acid (GABA) systems can be obtained. With correction for the random occurrence of gamma radiation it is possible to obtain semi-quantification of physiological and biochemical parameters. The production of isotopes with high specific activity can allow detection of sub-nanomolar concentrations of molecules, as for example dopamine receptors, in the brain.

TABLE 3.1 Single photon emission tomography (SPECT) radiotracers and their application

Radiotracers	Measurement
[^{99m}Tc]HMPAO	Blood flow
[^{123}I]IMP	Blood flow
[^{123}I]Iodobenzamide	Dopamine D_2/D_3 receptors
[^{123}I]Epidepride	Dopamine D_2/D_3 receptors
[^{123}I]Iomazenil	Benzodiapine receptors
[^{123}I]Nor-β-CIT	Dopamine and serotonin transporters

Since the isotopes used in SPECT are not normal constituents of organic molecules and have a relatively large molecular size, they may alter the property of the tracer molecule to which they are attached, which may influence the quantification of physiological parameters. The advantage is their long half-life, which makes it possible to ship radiotracer molecules from a synthesizing centre to the research site where the SPECT experiment is to be performed. The SPECT technique is only available for limited types of functional studies, such as blood flow and some receptor and transporter molecules. Compared to PET, SPECT has a lower sensitivity and resolution. Moreover, it has a lower potential for quantification.

Further refinement of emission tomographic methods came about when short-lived positron-emitting isotopes became generally available from the cyclotron industry in the 1950s. This allowed the synthesis of short-lived radiotracers and the development of the PET technique. Positron-emitting isotopes make possible a marked reduction of the effect of random noise from natural gamma radiation. These isotopes are produced by bombardment of natural elements with protons in a cyclotron. Positron-emitting isotopes are highly unstable. When disintegrating they emit positrons, i.e. positively charged electron-like particles (antimatter). The positron passes efficiently through the tissue until it encounters an electron. When these particles collide, they are both annihilated and simultaneously two gamma rays are emitted in opposite directions close to 180° from each other. It is possible to detect these two gamma rays by coincidence-coupled scintillation detectors in a ring (Figure 3.5). Using this procedure, only signals arising from the simultaneous activation of two detectors can be used for image reconstruction of the radiotracer distribution in the brain. Each coincidence-coupled detector pair detects the gamma radiation from isotope decays close to a line between the two detectors. By arranging rings of detectors

A. Positron emission in the brain   B. Positron camera, image generation

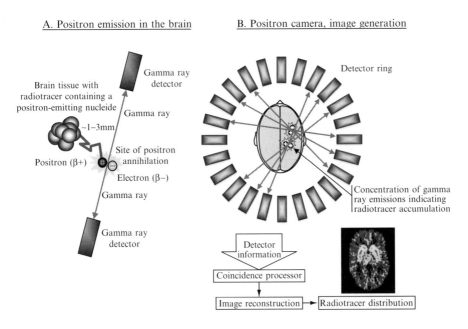

FIGURE 3.5 Principles of positron emission tomography (PET). **A** Radiotracer nucleide decays and emits a positron. The positron travels 1–3 mm and annihilates with an electron in the tissue, creating two gamma rays emitted in opposite directions. **B** The two gamma rays strike opposing detectors, mounted in a ring of many detectors, and a "coincidence event" is recorded. Image reconstruction yields the radiotracer distribution. See color plates

around the subject's head and using computer-based back projection techniques, the distribution of radiotracer can be obtained in two- or three-dimensional space. Initially, in the beginning of the 1970s, primitive PET cameras were developed that used only a few such coincidence-coupled detectors [55]. Over the years, the number of detectors placed in rings around the head has multiplied by more than a thousand-fold. An important historical event in PET was the use of 2-deoxyglucose labelled with the positron emitters fluorine-18 (^{18}F) or carbon-11 (^{11}C) as radiotracer to examine blood flow in local regions of the brain [56]. A second important step was the development by Wagner *et al.* of the first relatively selective neuroreceptor radioligand useful for PET [57]. This radioligand allowed for the first time the location of molecular components of specific neuronal signalling mechanisms to be visualized in the living human brain. These were also the first methods by which the molecular targets of neuroleptic drugs in regions of the human brain could be visualized and quantified [58, 59].

Several positron emitting isotopes useful for physiological studies can be produced by a cyclotron. The most common are oxygen-15 (^{15}O), carbon-11

(^{11}C) and fluorine-18 (^{18}F), with half-lives of about 2, 20 and 110 minutes respectively. These isotopes are highly versatile, because they are isotopes of normal constituents in organic molecules and drugs and their molecular sizes are close to those of the natural isotopes. Their short half-life is another advantage from the point of view of patient radiation exposure. However, the short half-life of these isotopes makes special demands on the possibility of having a cyclotron on site and a rapid and efficient radiosynthesis procedure to produce the radiotracer. The radiosynthesis procedure requires automated radiosynthesis facilities and quality control to estimate the specific activity and chemical purity of the radiotracer produced. The most recent cyclotrons can produce the positron isotopes to very high specific activities (>2000 Ci/mmol), which allows the use of very small mass amounts of the radiotracers, typically less than a few micrograms for a human subject. Thus, the radiotracers used in current PET experimentation are commonly used in such small amounts that they do not produce any pharmacological or mass effects on physiological mechanisms, which can be recorded with very high sensitivity. The rapid decay of the positron isotopes makes the radiation exposure brief (less than an hour). Table 3.2 presents a list of radiotracers useful for PET. Their research applications have expanded at an increasing rate in recent years.

Until the past few years, the PET technique has been most commonly used for recording regional changes of glucose metabolism and blood flow in research projects concerning cognition and psychiatric disorders. The rapid development of fMRI may lead to a diminution of these PET applications, although PET has the advantage of absolute quantification. On the other hand, PET appears to be the method of choice for examining radiotracer binding to explore signalling mechanisms in specific synaptic pathways of the brain. The availability of specific PET tracers for subtypes of dopamine and serotonin receptors as well as the transporters for serotonin, dopamine and noradrenaline in the brain represent new, intriguing developments (Figure 3.6) [60–62]. This has been made possible by the development of highly selective radioligands for various biochemical molecules participating in signal transmission in the brain. For example [^{11}C]raclopride, a highly selective D_2-dopamine receptor antagonist, when injected intravenously in tracer amounts, shows a highly reproducible profile of radioactivity accumulation over time in areas with a high density of D_2-class dopamine receptors. On the other hand, regions with a low density of these receptors, such as the cerebellum, will show little uptake. In this way, specific and non-specific binding can be distinguished using appropriate radiotracer models where the time–radioactivity curve can be used to quantify receptor number and affinity [58, 63]. The qualitative validity of this procedure has been demonstrated by showing the saturability and stereospecificity of radiotracer binding to dopamine receptors [59].

TABLE 3.2 Positron emission tomography (PET) radiotracers and their application

Radiotracer	Measurement
$C^{15}O_2/H_2^{15}O$	Blood flow
[^{11}C]SCH 23390	Dopamine D_1 receptor
[^{11}C]NNC112	Dopamine D_1 receptor
[^{11}C]Raclopride	Dopamine D_2 receptor
[^{11}C]FLB-457	Dopamine D_2 receptor
[^{11}C]RTI 121 and 32	Dopamine reuptake site markers
[^{18}F]Dopa and [^{18}F]Metatyrosine	Dopaminergic neuron density and integrity
[^{11}C]Dihydroxytetrabenazine	Vesicular monoamine transporter
[^{11}C]PE21	Dopamine transporter
[^{11}C]WAY 100635	Serotonin 5-HT$_{1A}$ receptor
[^{11}C]MDL-100907	Serotonin 5-HT$_{2A}$ receptor
[^{18}F]Altanserin	Serotonin 5-HT$_2$ receptor
[^{18}F]Setoperone	Serotonin 5-HT$_2$ receptor
[^{11}C]Methylspiperone	Cortical 5-HT$_2$ receptors and striatal D_2 receptors
[^{11}C]McN 5652	Serotonin transporter
[^{11}C]Methyltryptophan	Possible measure of serotonin synthesis rate
[^{11}C]Diprenorphine	Opiate μ, κ, and δ receptors
[^{11}C]Carfentanil	Opiate μ receptors
[^{11}C]Flumazenil	Central benzodiazepine receptors

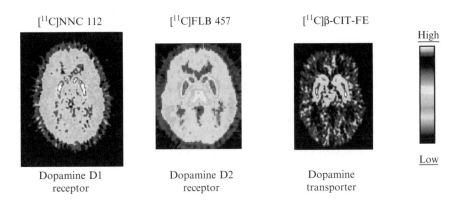

[^{11}C]NNC 112 — Dopamine D1 receptor

[^{11}C]FLB 457 — Dopamine D2 receptor

[^{11}C]β-CIT-FE — Dopamine transporter

High

Low

FIGURE 3.6 Examples of radioligands for positron emission tomography (PET) imaging of the dopamine system. See color plates

By courtesy of Lars Farde and Christer Halldin

The radiotracer binding approach has also been used in attempts to demonstrate alterations of amphetamine-induced transmitter release in the living human brain [64]. Although this approach cannot be used for quantitative purposes, due to the uncertainty of a number of assumptions for the kinetic models used, it has given interesting indications for increased dopamine release in studies on schizophrenia.

The great potential of the PET technology is its high specificity and sensitivity with regard to specific physiological and biochemical measurements. In these respects PET is unsurpassed by the other imaging modalities. The ability to obtain quantitative estimates of intracerebral mechanisms is another important feature. The limitation of PET is its rather low spatial resolution, currently of the order of 3–5 mm in the three dimensions. Currently, PET cameras with several thousands of detectors placed in rings around the head represent the state of the art.

As with other imaging techniques, SPECT and PET data are often presented and compared after transformation of the data into a standard brain space. The one commonly used for this purpose is the Talairach and Tournoux atlas [17].

A major advantage of PET blood flow measurements using oxygen-15 (^{15}O) labelled water is the ability to obtain quantitative data and also perform repeated measurements. Thus, several measurements of rCBF can be obtained over a three-hour period in a single subject. Previous studies were done predominantly by comparing subject groups at rest. In recent years subjects have been scanned while engaged in specific cognitive tasks. This is in principle similar to the experimental approaches used for fMRI. The major limitation of the PET technology, besides low resolution, is the very great expense involved, relating both to isotope production and radiosynthesis and to the cost of the cyclotron, the camera and the computer equipment required.

Studies of Glucose Metabolism and Blood Flow

As described above, SPECT and PET studies with radiotracers for glucose metabolism and blood flow reflect net neuronal activity in gross brain regions. To date, more than 700 articles have been published on psychiatric research using these methods. In this chapter, results obtained in schizophrenia and some other psychiatric disorders will be briefly summarized as relevant examples.

Schizophrenia In extensive series of studies using labelled deoxyglucose, Buchsbaum and his group have described abnormal regional glucose metabolism in schizophrenics both at rest and during specific cognitive tasks [65]. In these studies, reduced metabolism was primarily found in the frontal and temporal cortex. Patients with schizophrenia were also found to have lower metabolic rates in the anterior cingulate gyrus and higher rates in the posterior cingulate [66].

Rapoport and her group examined cerebral glucose metabolism by PET in childhood-onset schizophrenia. The results indicated reduced metabolic rate in the superior and middle frontal gyrus and increased rate in inferior frontal and supramarginal gyrus. There was also evidence for increased cerebellar metabolic rate in childhood-onset schizophrenia [67].

Using PET measurements of blood flow with [^{15}O]water, Andreasen and her group [68] also obtained evidence for reduced functional activity in frontal regions in neuroleptic naïve patients with schizophrenia. Three separate prefrontal regions (lateral, orbital, medial), as well as regions in inferior temporal and parietal cortex, had decreased perfusion. Regions with increased perfusion were also identified (thalamus, cerebellum, retrosplenial cingulate).

These findings are similar to data recently found by Kim *et al.* [69] in PET studies of blood flow in patients with chronic schizophrenia, and support the view that primary neural abnormalities in schizophrenia may be located to frontal, cerebellar and thalamic regions.

Martinot and his group [70] found evidence for cinguloparietal dysfunction and altered hemispheric functional dominance during working memory and word generation tasks in groups of patients with schizophrenia. Anterior cingulate gyrus dysfunction has also been implicated in attention deficits in schizophrenia by Carter *et al.* [71] and Dolan *et al.* [72].

Suzuki *et al.* [73] used SPECT to demonstrate increased blood flow in the left superior temporal area in hallucinating schizophrenic patients. Several groups examined regional blood flow by PET in relation to auditory verbal hallucinations. These authors also found alterations in brain areas normally involved in auditory perception such as mesotemporal regions [74, 75].

Liddle *et al.* [76] used PET to study the relationship between rCBF and symptom profiles in schizophrenic patients. The study confirmed predictions that psychomotor poverty and disorganization were associated with altered perfusion at different loci in the prefrontal cortex, and reality distortion with altered perfusion in the medial temporal lobe. Sabri *et al.* [77] examined blood flow with PET in schizophrenic patients and presented evidence that formal thought disorder and grandiosity correlated positively with bifrontal and bitemporal blood flow, whereas delusions and hallucinations were related to reduced flow in the cingulate, left thalamic, left frontal and left temporal regions.

Recent SPECT studies of blood flow in schizophrenic patients and their relatives found evidence of reduced perfusion in the left inferior prefrontal and anterior cingulate cortex in both patients and their relatives as compared to control subjects [78].

A recent more extensive review of PET studies in schizophrenia was published by Schultz and Andreasen [79]. The functional brain imaging studies with PET indicate that several frontal, temporal, cingulate, thalamic and cerebellar subregions exhibit altered activities in patients with schizophrenia.

Affective disorders. Ito *et al*. [80] examined blood flow with SPECT in groups of patients with unipolar and bipolar depression compared with controls. Both depressive groups showed significant reductions in blood flow in the prefrontal cortex, limbic system and paralimbic areas.

Drevets *et al*. [81] used PET to examine blood flow and glucose metabolism. They localized an area of abnormally decreased activity in the prefrontal cortex ventral to the genu of the corpus callosum in both familial bipolar depressives and familial unipolar depressives. The decrement in activity was at least partly explained by a reduction in cortical volume, since MRI demonstrated reductions in the grey matter volume in the same area in both patient samples.

Elliot *et al*. [82] used PET to measure blood flow in patients with unipolar depression and controls during cognitive performance. Depressed patients failed to show activation in the medial caudate and ventromedial orbitofrontal cortex. Blood flow was lower, and a differential response observed in normals under different task and feedback conditions was not seen in the patients.

In a PET study with [^{15}O]water to examine blood flow during provocation of transient sadness in depressed patients and controls, Mayberg *et al*. [83] found increases in limbic and paralimbic blood flow (subgenual cingulate, anterior insula) and decreases in neocortical regions (right dorsolateral prefrontal, inferior parietal).

Anxiety disorders. PET studies of blood flow in patients with phobia indicate that phobic fear might involve alterations of the anterior insular region, anterior cingulate, cerebellar vermis, amygdala, thalamus and striatum [84–86].

Studies of Transmitter Mechanisms

The possibility of using specific radioligands for neuroreceptors and transporters has allowed analysis of specific components of neurochemical signalling pathways in the living brains of psychiatric patients.

Schizophrenia. Most work has been done in the dopamine field. Such studies failed to consistently demonstrate alterations of D_1 and D_2 dopamine receptors in the basal ganglia of schizophrenic patients [87]. In some neocortical regions, too, results were equivocal. Two preliminary studies indicate reduced D_2 dopamine receptor binding in the thalamus of patients with schizophrenia (Farde L. and Suhara T., unpublished data).

The use of amphetamine challenge of radioligand binding to D_2 receptors has allowed the indirect estimation of dopamine release in schizophrenic patients by both SPECT and PET [64, 88]. Laruelle and Abi-Dargham [89] recently reviewed these studies where amphetamine-induced reduction of raclopride binding, as examined by PET, indicated elevated dopamine release in patients with schizophrenia as compared to control subjects.

Using the radiotracer [^{11}C]DTBZ (dihydrotetrabenazine) and PET to examine the vesicular monoamine transporter in patients with schizophrenia, euthymic patients with bipolar disorder type I and age-matched controls, Zubieta *et al.* [89] obtained interesting results: binding of the radiotracer in the thalamus was higher in the bipolar patients than in schizophrenic patients and in controls. Conversely, ventral brainstem binding was higher both in bipolar and in schizophrenic patients as compared to controls. These findings may indicate both similarities and differences regarding monoaminergic mechanisms in the thalamus and the ventral brainstem in these disorders.

PET studies of serotonin $5HT_{2A}$ receptors in patients with schizophrenia have also been published [91]. Several groups using the radioligand [^{18}F] setoperone or [^{11}C]NMSP (N-methylspiperone) failed to find major alterations of these receptors [92–94].

Studies of benzodiazepine receptors in schizophrenia have also been initiated. Thus, using SPECT with [^{123}I]iomazenil as radiotracer, Busatto *et al.* [95] found evidence for reduced benzodiazepine receptor binding in limbic cortical regions. This effect correlated to positive symptoms. Visualization and quantification of benzodiazepine receptor populations in three dimensions in the living human brain, using PET, [^{11}C]flumazenil and volume-rendering technique, was performed by Pauli *et al.* [96] and Pauli and Sedvall [97].

Affective disorders. Drevets *et al.* [98] used PET and [^{11}C]WAY-100635 as radiotracer to examine the radioligand binding potential (BP) to $5HT_{1A}$ receptors. The mean BP was reduced 42% in the raphe and 27% in the mesiotemporal cortex in depressed patients. The magnitude of these abnormalities was most prominent in bipolar depressives and unipolar depressives with relatives with bipolar disorder. Similar results were obtained by Sargent *et al.* [99].

$5HT_{2A}$ receptor binding was examined with PET by Biver *et al.* [100] in drug-free unipolar depressed patients and healthy subjects. [^{18}F]altanserin uptake was reduced in the posterolateral orbitofrontal cortex and the anterior insular cortex. Yatham *et al.* [101], using another radioligand for $5HT_{2A}$ receptors, [^{18}F]setoperone, demonstrated significantly lower $5HT_{2A}$

receptor binding in frontal, temporal, parietal and occipital cortical regions as compared to healthy controls. Meyer *et al.* [102], using the same radio-ligand, found no significant change of $5HT_{2A}$ receptors in depressed patients.

Studies of Antipsychotic Drug Action

Studies of treated schizophrenic patients have revealed the usefulness of radioligand studies with PET to explore pharmacokinetic aspects of neuro-leptic drug action on monoamine receptors in the brain [59, 103]. Such studies have demonstrated profound effects of conventional and atypical antipsychotic drugs on radioligand binding to D_2 dopamine and $5HT_{2A}$ serotonin receptors in the brain. High occupancy levels of dopamine D_2 receptors were obtained by conventional drugs [61, 103–105]. Clozapine produced a significantly lower degree of D_2 occupancy than the conven-tional drugs in patients treated with usual doses. Occupancy of $5HT_{2A}$ receptors was very high for clozapine and the new generation of atypical antipsychotics. Interestingly, several of the conventional antipsychotic drugs, such as chlorpromazine, were also found to induce a high level of occupancy of $5HT_{2A}$ receptors [91].

The PET studies of receptor occupancy by antipsychotic drugs have had profound practical implications. These studies demonstrated the specificity of antipsychotic drug targets in the living human brain. They also demon-strated quantitative relationships between D_2 dopamine receptor occupancy and antipsychotic as well as extrapyramidal side effects of neuroleptics [106]. These studies have also been instrumental in giving objective argu-ments for selection of lower antipsychotic drug doses for the treatment of schizophrenic patients than those previously used.

CONCLUSIONS

The brain imaging methods outlined in this chapter have brought new dimensions to research in psychiatry. The ability to examine structural, gross functional and neurosignalling mechanisms in the living human brain has allowed the initiation of an experimental analysis of brain–mind interaction in individual living human subjects. In disorders previously thought to be exclusively of a functional nature, such as schizophrenia, subtle alterations of brain structure have been consistently demonstrated. The functional imaging methods (fMRI, SPECT and PET) have demon-strated a variety of perturbations of functional activation levels during

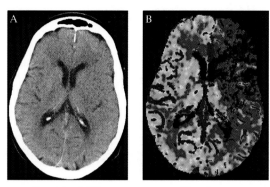

Precontrast CT   Flow Image

FIGURE 3.2 CT images of the brain of a 75-year-old woman with acute ischaemic stroke. **A** Precontrast CT (note visualization of the ventricular system and bone structure; note also poor contrast between grey and white matter). **B** CT image after injection of X-ray absorbing contrast medium reflecting blood flow.

Modified after Siemens-Elema AB. Copyright P-Åke PÅhlstorp

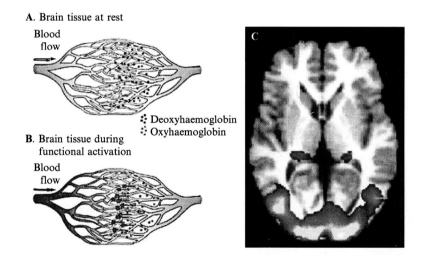

FIGURE 3.4 Functional magnetic resonance imaging (fMRI): blood oxygen level-dependent (BOLD) phenomenon reflecting blood flow. **A** Brain tissue at rest, containing a relatively low proportion of deoxyhaemoglobin in relation to oxyhaemoglobin. **B** After activation the proportion of deoxyhaemoglobin increases, giving a stronger signal from the tissue. **C** Image showing the increased signal in the visual cortex generated from a comparison of the cortex at rest and the activated cortex after visual stimulation.

Modified after [41]

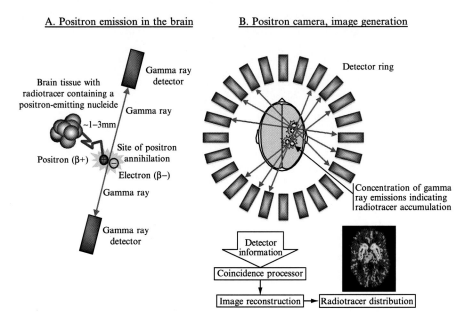

A. Positron emission in the brain

B. Positron camera, image generation

FIGURE 3.5 Principles of positron emission tomography (PET). **A** Radiotracer nucleide decays and emits a positron. The positron travels 1–3 mm and annihilates with an electron in the tissue, creating two gamma rays emitted in opposite directions. **B** The two gamma rays strike opposing detectors, mounted in a ring of many detectors, and a "coincidence event" is recorded. Image reconstruction yields the radiotracer distribution.

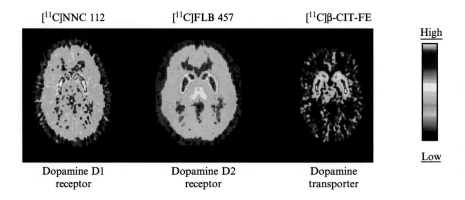

FIGURE 3.6 Examples of radioligands for positron emission tomography (PET) imaging of the dopamine system.

By courtesy of Lars Farde and Christer Halldin

cognitive tasks related to attention, speech, sensory and motor stimulation in particular groups of patients with schizophrenia and affective disorders.

In schizophrenia, evidence for altered structure and function in various prefrontal, temporal, cingular, thalamic and cerebellar regions has been collected. Radioligand studies indicate that presynaptic mechanisms for dopamine release may be perturbed in schizophrenia. The demonstration of such changes is of interest in relation to the antipsychotic actions of dopamine D_2 receptor antagonists.

In affective disorders, functional changes were observed in medial frontal, orbitofrontal and cingulate cortex and the amygdala. Clear evidence for reduced densities of serotonin $5HT_{1A}$ receptors has also been obtained in untreated depressed patients. These changes are of interest in relation to the mechanism for the antidepressant action of serotonin reuptake inhibitors.

The further use of these methods can be expected to dramatically alter and develop our conception of the biological substrates behind psychological phenomena produced by the human brain. This knowledge, when used in further systematic studies on all the different diagnostic categories of psychiatric disorders, will be a most fruitful dimension of clinical psychiatric research in the decades to come. The divergent results obtained so far with the functional imaging methods are in all probability partly related to heterogeneity of patient populations, experimental methods and paradigms. Experimental patient groups have generally been too small to reflect this heterogeneity. The fact that psychiatric symptoms and disorders are related to highly complex signalling neuronal networks within gross regions and between a large number of regions complicates the experimental and statistical analysis required to reveal significant signals and correlation patterns. For each imaging modality hundreds rather than tens of patients have to be examined in relation to a specific clinical question. Further research in the area has to take all this into account by standardizing experimental research paradigms between research groups and also by combining databases of results obtained in patient groups.

ACKNOWLEDGEMENT

General support was received from the National Institutes of Mental Health, Bethesda, MD, USA (NIMH 44814-12), the Swedish Medical Research Council (03560), The Wallenberg Foundation and the HUBIN Consortium, Karolinska Institute, Stockholm. Excellent secretarial support was supplied by Mrs. Marita Signarsson.

REFERENCES

1. Dandy W.E. (1919) Roentgenography of the brain after the injection of air into the spinal canal. *Ann. Surg.*, **70**: 397–403.
2. Cazzullo C.L. (1963) Biological and clinical studies on schizophrenia related to pharmacological treatment. *Rec. Adv. Biol. Psychiatry*, **5**: 114–143.
3. McCormac A.M. (1973) Reconstruction of densities from their projections, with application in radiological physics. *Phys. Med. Biol.*, **18**: 195–207.
4. Johnstone E.C., Crow T.J., Frith C.D., Husband J., Kreel L. (1976) Cerebral ventricular size and cognitive impairment in chronic schizophrenia. *Lancet*, 2: 924–926.
5. Vita A., Dieci M., Tenconi F. (1996) A meta-analysis of magnetic resonance imaging studies in schizophrenia. *Eur. Neuropsychopharmacol.*, **6**: S4–S45.
6. DeLisi L.E. (1999) Defining the course of brain structural change and plasticity in schizophrenia. *Psychiatry Res.*, **92**: 1–9.
7. Pearlson G.D., Marsh L. (1999) Structural brain imaging in schizophrenia: a selective review. *Biol. Psychiatry*, **46**: 627–649.
8. Supprian T., Ulmar G., Bauer M., Schuler M., Puschel K., Retz-Junginger P., Schmitt H.P., Heinsen H. (2000) Cerebellar vermis area in schizophrenic patients—a post-mortem study. *Schizophr. Res.*, 42: 19–28.
9. Zakzanis K.K., Poulin P., Hansen K.T., Jolic D. (2000) Searching the schizophrenic brain for temporal lobe deficits: a systematic review and meta-analysis. *Psychol. Med.*, **30**: 491–504.
10. Smith G.N., Flynn S.W., Kopala L.C., Bassett A.S., Lapointe J.S., Falkai P., Honer W.G. (1997) A comprehensive method of assessing routine CT scans in schizophrenia. *Acta Psychiatr. Scand.*, **96**: 395–401.
11. Bloch F. (1946) Nuclear induction. *Phys. Rev.*, **70**: 460.
12. Purcell E.M., Torrey H.C., Pound R.V. (1946) Resonance absorption by nuclear magnetic moments in a solid. *Phys. Rev.*, **69**: 37.
13. Hounsfield G.N. (1973) Computerized transverse axial scanning (tomography). 1. Description of system. *Br. J. Radiol.*, **46**: 1016–1022.
14. Kwong K.K., Belliveau J.W., Chesler D.A., Goldberg I.E., Weisskoff R.M., Poncelet B.P., Kennedy D.N., Hoppel B.E., Cohen M.S., Turner R. *et al.* (1992) Dynamic magnetic resonance imaging of human brain activity during primary sensory stimulation. *Proc. Natl. Acad. Sci. USA*, **89**: 5675–5679.
15. Stehling M.K., Turner R., Mansfield P. (1991) Echo-planar imaging: magnetic resonance imaging in a fraction of a second. *Science*, **254**: 43–50.
16. Andreasen N.C., Cohen G., Harris G., Cizadlo T., Parkkinen J., Rezai K., Swayze V.W. II (1992) Image processing for the study of brain structure and function: problems and programs. *J Neuropsychiatry Clin. Neurosci.*, **4**: 125–133.
17. Talairach J., Tournoux P. (1988) *Co-planar Stereotaxic Atlas of the Human Brain*, Thieme Medical, New York.
18. Okugawa G., Sedvall G., Nordström M., Andreasen N.C., Pierson R., Magnotta V., Agartz I. (2001) Selective reduction of the posterior superior vermis in men with chronic schizophrenia. *Schizophr Res.* (in press).
19. Lawrie S.M., Abukmeil S.S. (1998) Brain abnormality in schizophrenia. A systematic and quantitative review of volumetric magnetic resonance imaging studies. *Br. J. Psychiatry*, **172**: 110–120.
20. Baare W.F., van Oel C.J., Hulshoff Pol H.E., Schnack H.G., Durston S., Sitskoorn M.M., Kahn R.S. (2001) Volumes of brain structures in twins discordant for schizophrenia. *Arch. Gen. Psychiatry*, **58**: 33–40.

21. Giedd J.N., Jeffries N.O., Blumenthal J., Castellanos F.X., Vaituzis A.C., Fernandez T., Hamburger S.D., Liu H., Nelson J., Bedwell J. *et al.* (1999) Childhood-onset schizophrenia: progressive brain changes during adolescence. *Biol. Psychiatry*, **46**: 892–898.

22. Mathalon D.H., Sullivan E.V., Lim K.O., Pfefferbaum A. (2001) Progressive brain volume changes and the clinical course of schizophrenia in men: a longitudinal magnetic resonance imaging study. *Arch. Gen. Psychiatry*, **58**: 148–157.

23. Rapoport J.L., Giedd J.N., Blumenthal J., Hamburger S., Jeffries N., Fernandez T., Nicolson R., Bedwell J., Lenane M., Zijdenbos A. *et al.* (1999) Progressive cortical change during adolescence in childhood-onset schizophrenia. A longitudinal magnetic resonance imaging study. *Arch. Gen. Psychiatry*, **56**: 649–654.

24. Chua S.E., Wright I.C., Poline J.B., Liddle P.F., Murray R.M., Frackowiak R.S., Friston K.J., McGuire P.K. (1997) Grey matter correlates of syndromes in schizophrenia. A semi-automated analysis of structural magnetic resonance images. *Br. J. Psychiatry*, **170**: 406–410.

25. Pearlson G.D., Barta P.E., Powers R.E., Menon R.R., Richards S.S., Aylward E.H., Federman E.B., Chase G.A., Petty R.G., Tien A.Y. (1997) Medial and superior temporal gyral volumes and cerebral asymmetry in schizophrenia versus bipolar disorder. *Biol. Psychiatry*, **41**: 1–14.

26. Zipursky R.B., Marsh L., Lim K.O., DeMent S., Shear P.K., Sullivan E.V., Murphy G.M., Csernansky J.G., Pfefferbaum A. (1994) Volumetric MRI assessment of temporal lobe structures in schizophrenia. *Biol. Psychiatry*, **35**: 501–516.

27. Weinberger D.R., Berman K.F., Suddath R., Torrey E.F. (1992) Evidence of dysfunction of a prefrontal-limbic network in schizophrenia: a magnetic resonance imaging and regional cerebral blood flow study of discordant monozygotic twins. *Am. J. Psychiatry*, **149**: 890–897.

28. McNeil T.F., Cantor-Graae E., Weinberger D.R. (2000) Relationship of obstetric complications and differences in size of brain structures in monozygotic twin pairs discordant for schizophrenia. *Am. J. Psychiatry*, **157**: 203–212.

29. Agartz I., Andersson J.L., Skare S. (2001) Abnormal brain white matter in schizophrenia: a diffusion tensor imaging study. *Neuroreport*, **12**: 2251–2254.

30. Buchsbaum M.S., Tang C.Y., Peled S., Gudbjartsson H., Lu D., Hazlett E.A., Downhill J., Haznedar M., Fallon J.H., Atlas S.W. (1998) MRI white matter diffusion anisotropy and PET metabolic rate in schizophrenia. *Neuroreport*, **9**: 425–430.

31. Steel R.M., Bastin E.M., McConnell S., Marshall I., Cunningham-Owens D.G., Lawrie S.M., Johnstone E.C., Best J.J.K. (2001) Diffusion tensor imaging (DTI) and proton magnetic resonance spectroscopy (^{1}H MRS) in schizophrenic subjects and normal controls. *Psychiatry Res. Neuroimaging*, **106**: 161–170.

32. Harvey I., Persaud R., Ron M.A., Baker G., Murray R.M. (1994) Volumetric MRI measurements in bipolars compared with schizophrenics and healthy controls. *Psychol. Med.*, **24**: 689–699.

33. Sullivan E.V., Mathalon D.H., Lim K.O., Marsh L., Pfefferbaum A. (1998) Patterns of regional cortical dysmorphology distinguishing schizophrenia and chronic alcoholism. *Biol. Psychiatry*, **43**: 118–131.

34. Brown F.W., Lewine R.J., Hudgins P.A., Risch S.C. (1992) White matter hyperintensity signals in psychiatric and nonpsychiatric subjects. *Am. J. Psychiatry*, **149**: 620–625.

35. Hickie I., Scott E., Wilhelm K., Brodaty H. (1997) Subcortical hyperintensities on magnetic resonance imaging in patients with severe depression—A longitudinal evaluation. *Biol. Psychiatry*, **42**: 367–374.

36. Kumar A., Jin Z., Bilker W., Udupa J., Gottlieb G. (1998) Late-onset minor and major depression: early evidence for common neuroanatomical substrates detected by using MRI. *Proc. Natl. Acad. Sci. USA*, **95**: 7654–7658.
37. Mervaala E., Fohr J., Kononen M., Valkonen-Korhonen M., Vainio P., Partanen K., Partanen J., Tiihonen J., Viinamaki H., Karjalainen A.K. *et al.* (2000) Quantitative MRI of the hippocampus and amygdala in severe depression. *Psychol. Med.*, **30**: 117–125.
38. Steingard R.J., Renshaw P.F., Yurgelun-Todd D., Appelmans K.E., Lyoo I.K., Shorrock K.L., Bucci J.P., Cesena M., Abebe D., Zurakowski D. *et al.* (1996) Structural abnormalities in brain magnetic resonance images of depressed children. *J. Am. Acad. Child Adolesc. Psychiatry*, **35**: 307–311.
39. Shioiri T., Oshitani Y., Kato T., Murashita J., Hamakawa H., Inubushi T., Nagata T., Takahashi S. (1996) Prevalence of cavum septum pellucidum detected by MRI in patients with bipolar disorder, major depression and schizophrenia. *Psychol. Med.*, **26**: 431–434.
40. Raichle M.E. (1987) Circulatory and metabolic correlations of brain function in normal humans. In *Handbook of Physiology, Section 1, The Nervous System, Vol. 5, Higher Functions of the Brain* (Ed. V.B. Mountcastle), pp. 643–674, Oxford University Press, New York.
41. Kandel E.R., Schwartz J.H., Sessell T.M. (Eds) (2000) *Principles of Neural Science*, McGraw-Hill, New York.
42. Ogawa S., Menon R.S., Tank D.W., Kim S.G., Merkle H., Ellermann J.M., Ugurbil K. (1993) Functional brain mapping by blood oxygenation level-dependent contrast magnetic resonance imaging. A comparison of signal characteristics with a biophysical model. *Biophys. J.*, **64**: 803–812.
43. Cohen J., Forman S.D., Braver S., Casey B.J., Servan-Schreiber D., Noll D.C. (1995) Activation of prefrontal cortex in a non-spatial working memory task with functional MRI. *Hum. Brain Mapp.*, **1**: 291–304.
44. Martin A., Haxby J.V., Lalonde F.M., Wiggs C.L., Ungerleider L.G. (1995) Discrete cortical regions associated with knowledge of color and knowledge of action. *Science*, **270**: 102–105.
45. Stark C.E., Squire L.R. (2000) Functional magnetic resonance imaging (fMRI) activity in the hippocampal region during recognition memory. *J. Neurosci.*, **20**: 7776–7781.
46. Mattay V.S., Callicott J.H., Bertolino A., Santha A.K., Tallent K.A., Goldberg T.E., Frank J.A., Weinberger D.R. (1997) Abnormal functional lateralization of the sensorimotor cortex in patients with schizophrenia. *Neuroreport*, **8**: 2977–2984.
47. Menon V., Anagnoson R.T., Glover G.H., Pfefferbaum A. (2001) Functional magnetic resonance imaging evidence for disrupted basal ganglia function in schizophrenia. *Am. J. Psychiatry*, **158**: 646–649.
48. Woodruff P.W., Wright I.C., Bullmore E.T., Brammer M., Howard R.J., Williams S.C., Shapleske J., Rossell S., David A.S., McGuire P.K. *et al.* (1997) Auditory hallucinations and the temporal cortical response to speech in schizophrenia: a functional magnetic resonance imaging study. *Am. J. Psychiatry*, **154**: 1676–1682.
49. Beauregard M., Leroux J.M., Bergman S., Arzoumanian Y., Beaudoin G., Bourgouin P., Stip E. (1998) The functional neuroanatomy of major depression: an fMRI study using an emotional activation paradigm. *Neuroreport*, **9**: 3253–3258.
50. Birbaumer N., Grodd W., Diedrich O., Klose U., Erb M., Lotze M., Schneider F., Weiss U., Flor H. (1998) fMRI reveals amygdala activation to human faces in social phobics. *Neuroreport*, **9**: 1223–1226.

51. Schneider F., Weiss U., Kessler C., Muller-Gartner H.W., Posse S., Salloum J.B., Grodd W., Himmelmann F., Gaebel W., Birbaumer N. (1999) Subcortical correlates of differential classical conditioning of aversive emotional reactions in social phobia. *Biol. Psychiatry*, **45**: 863–871.

52. Lassen N.A., Ingvar D.H. (1961) The blood flow of the cerebral cortex determined by radioactive krypton-85. *Experientia*, **17**: 42.

53. Ingvar D.H., Franzen G. (1974) Abnormalities of cerebral blood flow distribution in patients with chronic schizophrenia. *Acta Psychiatr. Scand.*, **50**: 425–462.

54. Stokeley E.M., Sveinsdottir E., Lassen N.A., Rommer P. (1980) A single photon dynamic computer assisted tomograph (DCAT) for imaging brain function in multiple cross sections. *J. Comput. Assist. Tomogr.*, **4**: 230–240.

55. Phelps M.E., Hoffman E.J., Huang S.C., Kuhl D.E. (1978) ECAT: a new computerized tomographic imaging system for positron-emitting radiopharmaceuticals. *J. Nucl. Med.*, **19**: 635–647.

56. Sokoloff L. (1984) Modeling metabolic processes in the brain in vivo. *Ann. Neurol.*, **15**(Suppl. 6): S1–11.

57. Wagner H.N. Jr., Burns H.D., Dannals R.F., Wong D.F., Langstrom B., Duelfer T., Frost J.J., Ravert H.T., Links J.M., Rosenbloom S.B. *et al.* (1983) Imaging dopamine receptors in the human brain by positron tomography. *Science*, **221**: 1264–1266.

58. Farde L., Hall H., Ehrin E., Sedvall G. (1986) Quantitative analysis of D$_2$ dopamine receptor binding in the living human brain by PET. *Science*, **231**: 258–261.

59. Sedvall G., Farde L., Persson A., Wiesel F.A. (1986) Imaging of neurotransmitter receptors in the living human brain. *Arch. Gen. Psychiatry*, **43**: 995–1005.

60. Farde L., Suhara T., Nyberg S., Karlsson P., Nakashima Y., Hietala J., Halldin C. (1997) A PET-study of [^{11}C]FLB 457 binding to extrastriatal D$_2$-dopamine receptors in healthy subjects and antipsychotic drug-treated patients. *Psychopharmacology*, **133**: 396–404.

61. Farde L., Ginovart N., Halldin C., Chou Y.H., Olsson H., Swahn C.G. (2000) A PET study of [^{11}C]b-CIT-FE binding to the dopamine transporter in the monkey and human brain. *Int. J. Neuropsychopharmacol.*, **3**: 203–214.

62. Halldin C., Foged C., Chou Y.H., Karlsson P., Swahn C.G., Sandell J., Sedvall G., Farde L. (1998) Carbon-11-NNC 112: a radioligand for PET examination of striatal and neocortical D1-dopamine receptors. *J. Nucl. Med.*, **39**: 2061–2068.

63. Olsson H., Halldin C., Swahn C.G., Farde L. (1999) Quantification of [^{11}C]FLB 457 binding to extrastriatal dopamine receptors in the human brain. *J. Cereb. Blood Flow Metab.*, **19**: 1164–1173.

64. Laruelle M., Abi-Dargham A., van Dyck C.H., Gil R., D'Souza C.D., Erdos J., McCance E., Rosenblatt W., Fingado C., Zoghbi S.S. *et al.* (1996) Single photon emission computerized tomography imaging of amphetamine-induced dopamine release in drug-free schizophrenic subjects. *Proc. Natl. Acad. Sci. USA*, **93**: 9235–9240.

65. Buchsbaum M.S., Hazlett E.A. (1998) Positron emission tomography studies of abnormal glucose metabolism in schizophrenia. *Schizophr. Bull.*, **24**: 343–364.

66. Haznedar M.M., Buchsbaum M.S., Luu C., Hazlett E.A., Siegel B.V. Jr., Lohr J., Wu J., Haier R.J., Bunney W.E. Jr. (1997) Decreased anterior cingulate gyrus metabolic rate in schizophrenia. *Am. J. Psychiatry*, **154**: 682–684.

67. Jacobsen L.K., Hamburger S.D., Van Horn J.D., Vaituzis A.C., McKenna K., Frazier J.A., Gordon C.T., Lenane M.C., Rapoport J.L., Zametkin A.J. (1997) Cerebral glucose metabolism in childhood-onset schizophrenia. *Psychiatry Res.*, **75**: 131–144.

68. Andreasen N.C., O'Leary D.S., Flaum M., Nopoulos P., Watkins G.L., Boles Ponto L.L., Hichwa R.D. (1997) Hypofrontality in schizophrenia: distributed dysfunctional circuits in neuroleptic-naive patients. *Lancet*, **349**: 1730–1734.

69. Kim J.J., Mohamed S., Andreasen N.C., O'Leary D.S., Watkins G.L., Boles Ponto L.L., Hichwa R.D. (2000) Regional neural dysfunctions in chronic schizophrenia studied with positron emission tomography. *Am. J. Psychiatry*, **157**: 542–548.

70. Artiges E., Martinot J.L., Verdys M., Attar-Levy D., Mazoyer B., Tzourio N., Giraud M.J., Paillere-Martinot M.L. (2000) Altered hemispheric functional dominance during word generation in negative schizophrenia. *Schizophr. Bull.*, **26**: 709–721.

71. Carter C.S., Mintun M., Nichols T., Cohen J.D. (1997) Anterior cingulate gyrus dysfunction and selective attention deficits in schizophrenia: [^{15}O]H$_2$O PET study during single-trial Stroop task performance. *Am. J. Psychiatry*, **154**: 1670–1675.

72. Dolan R.J., Fletcher P.C., McKenna P., Friston K.J., Frith C.D. (1999) Abnormal neural integration related to cognition in schizophrenia. *Acta Psychiatr. Scand.*, **99**(Suppl. 395): 58–67.

73. Suzuki M., Yuasa S., Minabe Y., Murata M., Kurachi M. (1993) Left superior temporal blood flow increases in schizophrenic and schizophreniform patients with auditory hallucination: a longitudinal case study using ^{123}I-IMP SPECT. *Eur. Arch. Psychiatry Clin. Neurosci.*, **242**: 257–261.

74. David A.S. (1999) Auditory hallucinations: phenomenology, neuropsychology and neuroimaging update. *Acta Psychiatr. Scand.*, **99**(Suppl. 395): 95–104.

75. Epstein J., Stern E., Silbersweig D. (1999) Mesolimbic activity associated with psychosis in schizophrenia. Symptom-specific PET studies. *Ann. N.Y. Acad. Sci.*, **877**: 562–574.

76. Liddle P.F., Friston K.J., Frith C.D., Hirsch S.R., Jones T., Frackowiak R.S.J. (1992) Patterns of cerebral blood flow in schizophrenia. *Br. J. Psychiatry*, **160**: 179–186.

77. Sabri O., Erkwoh R., Schreckenberger M., Owega A., Sass H., Buell U. (1997) Correlation of positive symptoms exclusively to hyperperfusion or hypoperfusion of cerebral cortex in never-treated schizophrenics. *Lancet*, **349**: 1735–1739.

78. Blackwood D.H., Glabus M.F., Dunan J., O'Carroll R.E., Muir W.J., Ebmeier K.P. (1999) Altered cerebral perfusion measured by SPECT in relatives of patients with schizophrenia. Correlations with memory and P300. *Br. J. Psychiatry*, **175**: 357–366.

79. Schultz S.K., Andreasen N.C. (1999) Schizophrenia. *Lancet*, **353**: 1425–1430.

80. Ito H., Kawashima R., Awata S., Ono S., Sato K., Goto R., Koyama M., Sato M., Fukuda H. (1996) Hypoperfusion in the limbic system and prefrontal cortex in depression: SPECT with anatomic standardization technique. *J. Nucl. Med.*, **37**: 410–414.

81. Drevets W.C., Price J.L., Simpson J.R., Todd R.D., Reich T., Vannier M., Raichle M.E. (1997) Subgenual prefrontal cortex abnormalities in mood disorders. *Nature*, **386**: 824–827.

82. Elliott R., Sahakian B.J., Michael A., Paykel E.S., Dolan R.J. (1998) Abnormal neural response to feedback on planning and guessing tasks in patients with unipolar depression. *Psychol. Med.*, **28**: 559–571.

83. Mayberg H.S., Liotti M., Brannan S.K., McGinnis S., Mahurin R.K., Jerabek P.A., Silva J.A., Tekell J.L., Martin C.C., Lancaster J.L. *et al.* (1999) Reciprocal limbic-cortical function and negative mood: converging PET findings in depression and normal sadness. *Am. J. Psychiatry*, **156**: 675–682.

84. Bell C.J., Malizia A.L., Nutt D.J. The neurobiology of social phobia. *Eur. Arch. Psychiatry Clin. Neurosci.*, **249**(Suppl. 1): S11–18.

85. Reiman E.M. (1997) The application of positron emission tomography to the study of normal and pathologic emotions. *J. Clin. Psychiatry*, **58**(Suppl. 16): 4–12.

86. Wik G., Fredrikson M., Fischer H. (1997) Evidence of altered cerebral blood-flow relationships in acute phobia. *Int. J. Neurosci.*, **91**: 253–263.

87. Sedvall G., Farde, L. (1995) Chemical brain anatomy in schizophrenia. *Lancet*, **346**: 743–749.

88. Breier A., Su T.P., Saunders R., Carson R.E., Kolachana B.S., de Bartolomeis A., Weinberger D.R., Weisenfeld N., Malhotra A.K., Eckelman W.C. *et al.* (1997) Schizophrenia is associated with elevated amphetamine-induced synaptic dopamine concentrations: evidence from a novel positron emission tomography method. *Proc. Natl. Acad. Sci. USA*, **94**: 2569–2574.

89. Laruelle M., Abi-Dargham A. (1999) Dopamine as the wind of the psychotic fire: new evidence from brain imaging studies. *J. Psychopharmacol.*, **13**: 358–371.

90. Zubieta J.K., Taylor S.F., Huguelet P., Koeppe R.A., Kilbourn M.R., Frey K.A. (2001) Vesicular monoamine transporter concentrations in bipolar disorder type I, schizophrenia, and healthy subjects. *Biol. Psychiatry*, **49**: 110–116.

91. Trichard C., Paillere-Martinot M.L., Attar-Levy D., Recassens C., Monnet F., Martinot J.L. (1998) Binding of antipsychotic drugs to cortical 5-HT2A receptors: a PET study of chlorpromazine, clozapine, and amisulpride in schizophrenic patients. *Am. J. Psychiatry*, **155**: 505–508.

92. Lewis R., Kapur S., Jones C., DaSilva J., Brown G.M., Wilson A.A., Houle S., Zipursky R.B. (1999) Serotonin 5-HT2 receptors in schizophrenia: a PET study using [^{18}F]setoperone in neuroleptic-naive patients and normal subjects. *Am. J. Psychiatry*, **156**: 72–78.

93. Okubo Y., Suhara T., Suzuki K., Kobayashi K., Inoue O., Terasaki O., Someya Y., Sassa T., Sudo Y., Matsushima E. *et al.* (2000) Serotonin 5-HT2 receptors in schizophrenic patients studied by positron emission tomography. *Life Sci.*, **66**: 2455–2464.

94. Verhoeff N.P., Meyer J.H., Kecojevic A., Hussey D., Lewis R., Tauscher J., Zipursky R.B., Kapur S. (2000) A voxel-by-voxel analysis of [^{18}F]setoperone PET data shows no substantial serotonin 5-HT(2A) receptor changes in schizophrenia. *Psychiatry Res.*, **99**: 123–135.

95. Busatto G.F., Pilowsky L.S., Costa D.C., Ell P.J., David A.S., Lucey J.V., Kerwin R.W. (1997) Correlation between reduced in vivo benzodiazepine receptor binding and severity of psychotic symptoms in schizophrenia. *Am. J. Psychiatry*, **154**: 56–63.

96. Pauli S., Farde L., Halldin C., Sedvall G. (1994) Spatial neuroreceptor imaging in the living human brain. *Neuropsychopharmacology*, **10**: 29S.

97. Pauli S., Sedvall G. (1997) Three-dimensional visualization and quantification of the benzodiazepine receptor population within a living human brain using PET and MRI. *Eur. Arch. Psychiatry Clin. Neurosci.*, **247**: 61–70.

98. Drevets W.C., Frank E., Price J.C., Kupfer D.J., Holt D., Greer P.J., Huang Y., Gautier C., Mathis C. (1999) PET imaging of serotonin 1A receptor binding in depression. *Biol. Psychiatry*, **46**: 1375–1387.

99. Sargent P.A., Kjaer K.H., Bench C.J., Rabiner E.A., Messa C., Meyer J., Gunn R.N., Grasby P.M., Cowen P.J. (2000) Brain serotonin 1A receptor binding measured by positron emission tomography with [^{11}C]WAY-100635: effects of depression and antidepressant treatment. *Arch. Gen. Psychiatry*, **57**: 174–180.

100. Biver F., Wikler D., Lotstra F., Damhaut P., Goldman S., Mendlewicz J. (1997) Serotonin 5-HT2 receptor imaging in major depression: focal changes in orbito-insular cortex. *Br. J. Psychiatry*, **171**: 444–448.

101. Yatham L.N., Liddle P.F., Shiah I.S., Scarrow G., Lam R.W., Adam M.J., Zis A.P., Ruth T.J. (2000) Brain serotonin 2 receptors in major depression: a positron emission tomography study. *Arch. Gen. Psychiatry*, **57**: 850–858.

102. Meyer J.H., Kapur S., Houle S., DaSilva J., Owczarek B., Brown G.M., Wilson A.A., Kennedy S.H. (1999) Prefrontal cortex 5-HT2 receptors in depression: an [^{18}F]setoperone PET imaging study. *Am. J. Psychiatry*, **156**: 1029–1034.

103. Farde L., Nordstrom A.L., Wiesel F.A., Pauli S., Halldin C., Sedvall G. (1992) Positron emission tomographic analysis of central D_1 and D_2 dopamine receptor occupancy in patients treated with classical neuroleptics and clozapine. Relation to extrapyramidal side effects. *Arch. Gen. Psychiatry*, **49**: 538–544.

104. Kapur S., Zipursky R.B., Remington G. (1999) Clinical and theoretical implications of 5-HT2 and D_2 receptor occupancy of clozapine, risperidone, and olanzapine in schizophrenia. *Am. J. Psychiatry*, **156**: 286–293.

105. Kapur S., Zipursky R., Jones C., Remington G., Houle S. (2000) Relationship between dopamine D_2 occupancy, clinical response, and side effects: a double-blind PET study of first-episode schizophrenia. *Am. J. Psychiatry*, **157**: 514–520.

106. Nordstrom A.L., Farde L., Halldin C. (1993) High 5-HT2 receptor occupancy in clozapine treated patients demonstrated by PET. *Psychopharmacology*, **110**: 365–367.

4

Neuroendocrinological Research in Psychiatry

Charles B. Nemeroff and David A. Gutman

Department of Psychiatry and Behavioral Sciences, Emory University School of Medicine, 1639 Pierce Drive, Suite 4000, Atlanta, GA 30322-4990, USA

INTRODUCTION

The concept that neural tissue is capable of synthesizing and secreting hormones is now well established, but when first introduced in the 1950s it was remarkably controversial. This led to the establishment of the entire discipline of neuroendocrinology. The occurrence of prominent psychiatric symptoms associated with primary endocrine disorders including Cushing's disease and primary hypothyroidism provided a rationale for exploring the connection between hormones and both affective and cognitive function.

Bleuler was among the earliest researchers to systematically investigate the association between hormones, mood and behaviour. He first demonstrated that patients with primary endocrine disorders have higher than expected psychiatric comorbidity, which often resolved after correcting the primary hormonal abnormality. Work over the past 25 years has clearly demonstrated that endocrine gland secretion is tightly regulated by the central nervous system (CNS) and, further, that neurons are directly influenced by hormones.

As noted above, the concept that neurons are capable of synthesizing and releasing hormones sparked a controversy in endocrinology and neuroscience; namely, is it possible that certain neurons subserve endocrine functions? Two major findings fuelled this debate. First, neurohistologists working with mammalian as well as lower vertebrate and invertebrate species made several key observations. Led by a husband and wife team, the Scharrers, early researchers documented, by both light and electron microscopy, the presence of neurons that had all the characteristics of previously studied endocrine cells. These neurons stained positive with the Gomori's stain, which was believed to be specific to endocrine tissues, and

Psychiatry as a Neuroscience. Edited by Juan José López-Ibor, Wolfgang Gaebel, Mario Maj and Norman Sartorius. © 2002 John Wiley & Sons Ltd.

furthermore they contained granules or vesicles containing known endocrine substances. The second key area of research centred around the brain's control of the secretion of pituitary trophic hormones. These trophic hormones had long been known to control the secretion of peripheral target endocrine hormones, e.g. thyroid hormone, gonadal steroids, adrenal steroids, etc. These interactions were particularly compelling because of the earlier identification of an extremely important neuroendocrine system, namely the magnocellular cells of the paraventricular nucleus (PVN) of the hypothalamus, which synthesizes arginine-vasopressin (AVP) and oxytocin. These two nonapeptides were shown to be transported from PVN cell bodies down the axon to nerve terminals located in the posterior pituitary (neurohypophysis), and released in response to appropriate physiologic stimuli. AVP, also known as antidiuretic hormone, is a critical regulator of fluid balance, and oxytocin regulates the milk-letdown reflex during breast-feeding.

The ability of neurons to function as true endocrine tissues has now been clearly established. Neural tissue can both synthesize and release substances known as (neuro)hormones that are released directly into the circulatory system and have effects at sites far removed from the brain. One important example noted above is the action of AVP on the kidney. Although early in the development of the emerging discipline of neuroendocrinology it seemed important to document the ability of neurons to function as neuroendocrine cells, particularly those in the CNS, classification of specific chemical messengers as endocrine versus neuronal versus neuroendocrine soon lost its heuristic value. It is now recognized that the same substance can act as a neurotransmitter and a hormone depending on its location within the CNS and periphery. A good example of this is epinephrine (adrenaline), which functions as a classical hormone in the adrenal medulla but as a conventional neurotransmitter in the mammalian CNS. Similarly, it has been demonstrated that corticotropin-releasing factor (CRF) functions as a true peptide hormone in its role as a hypothalamic hypophysiotropic factor in promoting the release of adrenocorticotropin (ACTH) from the anterior pituitary, yet also functions as a "conventional" neurotransmitter in cortical and limbic areas. Thus the field now seeks to elucidate the role of particular chemical messengers in particular brain regions or endocrine axes.

The traditional endocrine and hormonal functions of several peptides discussed above have been well established, but many of these substances may possess paracrine roles as well, i.e. secretion of these substances from one cell acts upon proximal cells. These paracrine interactions remain largely unexplored. The importance of these paracrine effects has been well demonstrated in the gastrointestinal tract, where several peptides that act as hormones or neurotransmitter substances at other sites, including the CNS, have influences on local cellular function. Examples include vasoactive intestinal peptide, cholecystokinin and somatostatin.

Thus, neuroendocrinology comprises the study of the endocrine role of neuronal or glial cells as well as the neural regulation of endocrine secretion, with the latter focusing on the biology of the various hypothalamic–pituitary–end organ axes and the major neurohypophyseal hormones, vasopressin and oxytocin. Unravelling the intricate and elegant feedback systems of peripherally secreted hormones at pituitary, hypothalamic and other CNS sites is an integral part of this discipline. The role of the hypophysiotropic factors contained in the hypothalamus at extrahypothalamic sites is also of great interest.

OVERVIEW OF COMPONENTS AND CONTROL MECHANISMS

The hypothalamic–pituitary–end organ axes generally are organized in a hierarchical fashion (Figure 4.1). A large percentage of the neuroendocrine abnormalities in patients with psychiatric disorders are related to disturbances of target hormone feedback. A generic description is briefly outlined here. More comprehensive reviews on this topic are available [1]. In general, the hypothalamus contains neurons that synthesize and release factors that either promote or inhibit the release of anterior pituitary hormones, so-called release or release-inhibiting factors. These peptide hormones, as summarized in Table 4.1, are synthesized by transcription of the DNA sequence for the peptide prohormone. After translation in the endoplasmic reticulum, these prohormones are processed during axonal transport and packaged into vesicles destined for the nerve terminals. These now biologically active peptides are then released following appropriate physiological stimuli from the median eminence, the most ventral portion of the hypothalamus, and secreted into the primary plexus of the hypothalamo-hypophyseal portal vessels (Figure 4.2). These peptides are transported in high concentration to the sinusoids of the anterior pituitary (adenohypophysis), where they bind to specific membrane receptors on their targets, the pituitary trophic hormone-producing cells. Activation of these receptors promotes or inhibits the release of pituitary trophic hormones into the systemic circulation. The increase or decrease in the plasma concentrations of these pituitary trophic hormones produces a corresponding increase or decrease in their respective end-organ hormone secretion. The hormones of the end-organ axes, such as gonadal and adrenal steroids, feed back on both pituitary and hypothalamic cells to prevent further release, often referred to as "long-loop" negative feedback. Short-loop negative feedback circuits have also been identified in which pituitary hormones directly feed back on hypothalamic neurons to prevent further release of hypothalamic releasing factors.

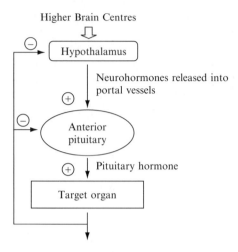

FIGURE 4.1 Overview of the common organizational motif of the neuroendocrine axis. The neurosecretion of hypothalamic factors into hypophyseal portal vessels is regulated by a set point of activity from higher brain centres. Neurohormones released from the hypothalamus into hypophyseal portal vessels in turn stimulate cells in the pituitary. These adenohypophyseal hormones then regulate the hormone output from the end organ. The end organ then exerts negative feedback effects at the pituitary and hypothalamus to prevent further neurohormone and pituitary hormone release via "long-loop" negative feedback. Short-loop negative feedback may also occur where pituitary hormones feed back directly on hypothalamic neurons to prevent further neurohormone release

TABLE 4.1 List of major releasing factors and their hormonal target

Neurohormone/releasing factor	Hormone stimulated
Corticotropin-releasing factor (CRF)	Adrenocorticotropic hormone (ACTH)
Thyrotropin-releasing hormone (TRH)	Thyroid-stimulating hormone (TSH)
Gonadotropin-releasing hormone (GnRH)	Follicle-stimulating hormone (FSH)
Somatostatin (SRIF)	Growth hormone (GH)
Growth hormone-releasing hormone (GHRH)	GH
Arginine vasopressin (AVP)	ACTH, prolactin
Oxytocin	Prolactin

Disturbances in the feedback regulation of the hypothalamic–pituitary–end organ axes are of considerable interest in psychiatry. The common occurrence of psychiatric symptoms in many primary endocrine disorders, such as hypothyroidism and Cushing's syndrome, served as an impetus for

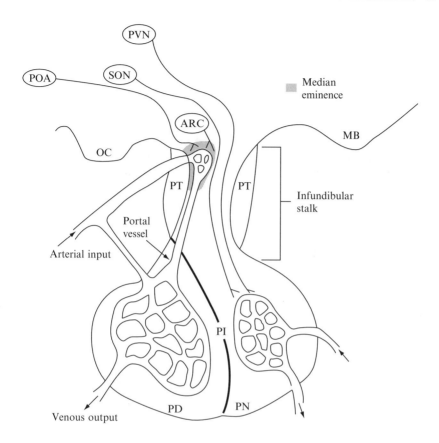

FIGURE 4.2   Diagram of the neurovascular anatomy of the hypothalamic–pituitary axis. PVN, paraventricular nucleus; SON, supraoptic nucleus; POA, preoptic area; ARC, arcuate nucleus; PT, pars tuberalis; PI, pars intermedia; PD, pars distalis; PN, pars nervosa; MB, mamillary body; OC, optic chiasm

investigation into the regulation of neuroendocrine systems in psychiatric disease states such as depression, schizophrenia and bipolar disorder. Thus, a large part of psychoneuroendocrinology has focused on identifying changes in basal levels of pituitary and end-organ hormones in patients with psychiatric disorders. For many of the axes discussed below, tests have been developed to assess the functional status of these feedback systems. In these so-called stimulation tests, hypothalamic and/or pituitary-derived factors or their synthetic analogues are exogenously administered, and the hormonal response to this "challenge" is assessed. For example, in the standard CRF stimulation test, a 1 μg/kg dose of CRF is administered intravenously, and the ACTH and cortisol response is measured over a period of two or three hours. This test is a very sensitive measure of hypothalamic–pituitary–adrenal

(HPA) axis activity, and changes in the magnitude and/or duration of the response relative to normal control values are characteristic of one or another type of dysregulation of the HPA axis.

Such studies, as outlined above, provide valuable information, but a brief discussion of some inherent limitations is warranted before a detailed review of the literature is presented. Normal circadian rhythms and the pulsatile release of many of the components of the hypothalamic–pituitary–end organ axes are often not taken into account when these stimulation tests are designed. Further, differences in assay sensitivity, gender differences, inclusion criteria for patients used in studies, and the severity of symptoms in the target patient population can potentially generate confounding or at least quite variable results. Nevertheless, a great deal about the neurobiology of psychiatric disorders has been discovered through such experiments. Although less commonly used today, an often-utilized strategy in the 1970s and 1980s was based on the perception that the neuroendocrine axes served as a "window" into CNS function. Peripheral neuroendocrine markers were often used to indirectly assess CNS function because the brain was relatively inaccessible to study, with the exception of cerebrospinal fluid (CSF) and post-mortem studies. With the emergence of the monoamine theories of mood disorders and schizophrenia, many investigators attempted to draw conclusions about the activity of noradrenergic, serotonergic and dopaminergic circuits in patients with various psychiatric disorders by measuring the basal and stimulated secretion of pituitary and end-organ hormones in plasma. Although these approaches have severe limitations, they have been useful in elucidating the pathophysiology of mood and anxiety disorders, and to a lesser extent, schizophrenia.

In summary, neuroendocrinology broadly encompasses the following:

- The neural regulation of the secretion of peripheral, target-organ hormones, pituitary trophic hormones, and hypothalamic–hypophysiotropic hormones.
- The effects of each of the hormones that comprise the various endocrine axes on the CNS. This includes, for example, the effects of synthetic glucocorticoids on memory processes.
- The study of alterations in the activity of the various endocrine axes in major psychiatric disorders, and, conversely, the behavioural consequences of endocrinopathies.

HYPOTHALAMIC–PITUITARY–THYROID AXIS

Components and Function

The thyroid gland, composed of two central lobes connected by an isthmus, synthesizes the hormones thyroxine (T_4) and triiodothyronine (T_3). These iodine-containing compounds serve as global regulators of the body's metabolic rate, and are also critical for brain development. The release and synthesis of these hormones is ultimately controlled by signals from the CNS.

The hypothalamic–pituitary–thyroid (HPT) axis is composed of three main parts, as its name suggests. The tripeptide (pGlu-His-Pro-NH$_2$) thyrotropin-releasing hormone (TRH) is synthesized predominantly in the PVN of the hypothalamus and stored in nerve terminals in the median eminence, where it is released into the vessels of the hypothalamo-hypophyseal portal system (Figure 4.3). TRH is then transported to the sinusoids in the anterior pituitary, where it binds to thyrotropes and releases the peptide thyroid-stimulating hormone (TSH) into the systemic circulation. TRH is heterogeneously distributed in the brain, which strongly suggests a role for this peptide as a neurotransmitter as well as a releasing hormone. Thus TRH itself can produce direct effects on the CNS independent of its actions on pituitary thyrotrophs. The HPT axis exhibits an ultradian rhythm, where TSH secretion, and consequently T$_3$ and T$_4$ levels, rise in the afternoon and evening, peak sometime after midnight and decline throughout the day [2].

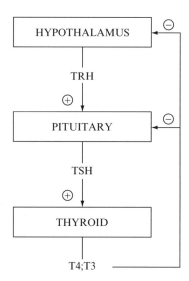

FIGURE 4.3 Overview of the feedback system of the hypothalamic–pituitary–thyroid (HPT) axis. Thyroid-releasing hormone (TRH) from the hypothalamus stimulates thyroid stimulating hormone (TSH) from the pituitary, which stimulates thyroid hormone release. As circulating thyroid hormone levels increase, they inhibit further release of TSH and TRH. Other hypothalamic–pituitary–end organ axes exhibit similar feedback control mechanisms

TSH is a 28-kDA glycoprotein composed of two non-covalently linked protein chains, TSH-α and TSH-β. The α subunit is identical to the α subunit contained in other pituitary hormones, including follicle-stimulating hormone, luteinizing hormone and human chorionic gonadotropin. Upon release from the pituitary, TSH circulates through the blood and exerts its effects via binding to the TSH receptor in the thyroid, a G-protein-coupled receptor that stimulates the activation of adenylate cyclase.

Upon stimulation by TSH, the thyroid gland releases the iodinated amino acids T_3 and T_4. Of the two hormones, T_3 is much more physiologically active. Although debate still exists in the literature, T_4 is often considered a prohormone that becomes active after monodeiodination in peripheral tissues. T_3 directly promotes gene expression through binding to thyroid response elements (TREs) located in the promoter regions of a diverse number of genes. T_3 also directly regulates the HPT axis by inhibiting TSH release and gene expression in the pituitary, and TRH gene expression in the hypothalamus [3]. This is characteristic of the end-product negative feedback seen in the hypothalamic–pituitary–end organ axes. In the circulation, these hormones are primarily bound to a carrier-protein, thyroglobulin, though it is the unbound form of these hormones that is metabolically active. Thyroid hormones have numerous effects on metabolism and increase heat production, oxygen consumption, lipid metabolism, intestinal absorption of carbohydrates, cardiac function and in regulating the activity of the $Na^+ - K^+$ ATPase. All of these functions are consistent with increasing metabolic rate.

Disorders of the HPT Axis

Disorders of the HPT axis lead to numerous psychiatric manifestations, ranging from mild depression to overt psychosis. Numerous conditions can lead to hypothyroid states, also known as myxoedema, including CNS causes of decreased TSH or TRH secretion, severe iodine deficiency, thyroid surgery, drugs, or autoimmune disorders. The most common cause of hypothyroidism is Hashimoto's thyroiditis, which is due to autoimmune destruction of thyroid tissue. Regardless of the aetiology, hypothyroidism leads to a number of clinical manifestations, including slowed mentation, forgetfulness, decreased hearing, cold intolerance and ataxia. Decreased energy, weight gain, depression, cognitive impairment or overt psychosis ("myxoedema madness") may also result. Due to the overlap of symptoms with clinical depression, thyroid hormone deficiency must be ruled out in the evaluation of patients with depression.

Hypothyroidism is frequently subclassified into the following four groups:

- Grade 1 hypothyroidism is classic primary hypothyroidism, with increased TSH, decreased peripheral thyroid hormone (T_3 and T_4) concentrations, and an increased TSH response to TRH.
- Grade 2 hypothyroidism is characterized by normal, basal thyroid hormone concentrations, but an increase in basal TSH concentrations and an exaggerated TSH response to TRH.
- Grade 3 hypothyroidism can only be detected by a TRH stimulation test; basal thyroid hormone and TSH concentrations are normal, but the TSH response to TRH is exaggerated.
- Grade 4 hypothyroidism is defined as normal findings on the three thyroid axis function tests noted above, but the patients have the abnormal presence of antithyroid antibodies.

Without treatment, most patients will progress from grade 4 to grade 1 hypothyroidism.

The first treatments for hypothyroidism became available in the 1890s; before that, many patients with this condition spent their final days in mental hospitals. One of the earliest descriptions of the effects of treatment with thyroid extracts was reported by Shaw and Stansfield in 1892. These physicians studied the effects of thyroid extracts given to a patient suffering from severe thyroid deficiency secondary to trauma to her thyroid gland. Within 10 weeks following treatment with a sheep thyroid extract, the mental signs associated with myxoedema disappeared and the patient was discharged [4]. Stansfield followed this patient's progress for several months, and five months after the last injection of thyroid extract, symptoms of hypothyroidism began to recur. Following ingestion of additional thyroid extracts, the symptoms were once again ameliorated. These results clearly demonstrated the profound psychiatric effects of thyroid deficiency, and provided an early demonstration that treatment of primary endocrine abnormalities can resolve the psychiatric manifestations of the disease [3].

The first prospective study that scrutinized psychiatric comorbidity in patients with hypothyroidism was carried out by Whybrow et al. [5]. In this seminal study, five of the seven patients manifested symptoms of depression at the time of the evaluation, while six of the seven displayed cognitive impairment. Interestingly, in all four of the patients with depression who were followed, thyroid replacement alone ameliorated the symptoms of depression. In a later study, Jain [6] studied 30 hypothyroid patients; in this study, 13 of 30 (43%) of the patients had a clinical depression, 10 (30%) had symptoms of anxiety, and 8 (27%) were confused. These symptoms were improved or resolved following treatment of the thyroid condition alone. These early studies clearly demonstrated that hypothyroid states have pronounced psychiatric manifestations, predominantly depression and dementia, which can be reversed following thyroid hormone replacement.

Later studies have demonstrated varying degrees of cognitive disturbance in up to 48% of psychiatrically ill hypothyroid cases, and approximately 50% of unselected hypothyroid patients have symptoms characteristic of depression [7]. Anxiety symptoms are also common, occurring in up to 30% of unselected patients. Mania and hypomanic states have been rarely reported in hypothyroid patients. Finally, although psychosis is the most common reported symptom in the case literature on hypothyroidism (52.9%), it accounts for only approximately 5% of the psychiatric morbidity in an unselected sample [7], presumably due to reporting bias.

HPT Axis Dysfunction in Patients with Primary Psychiatric Disorders

Excluding patients with primary endocrine disorders, a considerable amount of data has revealed an elevated rate of HPT axis dysfunction, predominantly hypothyroidism, in patients with major depression. More than 25 years ago, research groups led by Prange and Kastin demonstrated that approximately 25% of patients with major depression exhibit a blunted TSH response to TRH [8, 9]. Presumably this is due to hypersecretion of TRH from the median eminence, which leads to TRH receptor down-regulation in the anterior pituitary resulting in reduced sensitivity of the pituitary to exogenous TRH. This hypothesis seems plausible in the light of evidence showing elevated TRH concentrations in the CSF of drug-free depressed patients [10]. Depressed patients have also been shown to have an increased occurrence of symptomless autoimmune thyroiditis (SAT), defined by the abnormal presence of antithyroglobulin and/or antimicrosomal thyroid antibodies consistent with grade 4 hypothyroidism [11].

Recently, Duval et al. [12] performed a standard TSH stimulation test at both 8 a.m. and 11 p.m. in a depressed patient population and normal controls. The difference between the ΔTSH at 11 p.m. and the ΔTSH at the 8 a.m. timepoint was defined as $\Delta\Delta$TSH. These researchers demonstrated that depressed patients had a much lower $\Delta\Delta$TSH than controls. Normal HPT axis function returned following remission from depression, but patients who did not respond to antidepressant medications continued to show blunted $\Delta\Delta$TSH. This suggests that treatment with antidepressants per se is not responsible for the improvement in HPT axis function. Further, patients with the lowest pretreatment evening thyrotropin secretion also had the lowest rate of antidepressant response. This new methodology may serve as a more sensitive method to detect changes in HPT axis function.

Interestingly, Post's group measured both cerebral blood flow and cerebral glucose metabolism using positron emission tomography (PET) in both clinically depressed and bipolar patients. Both measures of cerebral activity were inversely correlated with serum TSH levels, and the authors suggested that HPT axis function contributes to primary and secondary mood disorders [13]. The current literature has also clearly demonstrated elevated TRH release in some depressed patients, but whether this is a causative factor in depression remains unknown. This same group proposed that elevated TRH levels might instead be a compensatory response to depression. In fact, they reported that a lumbar intrathecal infusion of 500 μg of TRH into medication-free inpatients with depression produced a clinically robust, but short-lived, improvement in mood and suicidality [14]. Although this work is preliminary, it does suggest that the development of a systemically administered TRH receptor agonist may represent a novel class of antidepressant agents.

HPT axis abnormalities have also been reported in bipolar disorders. Both elevated basal plasma concentrations of TSH and an exaggerated TSH response to TRH have been demonstrated [15, 16]. There is also evidence that bipolar patients with the rapid cycling subtype have a higher prevalence of hypothyroidism (grades 1, 2 and 3) than bipolar patients without rapid cycling [17, 18]. A blunted or absent evening surge of plasma TSH, a blunted TSH response to TRH [19, 20], and the presence of antithyroid microsomal and/or antithyroglobulin antibodies [21, 22] have also been demonstrated in bipolar patients.

Treatment of Hypothyroid States

As noted above, thyroid hormone extracts from sheep or cattle were the first treatments used that demonstrated efficacy in ameliorating the signs and symptoms of hypothyroidism. Several synthetic derivatives were introduced in the 1960s which quickly replaced desiccated thyroid tissue for the treatment of patients with thyroid disease. Among these are levothyroxine (Levoxyl, Levothroid, Synthroid), synthetic forms of thyroxine (T_4) and liothyronine (Cytomel), and the synthetic levorotatory isomer of triiodothyronine (T_3). Moreover, in part due to the seminal work carried out by Prange and collaborators in the United States in the 1960s, the use of thyroid hormones in augmenting antidepressant response in depression was established.

Hyperthyroid States

Although a number of conditions, including pituitary adenomas, can lead to hyperthyroid states, the most common non-iatrogenic cause of thyroid hormone excess is Graves' disease. In Graves' disease, the body generates an autoantibody to the TSH receptor which directly stimulates thyroid follicular cells to secrete excessive amounts of T_3 and T_4. In this state, the normal negative feedback exerted by T_3 and T_4 on TRH and TSH release is disrupted. The clinical manifestations of thyroid hormone excess are exaggerations of the normal physiologic effects of T_3 and T_4; they include diaphoresis, heat intolerance, fatigue, dyspnoea, palpitations, weakness (especially in proximal muscles), weight loss despite an increased appetite, hyperdefecation, increased psychomotor activity, and visual complaints. Psychiatric manifestations are also common and include anxiety (13% of unselected cases), depression (28% of patients) and cognitive changes (approximately 7% of patients). Psychotic manifestations and mania are less common, occurring in only 2% of unselected cases. Overall, psychiatric comorbidity is much less common in hyperthyroid states than it is in hypothyroid states [7].

Conclusions

Overall, there is clear evidence linking psychiatric symptomatology and thyroid disorders which extends back over 100 years. The observation that hypothyroid patients exhibit symptoms reminiscent of major depression led to a search for thyroid axis abnormalities in patients with affective illness. The efficacy of thyroid augmentation in the treatment of depression and other affective disorders provides further evidence linking HPT axis function and psychiatric illness [23, 24]. Although work over the past 40 years has demonstrated a number of HPT axis abnormalities in depressed and bipolar patients, the aetiological connection between these findings remains elusive.

HYPOTHALAMIC–PITUITARY–ADRENAL AXIS

Components and Function

The primary regulator of the hypothalamic–pituitary–adrenal (HPA) axis is CRF, a 41-amino-acid-containing peptide synthesized in parvocellular neurons located primarily in the PVN of the hypothalamus. CRF-containing cells in the PVN receive input from a variety of brain nuclei, including the amygdala, bed nucleus of the stria terminalis, and other brainstem nuclei [25]. These CRF-containing neurons in turn project to nerve terminals in the median eminence [26], and CRF is released into the hypophyseal–portal system, where it activates CRF receptors on corticotrophs in the anterior pituitary to promote the synthesis of pro-opiomelanocortin (POMC) and the

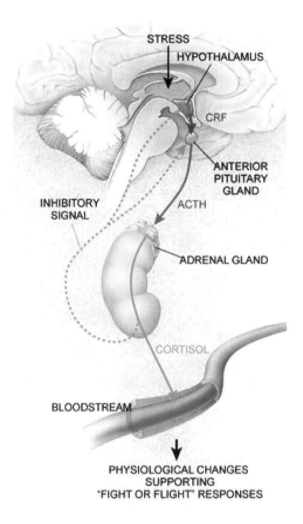

FIGURE 4.4 Overview of the feedback mechanisms of the hypothalamic–pituitary–adrenal axis. Following relevant stimuli, including stress, corticotropin-releasing factor (CRF) is released from the hypothalamus into hypophyseal portal vessels, where it is transported in high concentrations to the pituitary gland. CRF then promotes the release of adrenocorticotropin (ACTH), which in turn promotes the release of cortisol from the adrenal glands. Cortisol acts as an inhibitory signal at both the hypothalamus and pituitary, preventing further CRF and ACTH release, respectively. Mounting evidence suggests that chronic overactivity of the axis, and particularly overproduction of CRF, may contribute to the pathophysiology of depression. Reproduced from [82] with permission

release of its post-translational products: ACTH, β-endorphin and others (Figure 4.4). AVP can also promote the release of ACTH from the anterior pituitary, though CRF is necessary for AVP to exert this effect. ACTH released from the anterior pituitary in turn stimulates the production and release of cortisol, the primary glucocorticoid in humans, from the adrenal cortex (Figure 4.4).

The concentration of circulating glucocorticoids is modulated via long-loop negative feedback. An increase in circulating glucocorticoids inhibits hypothalamic CRF gene expression and ACTH secretion from the pituitary. This in turn prevents further glucocorticoid release. The HPA axis also exhibits a circadian rhythmicity in humans, whereby serum cortisol levels peak immediately before awakening and reach their nadir in the evening.

Discovery of CRF

Although Saffron and Schally identified a crude extract which promoted the release of ACTH from the pituitary in 1955 [27], it was not until 1981 that CRF was isolated and chemically characterized. Working with extracts derived from 500 000 sheep hypothalami, Vale et al. [28] at the Salk institute isolated, synthesized and elucidated the structure of CRF. This discovery led to the availability of synthetic CRF, which allowed a comprehensive assessment of the HPA axis to proceed. It is now clear that CRF coordinates the endocrine, immune, autonomic and behavioural responses of mammals to stress.

Two CRF receptor subtypes, CRF_1 and CRF_2, with distinct anatomical localization and receptor pharmacology, have been identified [29–33]. Both are G-protein-coupled receptors and are positively coupled to adenylyl cyclase via G_s. CRF_1 is the predominant receptor in the pituitary, cerebellum and neocortex in the rat [34]. A growing body of evidence from animal studies has shown that the CRF_1 receptor may specifically mediate some of the anxiogenic-like behaviours observed after administration of CRF [35]. The CRF_2 receptor family is composed of two primary splice variants, CRF_{2A} and CRF_{2B}. The CRF_{2A} receptor is more prevalent in subcortical regions, such as the ventromedial hypothalamus, lateral septum and dorsal raphe nucleus, whereas CRF_{2B} is more abundantly expressed in the periphery. A structurally related member of the CRF peptide family, urocortin, has also been identified in the mammalian brain. The endogenous neuropeptide urocortin has equally high affinity for both the CRF_1 and CRF_2 receptor subtypes [36], whereas CRF displays a higher affinity at CRF_1 receptors than it does at CRF_2 receptors. This fact, along with the distribution of urocortin and CRF_2 receptors, suggests that urocortin is the preferred endogenous ligand at CRF_2 receptors.

The Effects of Changes in Glucocorticoid Availability

A deficiency of endogenous glucocorticoids produces overt clinical symptoms, including weakness, fatigue, hypoglycemia, hyponatremia, hyperkalemia, fever, diarrhoea, nausea and shock. This condition, also known as Addison's disease, is most often caused by autoimmune destruction of the adrenal cortex. However, it is important to note that abrupt withdrawal from exogenous corticosteroids or ACTH can also induce an Addisonian crisis, because the exogenous administration of these compounds suppresses endogenous HPA axis activity. This is why tapering of the dose of adrenal steroids is essential before discontinuation. Glucocorticoid deficiency may also produce mild to severe depression or, less commonly, psychosis.

Excessive glucocorticoid secretion leads to a number of characteristic symptoms, including moon facies, plethoric appearance, truncal obesity, purple abdominal striae, hypertension, protein depletion and signs of glucose intolerance or overt diabetes mellitus. Psychiatric symptoms, specifically depression and anxiety, are also associated with glucocorticoid excess. Cognitive impairment, especially decrements in memory function and attention, are also common, and may be due to the direct effects of corticosteroids on the hippocampal formation [37].

The most common form of non-iatrogenic hypercortisolism is due to an ACTH-secreting pituitary adenoma, also known as Cushing's disease. Harvey Cushing, from whom the disease is named, first documented the occurrence of psychiatric symptoms, particularly depression, in his description of the illness in 1913. Hypercortisolism from other causes is often referred to as Cushing's syndrome. Since Cushing's initial description, the occurrence of depression in Cushing's syndrome has been well documented [38, 39].

HPA Axis Abnormalities in Depression

The occurrence of depression and other psychiatric symptoms in both Cushing's and Addison's disease served as an impetus for researchers to scrutinize HPA axis abnormalities in depression and other psychiatric disorders. Most investigators would agree that one of the most venerable findings in all of psychiatry is the hyperactivity of the HPA axis observed in a significant subset of patients with major depression. Based on the work of research groups led by Board, Bunney and Hamburg, as well as by Carroll, Sachar, Stokes and Besser, literally thousands of studies have been conducted in this area.

The earliest studies in this field demonstrated elevated plasma cortisol concentrations in depressed patients [40, 41]. Other markers of hypercortisolism that have been reliably demonstrated in depressed patients include elevated 24-hour urinary free cortisol concentrations and increased levels of cortisol metabolites in urine [42]. One commonly used test to measure HPA axis function is the dexamethasone suppression test (DST). In this test, 1 mg dexamethasone is given at 11 p.m., blood is then drawn at 8 a.m. the following morning and cortisol levels measured. Dexamethasone is a synthetic steroid similar to cortisol and suppresses ACTH secretion, and subsequently cortisol release, in healthy volunteers. Non-suppression of plasma glucocorticoid levels following the administration of dexamethasone is common in depression. The rate of cortisol non-suppression after dexamethasone administration generally correlates with the severity of depression [43]; in fact, nearly all patients with major depression with psychotic features exhibit non-suppression in the DST [44, 45]. Since Carroll's initial report [46, 47] and subsequent claims for diagnostic utility [48], the DST has generated considerable controversy [49] as to its diagnostic utility. Diagnostic issues notwithstanding, the overwhelming conclusion from the myriad of studies demonstrates that a sizeable percentage of depressed patients exhibit HPA axis abnormalities.

Another method used to assess HPA axis activity is the CRF stimulation test, which became available shortly after CRF was synthesized. In this paradigm, CRF is administered intravenously (usually a 1 µg/kg dose), and the ensuing ACTH and cortisol response is measured at 30-minute intervals over a two- to three-hour period [50]. Numerous studies have now demonstrated a blunted ACTH and β-endorphin response to exogenously administered ovine CRF (oCRF) or human CRF (hCRF) in depressed patients compared to non-depressed subjects, though the cortisol response in depressed patients and non-depressed control subjects did not differ consistently [51–55]. The attenuated ACTH response to CRF is presumably due to either chronic hypersecretion of CRF from nerve terminals in the median eminence, which results in down-regulation of CRF receptors in the anterior pituitary, and/or to the chronic hypercortisolemia. This receptor down-regulation results in a reduced responsivity of the anterior pituitary to CRF, as has been demonstrated in laboratory animals [56–60]. Following recovery from depression, the documented disturbances in the HPA axis generally remit.

A combined dexamethasone/CRF test has also been developed. In this test, 1.5 mg dexamethasone is administered orally at night (11 p.m.) and subjects receive an intravenous bolus of 100 µg hCRF at 3 p.m. the following day. Patients with HPA axis dysfunction display a paradoxically increased release of ACTH and cortisol relative to controls. These abnormalities, which are frequently encountered in depressed patients, disappear following remission of depressive symptoms, and normalization of HPA axis function seems to precede full clinical remission [61, 62]. The combined test appears to have much higher sensitivity for detecting subtle alterations in HPA axis function: approximately 80% of patients with major depression produce an abnormal response, whereas only about 44% of patients with major depression have an abnormal response when the DST is administered alone [61, 62]. Furthermore, otherwise healthy individuals with first-degree relatives suffering from an affective illness demonstrated cortisol and ACTH responses to the combined test which were higher than those in a control group, but less than those in patients currently suffering from major depression. This suggests that a genetically transmissible defect in corticosteroid receptor function may render these individuals more susceptible to developing affective disorders [63].

Structural changes in the components of the HPA axis have also been documented in depressed patients. Perhaps in part due to the trophic effects of CRF, pituitary gland enlargement has been documented in depressed patients as measured by magnetic resonance imaging (MRI) [64]. Enlargement of the adrenal glands, presumably due to ACTH hypersecretion, has repeatedly been demonstrated both in depressed patients post mortem [65, 66] and in suicide victims [67]. It is reasonable to hypothesize that the normal plasma cortisol response to CRF seen in depressed patients is due to adrenocortical hypertrophy, in light of the blunted ACTH and β-endorphin responses to CRF seen in these same patients [52, 54, 65, 68, 69]. Presumably, although the ACTH response to CRF is decreased in depressed patients, the enlarged adrenal cortex may secrete relatively greater quantities of cortisol compared to control subjects in response to a given amount of ACTH. There are reports of increased cortisol responses to pharmacological doses of ACTH that support this hypothesis [70–74], though discordant findings have also been reported [75].

The studies thus far discussed focused primarily on dysregulations of the HPA axis, but, as mentioned earlier, CRF controls not only the neuroendocrine, but also the autonomic, immune, and behavioural responses to stress in mammals. Moreover, results from clinical studies and a rich body of literature on research conducted primarily in rodents and lower primates have both indicated the importance of CRF at extrahypothalamic sites. In rodents, primates and humans, CRF and its receptors have been heterogeneously localized in a variety of regions, including the amygdala, thalamus, hippocampus and prefrontal cortex, among others [76–79]. These brain regions are important in regulating many aspects of the mammalian stress response, and in regulating affect. The presence of CRF receptors in both the dorsal raphe (DR) and locus coeruleus (LC), the major serotonergic- and noradrenergic-containing regions in the brain, respectively, also deserves comment. Because most available antidepressants, including tricyclics and selective serotonin reuptake inhibitors, are believed to work via modulation of noradrenergic and/or serotonergic systems, the neuroanatomical proximity of CRF and monoaminergic systems suggests a possible site of interaction between CRF systems and antidepressants.

Involvement of extrahypothalamic CRF systems in the pathophysiology of depression is suggested by numerous studies showing elevated CRF concentration in the CSF of patients suffering from depression [10, 80–83], though discrepant results have been reported [84]. Elevated CSF levels of CRF have also been detected in depressed people who committed suicide [80]. A reduction in concentrations of CRF in CSF has been reported in healthy volunteers treated with the tricyclic antidepressant desipramine [85], providing further evidence of a possible interconnection between anti-depressants, noradrenergic neurons and CRF systems. Similar effects have been reported with fluoxetine and electroconvulsive therapy in depressed patients [86].

Depressed patients who are non-suppressors in the DST also have significantly higher CSF levels of CRF than do depressed patients with normal DST results. Presumably the elevated CSF concentrations of CRF are due to hypersecretion of CRF in the CNS [87]; the CRF may be acting at sites throughout the brain and contribute to many of the behaviours characteristic of depression. A reduction in the density of CRF receptors in the frontal cortex has also been reported in the frontal cortex of suicide victims [88]. Presumably hypersecretion of CRF results in a down-regulation of CRF receptors in the frontal cortex.

While the exact mechanism that lies behind CRF hyperactivity remains obscure, studies from our group and others have documented long-term persistent increases in HPA axis activity and extrahypothalamic CRF neuronal activity after exposure to early untoward life events—for example, neglect and child abuse respectively in both laboratory animals (rat and non-human primates) and patients [63, 89–91]. Early life stress apparently permanently sensitizes the HPA axis and leads to a greater risk of developing depression later in life. In one schema, early sensitization of CRF systems results in heightened responses to stress later in life. To measure HPA responsivity to stress, the Trier Social Stress Test (TSST) was developed. This laboratory paradigm involves a simulated 10-minute public speech and a mental arithmetic task. The TSST has been validated as a potent activator of the HPA axis in humans [92]. Recently, our group has reported increased plasma ACTH and cortisol concentrations, presumably due to hypersecretion of CRF, after exposure to the TSST in women (both depressed and non-depressed) who were exposed to severe physical and emotional trauma as children [93]. These data provide evidence for functional hyperactivity of CRF systems that may be influenced by early adverse life events.

Space constraints do not permit an extensive review of the preclinical literature. However, several additional points are worth interjecting. Numerous studies have documented that when CRF is injected directly into the CNS of laboratory animals it produces effects reminiscent of the cardinal symptoms of depression, including decreased libido, reduced appetite and weight loss, sleep disturbances and neophobia. Indeed, newly developed CRF_1 receptor antagonists represent a novel putative class of antidepressants. Such compounds show activity in nearly every preclinical screen for antidepressants and anxiolytics currently employed. Recently, a small open-label study examining the effectiveness of R121919, a CRF_1 receptor antagonist, in major depression was completed [94]. Severity measures of both anxiety and depression were reduced in the depressed patients. Although this drug is no longer in clinical development, it is clear that CRF_1 receptor antagonists may represent a new class of agents to treat anxiety and affective disorders.

HPA Axis Alterations in Other Psychiatric Disorders

When depression is comorbid with a variety of other disorders, such as multiple sclerosis, Alzheimer's disease, multi-infarct dementia, Huntington's disease, and others, both CRF hypersecretion and HPA axis hyperactivity are common. In contrast, HPA axis dysfunction has rarely been reported in schizophrenia. Consistent with the role of CRF in both depression-like and anxiety-like behaviours in preclinical animal studies, increased CSF concentrations of CRF have been reported in post-traumatic stress disorder (PTSD) [95]. A recent elegant study that used an in-dwelling cannula in the lumbar space, allowing repeated sampling of CSF several hours after the initial, and presumably stressful, lumbar puncture, demonstrated elevated CSF levels of CRF in combat veterans suffering from PTSD [96]. In contrast, low serum cortisol and urinary free cortisol levels have been repeatedly, yet unexpectedly, detected in PTSD. One possible mechanism that has been proposed by Yehuda *et al.* [97] suggests heightened negative feedback within the HPA axis in patients with chronic PTSD. Finally, CRF neuronal degeneration is now well known to occur in the cerebral cortex of patients with Alzheimer's disease, with compensatory up-regulation of CRF receptor numbers, and this effect precedes the better-studied cholinergic neuronal involvement [98].

HYPOTHALAMIC–PITUITARY–GONAD AXIS

The overall organization of the hypothalamic–pituitary–gonad (HPG) axis is similar to the other major neuroendocrine axes. A "pulse" generator in the arcuate nucleus of the hypothalamus controls gonadotropin-releasing hormone (GnRH) secretion, which occurs in a pulsatile fashion [99]. GnRH is released into the portal circulation connecting the hypothalamus and anterior pituitary, where it binds to gonadotrophs and promotes the release of luteinizing hormone (LH) and follicle-stimulating hormone (FSH) into the systemic circulation [100]. These hormones then bind to Leydig's cells in the testes to promote testosterone secretion or the ovaries to promote oestrogen secretion. In females, FSH also promotes the development of ovarian follicles and the synthesis and secretion of androgen-binding proteins and inhibin. Inhibin acts directly on the anterior pituitary to inhibit FSH secretion without affecting LH release. In both sexes, testosterone/estradiol generated by the testes/ovaries feed back on the pituitary and hypothalamus to inhibit further FSH, LH and GnRH release.

Despite the significantly higher rates of depression in women, data on HPG abnormalities in psychiatric disorders remain remarkably limited. Early studies showed no differences in plasma concentrations of LH and FSH in depressed postmenopausal women compared with non-depressed matched control subjects [101]. However, a later study showed decreased plasma LH concentrations in depressed postmenopausal women compared to matched controls [102]. In a more recent study, significantly lower estradiol levels were detected in women with depression, but the blood levels of other reproductive hormones fell within the normal range [103]. Because estradiol affects a number of neurotransmitter systems, including norepinephrine and serotonin, these results merit further study.

The response to administration of exogenous GnRH in depressed patients has also been investigated. Normal LH and FSH responses to a high dose of GnRH (250 µg) have been reported in male depressed and female depressed (pre- and postmenopausal) patients [104], whereas a decreased LH response to a lower dose of GnRH (150 µg) has been reported in pre- and postmenopausal depressed patients [102]. Unden et al. [105] observed no change in basal or TRH/luteinizing hormone-releasing hormone (LHRH)-stimulated LH concentrations in a depressed cohort including both sexes, though depressed males with an abnormal DST response showed a significantly higher increase in FSH compared to the controls.

The prevalence of mood disorders in women, including premenstrual syndrome (PMS) and post-partum depression, also deserves mention. PMS is a cyclic recurrence of symptoms both somatic (oedema, fatigue, breast tenderness, headaches) and psychological (depression, irritability, and affective lability). The symptoms start following ovulation and disappear within the first day or two of menses, followed by a symptom-free interval between menses and the next ovulation. In some cases (5–10%), symptoms may be severe enough to interfere with normal functioning, leading to the diagnosis of premenstrual dysphoric disorder (PMDD) [106]. GnRH agonists, which produce a "clinical ovariectomy" by down-regulation of GnRH receptors in the pituitary and reduced gonadotropin secretions, have been shown to be an effective treatment for PMS, suggesting that the HPG axis is involved in the manifestation of symptoms [107]. However, significant variations in HPG axis function have yet to be identified in women especially susceptible to PMS.

Post-partum mood disorders are also common, occurring in approximately 10% of women after childbirth. Both post-partum depression and the less frequent post-partum psychosis show their highest prevalence in the first three months after childbirth [108]. The timing of these syndromes would suggest that neuroendocrine dysregulation may contribute to their expression, but no major abnormalities in HPG axis function were detected in a prospective investigation of post-partum disorders [109]. Additional research on the HPG axis in depression and in other mood states is needed.

HYPOTHALAMIC–PROLACTIN AXIS

Unlike other anterior pituitary hormones, prolactin release is regulated via tonic inhibition by prolactin-inhibitory factor (PIF), which was later determined to be dopamine. Dopamine neurons in the tuberoinfundibular system of the hypothalamus directly inhibit prolactin release. Prolactin can also inhibit its own release by a short-loop negative feedback to the hypothalamus. TRH, oxytocin, serotonin, oestrogen and other neuroregulators also have prolactin-releasing factor activity [110]. Prolactin primarily regulates the behavioural aspects of reproduction and infant care. Basal prolactin levels increase in females following parturition, and suckling stimulates prolactin release. Prolactin itself stimulates breast growth and milk synthesis.

Excess circulating prolactin can lead to a number of clinical symptoms. Hyperprolactinemia often leads to reduced testosterone secretion in men and a decreased libido in both men and women. Patients may also complain of depression, stress intolerance, anxiety and increased irritability, which usually resolve following treatments that reduce serum prolactin levels. Despite these effects, alterations in the hypothalamic–prolactin axis have not been clearly demonstrated in psychiatric disorders [111]. Hyperprolactinemia also frequently occurs following treatment with conventional antipsychotic medications, because of their potent blockade of dopamine receptors. Because prolactin release is inhibited by dopamine, the prolactin response to infusions of dopaminergic agonists has also been used to estimate CNS dopaminergic tone, though it probably only reflects hypothalamic dopamine neuronal function.

Although abnormalities in prolactin secretion have not been clearly demonstrated in depression per se, a large number of reports have used provocative tests of prolactin secretion in patients with psychiatric disorders (for a review see [112]). Briefly, these tests use agents that increase serotonergic transmission, for example L-tryptophan, 5-hydroxytryptophan (5HTP), and fenfluramine, among others. In general, the prolactin response to agents that increase serotonergic activity is blunted in depression [113, 114], as well as in patients with cluster B personality disorders [115]. These data suggest that the blunted prolactin response is mediated by alteration in $5HT_{1A}$ receptor responsiveness, and that serotonergic transmission in these patients is abnormal.

OXYTOCIN AND ARGININE–VASOPRESSIN

Oxytocin and AVP are nonapeptides synthesized in the magnocellular neurons of the PVN of the hypothalamus and released directly into the bloodstream from axon terminals in the posterior pituitary. This is in contrast to the hypothalamic releasing factors we have discussed thus far, which are released in the portal system from the median eminence, and distinct from the anterior pituitary hormones, which are released following the activation of pituicytes by the releasing factors synthesized in the hypothalamus.

AVP has prominent roles in controlling fluid balance via its effects on the kidney and regulating blood pressure via its vasoconstrictive effects on blood vessels, and can directly promote the sensation of thirst. AVP also promotes the release of ACTH from the anterior pituitary in the presence of CRF, and is released following stressful stimuli [116]. In humans, oxytocin is predominantly involved in controlling smooth muscle contraction during both breast-feeding and parturition (myometrium). In rodents, oxytocin promotes a number of reproductive (grooming, arousal, lordosis, orgasm, nesting, birthing) and maternal behaviours. Although there are marked species differences in the effects of oxytocin, central infusion of this peptide in females of a monogamous prairie vole species promotes lifelong pair bonding in the absence of mating. Furthermore, pair bonding in this species, which normally accompanies mating, can be blocked by oxytocin antagonists, thus implying a key role for oxytocin in the expression of this lifelong behaviour. Rodent studies have also demonstrated that AVP has a pair-bonding function in males, analogous to the pair-bond-promoting behaviours induced by oxytocin administration in females. AVP promotes monogamy and paternal behaviour in some species of male prairie voles. These studies have led some researchers to speculate that oxytocin and AVP may play a role in psychiatric disorders characterized by disrupted affiliative behaviours, such as Asperger's disease and autism [116]. Clearly, more work is needed in order to better understand the function of these two hormones in the human brain.

PITUITARY–GROWTH HORMONE AXIS

Growth hormone (GH) is synthesized and secreted from somatotrophs located in the anterior pituitary. Its release is unique in that it is controlled by two peptide hypothalamic hypophysiotropic hormones, growth hormone-releasing factor (GHRF) and somatostatin (SRIF). SRIF, also known as growth hormone-release-inhibiting hormone (GHIH), was first isolated from ovine hypothalamus in 1974. It is a tetradecapeptide, containing a disulfide bridge linking the two cysteine residues. It is released predominantly from the periventricular and the PVN of the hypothalamus and inhibits GH release. SRIF has a wide extrahypothalamic distribution in brain regions, including the cerebral cortex, hippocampus and amygdala.

GHRF was characterized and sequenced in 1981, after considerable difficulty, from extracts of an ectopic tumour associated with acromegaly. GHRF is a 44-amino-acid peptide and has the most limited CNS distribution of all the hypothalamic-releasing hormones so far identified. GHRF-containing neurons are concentrated in the arcuate nucleus of the hypothalamus and stimulate the synthesis and release of GH. Dopamine, norepinephrine and serotonin innervate GHRF-containing neurons to modulate GH release. Both GHRF and SRIF are released from the median eminence into the hypothalamo-hypophyseal portal system, where they act on somatotrophs in the anterior pituitary to regulate GH release. The GH axis is unique in that it does not have a single target endocrine gland; instead, GH acts directly on targets including bone, muscle and liver. GH also stimulates the release of somatomedin from the liver and insulin-like growth factors. GH shows pulsatile release, with highest release occurring around the time of sleep onset and extending into the first non-REM period of sleep [117].

GH release response to a variety of stimuli, including L-DOPA, a dopamine precursor [118], apomorphine, a centrally active dopamine agonist [110], and the serotonin precursors L-tryptophan [119] and 5HTP [120], has been demonstrated. Several findings indicate dysregulation of GH secretion in depression. Studies have demonstrated a blunted nocturnal GH surge in depression [121], whereas daylight GH secretion seems to be exaggerated in both unipolar and bipolar depressed patients [122]. A number of studies have also demonstrated a blunted GH response to the α-adrenergic agonist clonidine in depressed patients [123, 124]. Siever et al. [125] demonstrated that the blunted GH response to clonidine was not related to age or sex, and this study provided evidence that the diminished GH response to clonidine may be secondary to decreased α_2-adrenergic receptor sensitivity in depression. Using a GHRF stimulation test, our group later demonstrated a slight exaggeration of GH response to GHRH in depressed patients compared to controls, although this difference was mainly attributable to 3 of the 19 depressed patients, who exhibited markedly high GH responses to GHRF [126]. Others, however, have reported a blunted GH response to GHRH in depressed patients. Thus, it is unclear whether the blunted GH response to clonidine seen in depression is due to a pituitary defect in GH secretion, further implying the existence of a subsensitivity of α-adrenergic receptors in depression, or to a GHRH deficit. Recently, a diminished GH response to clonidine was demonstrated in children and adolescents at high risk for major depressive disorder. In the light of evidence demonstrating GH dysregulation in childhood depression [127], the blunted GH response seen in high-risk adolescents may represent a trait marker for depression in children and adolescents [128]. Arguably, the blunted GH response to clonidine seen in depression may be the most reproducible and specific finding in the biology of affective disorders.

A GHRH stimulation test has also been developed and employed in depressed patients. Two groups have shown a blunted GH response to GHRH in depressed patients [129–131]. However, Krishnan *et al.* [126, 132] found minimal differences in serum GH response to GHRH between depressed and control patients. A comprehensive review of GHRH stimulation tests in depression, anorexia nervosa, bulimia, panic disorder, schizophrenia and Alzheimer's disease concluded that the results of this test are not consistent and in some cases are contradictory [133]. Factors including the variability of GHRH-stimulated GH among controls, lack of standard outcome measures, and age and gender-related effects may account for some of this variability. Further studies using GHRH will help develop a standard stimulation test to clarify further the response to GHRH in depression and other psychiatric disorders.

Several studies have demonstrated decreased SRIF levels in the CSF of patients suffering from depression [134, 135], dementia, schizophrenia [136] and Alzheimer's disease [98, 137]. SRIF concentrations are also markedly elevated in the basal ganglia of patients with Huntington's disease [138], though the implications of this finding are unknown. SRIF also inhibits the release of both CRF and ACTH [139–141], indicating a direct interaction between the GH and HPA axes. No published studies measuring GHRH concentration and GHRH mRNA expression have been conducted in post-mortem tissue from depressed patients and matched controls, which, in view of the evidence presented here, is of interest. Similarly, CSF studies of GHRH are lacking.

CONCLUSIONS

Basic clinical observations of psychiatric disorders associated with primary endocrine disorders, such as Cushing's syndrome and hypothyroidism, have led us to a broader understanding of the role of neuroendocrine disturbances in a variety of psychiatric disorders, including depression and bipolar disorders. These studies have allowed major advances in biological psychiatry by helping us to understand the brain circuits involved in the pathophysiology of mood and anxiety disorders. Foremost among these is the CRF theory of depression, which is supported by studies from a variety of disciplines, and which has led to the development of a novel therapeutic approach, namely using CRF receptor antagonists. Further, this work has provided a mechanism to explain the increase in the prevalence of depression seen in patients exposed to trauma early in life (first postulated by Freud in the early part of the twentieth century). If CRF truly is the "black bile" of depression, CRF antagonists may represent a novel class of antidepressants with a unique mechanism of action. Indeed, a number of CRF receptor antagonists are now in clinical development as novel anxiolytics and antidepressants.

In addition to the HPA axis and CRF alterations observed in depression, HPT axis abnormalities are also very common; the majority of depressed patients, in fact, exhibit alterations in one of these two axes. Furthermore, there is a widely replicated blunting of GH response to clonidine and a blunted prolactin response to serotonergic stimuli in depressed patients. Although these studies have not added much understanding to the prevailing monoamine theory of depression, the mechanistic studies that have followed have been remarkably fruitful. Is it obvious that the vast majority of studies have been focused on patients with mood disorders, particularly unipolar depression. Clearly, other disorders including eating disorders, anxiety disorders, schizophrenia and axis II diagnoses should be similarly scrutinized.

The availability of selective ligands that can be used with PET will mark the next major leap in our understanding of the neuroendocrine axes in psychiatric disorders. The ability to determine peptide receptor alterations in the brain and pituitary of patients with psychiatric disorders will contribute immensely to our understanding of the neurobiological underpinnings of such disorders.

Finally, a growing number of studies have demonstrated that depression is a systemic disease that increases vulnerability to other disorders. Depressed patients demonstrate increased incidence of coronary artery disease and stroke, osteoporosis and perhaps cancer. These observations may at least be partly attributed to the endocrine alterations observed in depression.

ACKNOWLEDGEMENTS

We would like to acknowledge support from the National Institutes of Health (MH-42088) and Conte Center for Neuroscience of Mental Disorders (MH-58922).

REFERENCES

1. Levine J. (2000) The hypothalamus as a major integrating center. In *Neuroendo-crinology in Physiology and Medicine* (Eds P. Conn, M.E. Freeman), pp. 75–95, Humana Press, Totowa, New Jersey.
2. Veldhuis D. (2000) The neuroendocrine control of ultradian rhythms. In *Neuroendocrinology in Physiology and Medicine* (Eds P. Conn, M.E. Freeman), pp. 453–475, Humana Press, Totowa, New Jersey.
3. DeVito W. (2000) Neuroendocrine regulation of thyroid function. In *Neuroendo-crinology in Physiology and Medicine* (Eds P. Conn, M.E. Freeman), pp. 225–241, Humana Press, Totowa, New Jersey.
4. Shaw C. (1892) Case of myxedema with restless melancholia treated by injections of thyroid juice: recovery. *Br. J. Med.*, 451.
5. Whybrow P.C., Prange A.J. Jr., Treadway C.R. (1969) Mental changes accompanying thyroid gland dysfunction. A reappraisal using objective psychological measurement. *Arch. Gen. Psychiatry*, **20**: 48–63.
6. Jain V.K. (1972) A psychiatric study of hypothyroidism. *Psychiatr. Clin.*, **5**: 121–130.
7. Boswell E., Anfinson, T.J., Nemeroff, C.B. (2001) Neuropsychiatric aspects of endocrine disorders. In *Textbook of Neuropsychiatry*, Vol. 3, 3rd ed. (Eds S. Yudofsky, R. Hales), American Psychiatric Association Press, Washington (in press).
8. Kastin A.J., Ehrensing R.H., Schalch D.S., Anderson M.S. (1972) Improvement in mental depression with decreased thyrotropin response after administration of thyrotropin-releasing hormone. *Lancet*, **2**: 740–742.
9. Prange A.J. Jr., Lara P.P., Wilson I.C., Alltop L.B., Breese G.R. (1972) Effects of thyrotropin-releasing hormone in depression. *Lancet*, **2**: 999–1002.
10. Banki C.M., Bissette G., Arato M., Nemeroff C.B. (1988) Elevation of immunor-eactive CSF TRH in depressed patients. *Am. J. Psychiatry*, **145**: 1526–1531.
11. Nemeroff C.B., Simon J.S., Haggerty J.J. Jr., Evans D.L. (1985) Antithyroid antibodies in depressed patients. *Am. J. Psychiatry*, **142**: 840–843.
12. Duval F., Mokrani M.C., Crocq M.A., Jautz M., Bailey P., Diep T.S., Macher J.P. (1996) Effect of antidepressant medication on morning and evening thyroid function tests during a major depressive episode. *Arch. Gen. Psychiatry*, **53**: 833–840.
13. Marangell L.B., Ketter T.A., George M.S., Pazzaglia P.J., Callahan A.M., Parekh P., Andreason P.J., Horwitz B., Herscovitch P., Post R.M. (1997) Inverse relationship of peripheral thyrotropin-stimulating hormone levels to brain activity in mood disorders. *Am. J. Psychiatry*, **154**: 224–230.
14. Marangell L.B., George M.S., Callahan A.M., Ketter T.A., Pazzaglia P.J., L'Herrou T.A., Leverich G.S., Post R.M. (1997) Effects of intrathecal thyrotropin-releasing hormone (protirelin) in refractory depressed patients. *Arch. Gen. Psychiatry*, **54**: 214–222.
15. Loosen P.T., Prange A.J. Jr. (1982) Serum thyrotropin response to thyrotropin-releasing hormone in psychiatric patients: a review. *Am. J. Psychiatry*, **139**: 405–416.
16. Haggerty J.J. Jr., Simon J.S., Evans D.L., Nemeroff C.B. (1987) Relationship of serum TSH concentration and antithyroid antibodies to diagnosis and DST response in psychiatric inpatients. *Am. J. Psychiatry*, **144**: 1491–1493.
17. Cowdry R.W., Wehr T.A., Zis A.P., Goodwin F.K. (1983) Thyroid abnormalities associated with rapid-cycling bipolar illness. *Arch. Gen. Psychiatry*, **40**: 414–420.

18. Bauer M.S., Whybrow P.C., Winokur A. (1990) Rapid cycling bipolar affective disorder. I. Association with grade I hypothyroidism. *Arch. Gen. Psychiatry*, **47**: 427–432.

19. Sack D.A., James S.P., Rosenthal N.E., Wehr T.A. (1988) Deficient nocturnal surge of TSH secretion during sleep and sleep deprivation in rapid-cycling bipolar illness. *Psychiatry Res.*, **23**: 179–191.

20. Souetre E., Salvati E., Wehr T.A., Sack D.A., Krebs B., Darcourt G. (1988) Twenty-four-hour profiles of body temperature and plasma TSH in bipolar patients during depression and during remission and in normal control subjects. *Am. J. Psychiatry*, **145**: 1133–1137.

21. Myers D.H., Carter R.A., Burns B.H., Armond A., Hussain S.B., Chengapa V.K. (1985) A prospective study of the effects of lithium on thyroid function and on the prevalence of antithyroid antibodies. *Psychol. Med.*, **15**: 55–61.

22. Lazarus J.H., McGregor A.M., Ludgate M., Darke C., Creagh F.M., Kingswood C.J. (1986) Effect of lithium carbonate therapy on thyroid immune status in manic depressive patients: a prospective study. *J. Affect. Disord.*, **11**: 155–160.

23. Dording C.M. (2000) Antidepressant augmentation and combinations. *Psychiatr. Clin. North Am.*, **23**: 743–755.

24. Prange A.J. (1996) Novel uses of thyroid hormones in patients with affective disorders. *Thyroid*, **6**: 537–543.

25. Hauger R., Dautzenberg F.M. (2000) Regulation of the stress response by corticotropin releasing factor. In *Neuroendocrinology in Physiology and Medicine* (Eds P. Conn, M.E. Freeman), pp. 267–293, Humana Press, Totowa, New Jersey.

26. Swanson L.W., Sawchenko P.E., Rivier J., Vale W.W. (1983) Organization of ovine corticotropin-releasing factor immunoreactive cells and fibers in the rat brain: an immunohistochemical study. *Neuroendocrinology*, **36**: 165–186.

27. Saffran M., Schally A.V., Benfey B.G. (1955) Stimulation of the release of corticotropin from the adenohypophysis by a neurohypophysial factor. *Endocrinology*, **57**: 439–444.

28. Vale W., Spiess J., Rivier C., Rivier J. (1981) Characterization of a 41-residue ovine hypothalamic peptide that stimulates secretion of corticotropin and beta-endorphin. *Science*, **213**: 1394–1397.

29. Chalmers D.T., Lovenberg T.W., Grigoriadis D.E., Behan D.P., De Souza E.B. (1996) Corticotrophin-releasing factor receptors: from molecular biology to drug design. *Trends Pharmacol. Sci.*, **17**: 166–172.

30. Lovenberg T.W., Liaw C.W., Grigoriadis D.E., Clevenger W., Chalmers D.T., De Souza E.B., Oltersdorf T. (1995) Cloning and characterization of a functionally distinct corticotropin-releasing factor receptor subtype from rat brain. *Proc. Natl. Acad. Sci. USA*, **92**: 836–840.

31. Grigoriadis D.E., Lovenberg T.W., Chalmers D.T., Liaw C., De Souza E.B. (1996) Characterization of corticotropin-releasing factor receptor subtypes. *Ann. NY Acad. Sci.*, **780**: 60–80.

32. Chang C.P., Pearse R.V.D., O'Connell S., Rosenfeld M.G. (1993) Identification of a seven transmembrane helix receptor for corticotropin-releasing factor and sauvagine in mammalian brain. *Neuron*, **11**: 1187–1195.

33. Chen R., Lewis K.A., Perrin M.H., Vale W.W. (1993) Expression cloning of a human corticotropin-releasing-factor receptor. *Proc. Natl. Acad. Sci. USA*, **90**: 8967–8971.

34. Primus R.J., Yevich E., Baltazar C., Gallager D.W. (1997) Autoradiographic localization of CRF1 and CRF2 binding sites in adult rat brain. *Neuropsychopharmacology*, **17**: 308–316.

35. Heinrichs S.C., Lapsansky J., Lovenberg T.W., De Souza E.B., Chalmers D.T. (1997) Corticotropin-releasing factor CRF1, but not CRF2, receptors mediate anxiogenic-like behavior. *Regul. Pept.*, **71**: 15–21.
36. Vaughan J., Donaldson C., Bittencourt J., Perrin M.H., Lewis K., Sutton S., Chan R., Turnbull A.V., Lovejoy D., Rivier C. (1995) Urocortin, a mammalian neuropeptide related to fish urotensin I and to corticotropin-releasing factor. *Nature*, **378**: 287–292.
37. Sadock B., Sadock, V. (2000) *Comprehensive Textbook of Psychiatry*, 7th ed., Lippincott Williams & Williams, Philadelphia.
38. Spillane J. (1951) Nervous and mental disorders in Cushing's syndrome. *Brain*, **74**: 72–94.
39. Zeiger M.A., Fraker D.L., Pass H.I., Nieman L.K., Cutler G.B. Jr., Chrousos G.P., Norton J.A. (1993) Effective reversibility of the signs and symptoms of hypercortisolism by bilateral adrenalectomy. *Surgery*, **114**: 1138–1143.
40. Carpenter W.T. Jr., Bunney W.E. Jr. (1971) Adrenal cortical activity in depressive illness. *Am. J. Psychiatry*, **128**: 31–40.
41. Gibbons J., McHugh P.R. (1962) Plasma cortisol in depressive illness. *J. Psychiatr. Res.*, **1**: 162–171.
42. Sachar E.J., Hellman L., Fukushima D.K., Gallagher T.F. (1970) Cortisol production in depressive illness. A clinical and biochemical clarification. *Arch. Gen. Psychiatry*, **23**: 289–298.
43. Evans D.L., Nemeroff C.B. (1987) The clinical use of the dexamethasone suppression test in DSM-III affective disorders: correlation with the severe depressive subtypes of melancholia and psychosis. *J. Psychiatr. Res.*, **21**: 185–194.
44. Evans D.L., Nemeroff C.B. (1983) Use of the dexamethasone suppression test using DSM-III criteria on an inpatient psychiatric unit. *Biol. Psychiatry*, **18**: 505–511.
45. Arana G.W., Baldessarini R.J., Ornsteen M. (1985) The dexamethasone suppression test for diagnosis and prognosis in psychiatry. Commentary and review. *Arch. Gen. Psychiatry*, **42**: 1193–1204.
46. Carroll B.J., Martin F.I., Davies B. (1968) Pituitary-adrenal function in depression. *Lancet*, **1**: 1373–1374.
47. Carroll B.J., Martin F.I., Davies B. (1968) Resistance to suppression by dexamethasone of plasma 11-O.H.C.S. levels in severe depressive illness. *Br. Med. J.*, **3**: 285–287.
48. Carroll B.J. (1982) Use of the dexamethasone suppression test in depression. *J. Clin. Psychiatry*, **43**: 44–50.
49. Arana G.W., Mossman D. (1988) The dexamethasone suppression test and depression. Approaches to the use of a laboratory test in psychiatry. *Neurol. Clin.*, **6**: 21–39.
50. Hermus A.R., Pieters G.F., Smals A.G., Benraad T.J., Kloppenborg P.W. (1984) Plasma adrenocorticotropin, cortisol, and aldosterone responses to corticotropin-releasing factor: modulatory effect of basal cortisol levels. *J. Clin. Endocrinol. Metab.*, **58**: 187–191.
51. Amsterdam J.D., Maislin G., Winokur A., Berwish N., Kling M., Gold P. (1988) The oCRH stimulation test before and after clinical recovery from depression. *J. Affect. Disord.*, **14**: 213–222.
52. Gold P.W., Chrousos G., Kellner C., Post R., Roy A., Augerinos P., Schulte H., Oldfield E., Loriaux D.L. (1984) Psychiatric implications of basic and clinical studies with corticotropin-releasing factor. *Am. J. Psychiatry*, **141**: 619–627.

53. Holsboer F., Muller O.A., Doerr H.G., Sippell W.G., Stalla G.K., Gerken A., Steiger A., Boll E., Benkert O. (1984) ACTH and multisteroid responses to corticotropin-releasing factor in depressive illness: relationship to multisteroid responses after ACTH stimulation and dexamethasone suppression. *Psycho-neuroendocrinology*, **9**: 147–160.

54. Kathol R.G., Jaeckle R.S., Lopez J.F., Meller W.H. (1989) Consistent reduction of ACTH responses to stimulation with CRH, vasopressin and hypoglycaemia in patients with major depression. *Br. J. Psychiatry*, **155**: 468–478.

55. Young E.A., Watson S.J., Kotun J., Haskett R.F., Grunhaus L., Murphy-Wein-berg V., Vale W., Rivier J., Akil H. (1990) Beta-lipotropin-beta-endorphin response to low-dose ovine corticotropin releasing factor in endogenous depression. Preliminary studies. *Arch. Gen. Psychiatry*, **47**: 449–457.

56. Wynn P.C., Aguilera G., Morell J., Catt K.J. (1983) Properties and regulation of high-affinity pituitary receptors for corticotropin-releasing factor. *Biochem. Biophys. Res. Commun.*, **110**: 602–608.

57. Wynn P.C., Hauger R.L., Holmes M.C., Millan M.A., Catt K.J., Aguilera G. (1984) Brain and pituitary receptors for corticotropin releasing factor: localization and differential regulation after adrenalectomy. *Peptides*, **5**: 1077–1084.

58. Aguilera G., Wynn P.C., Harwood J.P., Hauger R.L., Millan M.A., Grewe C., Catt K.J. (1986) Receptor-mediated actions of corticotropin-releasing factor in pituitary gland and nervous system. *Neuroendocrinology*, **43**: 79–88.

59. Holmes M.C., Catt K.J., Aguilera G. (1987) Involvement of vasopressin in the down-regulation of pituitary corticotropin-releasing factor receptors after adrenalectomy. *Endocrinology*, **121**: 2093–2098.

60. Wynn P.C., Harwood J.P., Catt K.J., Aguilera G. (1988) Corticotropin-releasing factor (CRF) induces desensitization of the rat pituitary CRF receptor-adenylate cyclase complex. *Endocrinology*, **122**: 351–358.

61. Heuser I., Yassouridis A., Holsboer F. (1994) The combined dexamethasone/CRH test: a refined laboratory test for psychiatric disorders. *J. Psychiatr. Res.*, **28**: 341–356.

62. Holsboer F. (2000) The corticosteroid receptor hypothesis of depression. *Neuropsychopharmacology*, **23**: 477–501.

63. Holsboer F., Lauer C.J., Schreiber W., Krieg J.C. (1995) Altered hypothalamic-pituitary-adrenocortical regulation in healthy subjects at high familial risk for affective disorders. *Neuroendocrinology*, **62**: 340–347.

64. Krishnan K.R., Doraiswamy P.M., Lurie S.N., Figiel G.S., Husain M.M., Boyko O.B., Ellinwood E.H. Jr., Nemeroff C.B. (1991) Pituitary size in depression. *J. Clin. Endocrinol. Metab.*, **72**: 256–259.

65. Amsterdam J.D., Marinelli D.L., Arger P., Winokur A. (1987) Assessment of adrenal gland volume by computed tomography in depressed patients and healthy volunteers: a pilot study. *Psychiatry Res.*, **21**: 189–197.

66. Nemeroff C.B., Krishnan K.R., Reed D., Leder R., Beam C., Dunnick N.R. (1992) Adrenal gland enlargement in major depression. A computed tomographic study. *Arch. Gen. Psychiatry*, **49**: 384–387.

67. Dorovini-Zis K., Zis A.P. (1987) Increased adrenal weight in victims of violent suicide. *Am. J. Psychiatry*, **144**: 1214–1215.

68. Holsboer F., Von Bardeleben U., Gerken A., Stalla G.K., Muller O.A. (1984) Blunted corticotropin and normal cortisol response to human corticotropin-releasing factor in depression. *N. Engl. J. Med.*, **311**: 1127.

69. Gold P.W., Loriaux D.L., Roy A., Kling M.A., Calabrese J.R., Kellner C.H., Nieman L.K., Post R.M., Pickar D., Gallucci W. (1986) Responses to

corticotropin-releasing hormone in the hypercortisolism of depression and Cushing's disease. Pathophysiologic and diagnostic implications. *N. Engl. J. Med.*, **314**: 1329–1335.

70. Kalin N.H., Weiler S.J., Shelton S.E. (1982) Plasma ACTH and cortisol concentrations before and after dexamethasone. *Psychiatry Res*, **7**: 87–92.

71. Amsterdam J.D., Winokur A., Abelman E., Lucki I., Rickels K. (1983) Cosyntropin (ACTH alpha 1–24) stimulation test in depressed patients and healthy subjects. *Am. J. Psychiatry*, **140**: 907–909.

72. Linkowski P., Mendlewicz J., Leclercq R., Brasseur M., Hubain P., Golstein J., Copinschi G., Van Cauter E. (1985) The 24-hour profile of adrenocorticotropin and cortisol in major depressive illness. *J. Clin. Endocrinol. Metab.*, **61**: 429–438.

73. Jaeckle R.S., Kathol R.G., Lopez J.F., Meller W.H., Krummel S.J. (1987) Enhanced adrenal sensitivity to exogenous cosyntropin (ACTH alpha 1–24) stimulation in major depression. Relationship to dexamethasone suppression test results. *Arch. Gen. Psychiatry*, **44**: 233–240.

74. Krishnan K.R., Ritchie J.C., Saunders W.B., Nemeroff C.B., Carroll B.J. (1990) Adrenocortical sensitivity to low-dose ACTH administration in depressed patients. *Biol. Psychiatry*, **27**: 930–933.

75. Heim C., Newport D.J., Bonsall R., Miller A.H., Nemeroff C.B. (2001) Altered pituitary-adrenal axis responses to provocative challenge tests in adult survivors of childhood abuse. *Am. J. Psychiatry*, **158**: 575–581.

76. Suda T., Tomori N., Tozawa F., Mouri T., Demura H., Shizume K. (1984) Distribution and characterization of immunoreactive corticotropin-releasing factor in human tissues. *J. Clin. Endocrinol. Metab.*, **59**: 861–866.

77. Sanchez M.M., Young L.J., Plotsky P.M., Insel T.R. (1999) Autoradiographic and in situ hybridization localization of corticotropin-releasing factor 1 and 2 receptors in nonhuman primate brain. *J. Comp. Neurol.*, **408**: 365–377.

78. Van Pett K., Viau V., Bittencourt J.C., Chan R.K., Li H.Y., Arias C., Prins G.S., Perrin M., Vale W., Sawchenko P.E. (2000) Distribution of mRNAs encoding CRF receptors in brain and pituitary of rat and mouse. *J. Comp. Neurol.*, **428**: 191–212.

79. Charlton B.G., Ferrier I.N., Perry R.H. (1987) Distribution of corticotropin-releasing factor-like immunoreactivity in human brain. *Neuropeptides*, **10**: 329–334.

80. Arato M., Banki C.M., Bissette G., Nemeroff C.B. (1989) Elevated CSF CRF in suicide victims. *Biol. Psychiatry*, **25**: 355–359.

81. France R.D., Urban B., Krishnan K.R., Bissett G., Banki C.M., Nemeroff C., Speilman F.J. (1988) CSF corticotropin-releasing factor-like immunoactivity in chronic pain patients with and without major depression. *Biol. Psychiatry*, **23**: 86–88.

82. Nemeroff C.B. (1988) The role of corticotropin-releasing factor in the pathogenesis of major depression. *Pharmacopsychiatry*, **21**: 76–82.

83. Risch S.C., Lewine R.J., Kalin N.H., Jewart R.D., Risby E.D., Caudle J.M., Stipetic M., Turner J., Eccard M.B., Pollard W.E. (1992) Limbic-hypothalamic-pituitary-adrenal axis activity and ventricular-to-brain ratio studies in affective illness and schizophrenia. *Neuropsychopharmacology*, **6**: 95–100.

84. Roy A., Pickar D., Paul S., Doran A., Chrousos G.P., Gold P.W. (1987) CSF corticotropin-releasing hormone in depressed patients and normal control subjects. *Am. J. Psychiatry*, **144**: 641–645.

85. Veith R.C., Lewis N., Langohr J.I., Murburg M.M., Ashleigh E.A., Castillo S., Peskind E.R., Pascualy M., Bissette G., Nemeroff C.B. (1993) Effect of desipra-

mine on cerebrospinal fluid concentrations of corticotropin-releasing factor in human subjects. *Psychiatry Res.*, **46**: 1–8.

86. Nemeroff C.B., Bissette G., Akil H., Fink M. (1991) Neuropeptide concentrations in the cerebrospinal fluid of depressed patients treated with electroconvulsive therapy. Corticotrophin-releasing factor, beta-endorphin and somatostatin. *Br. J. Psychiatry*, **158**: 59–63.

87. Post R.M., Gold P., Rubinow D.R., Ballenger J.C., Bunney W.E. Jr., Goodwin F.K. (1982) Peptides in the cerebrospinal fluid of neuropsychiatric patients: an approach to central nervous system peptide function. *Life Sci.*, **31**: 1–15.

88. Nemeroff C.B., Owens M.J., Bissette G., Andorn A.C., Stanley M. (1988) Reduced corticotropin releasing factor binding sites in the frontal cortex of suicide victims. *Arch. Gen. Psychiatry*, **45**: 577–579.

89. Holsboer F., von Bardeleben U., Wiedemann K., Muller O.A., Stalla G.K. (1987) Serial assessment of corticotropin-releasing hormone response after dexamethasone in depression. Implications for pathophysiology of DST nonsuppression. *Biol. Psychiatry*, **22**: 228–234.

90. Coplan J.D., Andrews M.W., Rosenblum L.A., Owens M.J., Friedman S., Gorman J.M., Nemeroff C.B. (1996) Persistent elevations of cerebrospinal fluid concentrations of corticotropin-releasing factor in adult nonhuman primates exposed to early-life stressors: implications for the pathophysiology of mood and anxiety disorders. *Proc. Natl. Acad. Sci. USA.*, **93**: 1619–1623.

91. Nemeroff C.B. (1999) The preeminent role of early untoward experience on vulnerability to major psychiatric disorders: the nature–nurture controversy revisited and soon to be resolved. *Mol. Psychiatry*, **4**: 106–108.

92. Kirschbaum C., Pirke K.M., Hellhammer D.H. (1993) The 'Trier Social Stress Test'—A tool for investigating psychobiological stress responses in a laboratory setting. *Neuropsychobiology*, **28**: 76–81.

93. Heim C., Newport D.J., Heit S., Graham Y.P., Wilcox M., Bonsall R., Miller A.H., Nemeroff C.B. (2000) Pituitary-adrenal and autonomic responses to stress in women after sexual and physical abuse in childhood. *JAMA*, **284**: 592–597.

94. Zobel A.W., Nickel T., Kunzel H.E., Ackl N., Sonntag A., Ising M., Holsboer F. (2000) Effects of the high-affinity corticotropin-releasing hormone receptor 1 antagonist R121919 in major depression: the first 20 patients treated. *J. Psychiatr. Res.*, **34**: 171–181.

95. Bremner J.D., Licinio J., Darnell A., Krystal J.H., Owens M.J., Southwick S.M., Nemeroff C.B., Charney D.S. (1997) Elevated CSF corticotropin-releasing factor concentrations in posttraumatic stress disorder. *Am. J. Psychiatry*, **154**: 624–629.

96. Baker D.G., West S.A., Nicholson W.E., Ekhator N.N., Kasckow J.W., Hill K.K., Bruce A.B., Orth D.N., Geracioti T.D. Jr. (1999) Serial CSF corticotropin-releasing hormone levels and adrenocortical activity in combat veterans with posttraumatic stress disorder. *Am. J. Psychiatry*, **156**: 585–588.

97. Yehuda R., Teicher M.H., Trestman R.L., Levengood R.A., Siever L.J. (1996) Cortisol regulation in posttraumatic stress disorder and major depression: a chronobiological analysis. *Biol. Psychiatry*, **40**: 79–88.

98. Bissette G., Cook L., Smith W., Dole K.C., Crain B., Nemeroff C.B. (1998) Regional neuropeptide pathology in Alzheimer's disease: corticotropin-releasing factor and somatostatin. *J. Alzheim. Dis.*, **1**: 1–15.

99. Knobil E. (1990) The GnRH pulse generator. *Am. J. Obstet. Gynecol.*, **163**: 1721–1727.

100. Midgley A.R. Jr., Jaffe R.B. (1971) Regulation of human gonadotropins. X. Episodic fluctuation of LH during the menstrual cycle. *J. Clin. Endocrinol. Metab.*, **33**: 962–969.
101. Nathan K.I., Musselman D.L., Schatzberg A.F., Nemeroff C.B. (1995) Biology of mood disorders. In *The American Psychiatric Press Textbook of Psychopharmacology* (Eds A.F. Schatzberg, C.B. Nemeroff), pp. 439–449, American Psychiatric Press, Washington.
102. Brambilla F., Maggioni M., Ferrari E., Scarone S., Catalano M. (1990) Tonic and dynamic gonadotropin secretion in depressive and normothymic phases of affective disorders. *Psychiatry Res.*, **32**: 229–239.
103. Young E.A., Midgley A.R., Carlson N.E., Brown M.B. (2000) Alteration in the hypothalamic–pituitary–ovarian axis in depressed women. *Arch. Gen. Psychiatry*, **57**: 1157–1162.
104. Winokur A., Amsterdam J., Caroff S., Snyder P.J., Brunswick D. (1982) Variability of hormonal responses to a series of neuroendocrine challenges in depressed patients. *Am. J. Psychiatry*, **139**: 39–44.
105. Unden F., Ljunggren J.G., Beck-Friis J., Kjellman B.F., Wetterberg L. (1988) Hypothalamic–pituitary–gonadal axis in major depressive disorders. *Acta. Psychiatr. Scand.*, **78**: 138–146.
106. Altshuler L.L., Hendrick V., Parry B. (1995) Pharmacological management of premenstrual disorder. *Harvard Rev. Psychiatry*, **2**: 233–245.
107. Freeman E.W., Sondheimer S.J., Rickels K. (1997) Gonadotropin-releasing hormone agonist in the treatment of premenstrual symptoms with and without ongoing dysphoria: a controlled study. *Psychopharmacol Bull.*, **33**: 303–309.
108. Wisner K.L., Stowe Z.N. (1997) Psychobiology of postpartum mood disorders. *Semin. Reprod. Endocrinol.*, **15**: 77–89.
109. O'Hara M.W., Zekoski E.M., Philipps L.H., Wright E.J. (1990) Controlled prospective study of postpartum mood disorders: comparison of childbearing and nonchildbearing women. *J. Abnorm. Psychol.*, **99**: 3–15.
110. Fink G. (2000) Neuroendocrine regulation of pituitary function: general principles. In *Neuroendocrinology in Physiology and Medicine* (Eds P. Conn, M.E. Freeman), pp. 112–120. Humana Press, Totowa, New Jersey.
111. Nicholas L., Dawkins K., Golden R.N. (1998) Psychoneuroendocrinology of depression. Prolactin. *Psychiatr. Clin. North Am.*, **21**: 341–358.
112. Van de Kar L.D. (1989) Neuroendocrine aspects of the serotonergic hypothesis of depression. *Neurosci. Biobehav. Rev.*, **13**: 237–246.
113. Mann J.J., McBride P.A., Malone K.M., DeMeo M., Keilp J. (1995) Blunted serotonergic responsivity in depressed inpatients. *Neuropsychopharmacology*, **13**: 53–64.
114. Golden R.N., Ekstrom D., Brown T.M., Ruegg R., Evans D.L., Haggerty J.J. Jr., Garbutt J.C., Pedersen C.A., Mason G.A., Browne J. (1992) Neuroendocrine effects of intravenous clomipramine in depressed patients and healthy subjects. *Am. J. Psychiatry*, **149**: 1168–1175.
115. Coccaro E.F., Kavoussi R.J., Hauger R.L. (1997) Serotonin function and antiaggressive response to fluoxetine: a pilot study. *Biol. Psychiatry*, **42**: 546–552.
116. Insel T.R. (1997) A neurobiological basis of social attachment. *Am. J. Psychiatry*, **154**: 726–735.
117. Finkelstein J.W., Roffwarg H.P., Boyar R.M., Kream J., Hellman L. (1972) Age-related change in the twenty-four-hour spontaneous secretion of growth hormone. *J. Clin. Endocrinol. Metab.*, **35**: 665–670.

118. Boyd A.E.D., Lebovitz H.E., Pfeiffer J.B. (1970) Stimulation of human-growth-hormone secretion by L-dopa. *N. Engl. J. Med.*, **283**: 1425–1429.
119. Muller E.E., Brambilla F., Cavagnini F., Peracchi M., Panerai A. (1974) Slight effect of L-tryptophan on growth hormone release in normal human subjects. *J. Clin. Endocrinol. Metab.*, **39**: 1–5.
120. Imura H., Nakai Y., Yoshimi T. (1973) Effect of 5-hydroxytryptophan (5-HTP) on growth hormone and ACTH release in man. *J. Clin. Endocrinol. Metab.*, **36**: 204–206.
121. Schilkrut R., Chandra O., Osswald M., Ruther E., Baafusser B., Matussek N. (1975) Growth hormone release during sleep and with thermal stimulation in depressed patients. *Neuropsychobiology*, **1**: 70–79.
122. Mendlewicz J., Linkowski P., Kerkhofs M., Desmedt D., Golstein J., Copinschi G., Van Cauter E. (1985) Diurnal hypersecretion of growth hormone in depression. *J. Clin. Endocrinol. Metab.*, **60**: 505–512.
123. Charney D.S., Heninger G.R., Sternberg D.E., Hafstad K.M., Giddings S., Landis D.H. (1982) Adrenergic receptor sensitivity in depression. Effects of clonidine in depressed patients and healthy subjects. *Arch. Gen. Psychiatry*, **39**: 290–294.
124. Siever L.J., Uhde T.W., Silberman E.K., Lake C.R., Jimerson D.C., Risch S.C., Kalin N.H., Murphy D.L. (1982) Evaluation of alpha-adrenergic responsiveness to clonidine challenge and noradrenergic metabolism in the affective disorders and their treatment. *Psychopharmacol. Bull.*, **18**: 118–119.
125. Siever L.J., Uhde T.W., Silberman E.K., Jimerson D.C., Aloi J.A., Post R.M., Murphy D.L. (1982) Growth hormone response to clonidine as a probe of noradrenergic receptor responsiveness in affective disorder patients and controls. *Psychiatry Res.*, **6**: 171–183.
126. Krishnan K.R., Manepalli A.N., Ritchie J.C., Rayasam K., Melville M.L., Thorner M.O., Rivier J.E., Vale W.W., Nemeroff C.B. (1988) Growth hormone response to growth hormone-releasing factor in depression. *Peptides*, **9**, (Suppl. 1): 113–116.
127. Ryan N.D., Dahl R.E., Birmaher B., Williamson D.E., Iyengar S., Nelson B., Puig-Antich J., Perel J.M. (1994) Stimulatory tests of growth hormone secretion in prepubertal major depression: depressed versus normal children. *J. Am. Acad. Child Adolesc. Psychiatry*, **33**: 824–833.
128. Birmaher B., Dahl R.E., Williamson D.E., Perel J.M., Brent D.A., Axelson D.A., Kaufman J., Dorn L.D., Stull S., Rao U. *et al.* (2000) Growth hormone secretion in children and adolescents at high risk for major depressive disorder. *Arch. Gen. Psychiatry*, **57**: 867–872.
129. Lesch K.P., Laux G., Erb A., Pfuller H., Beckmann H. (1987) Attenuated growth hormone response to growth hormone-releasing hormone in major depressive disorder. *Biol. Psychiatry*, **22**: 1495–1499.
130. Lesch K.P., Laux G., Pfuller H., Erb A., Beckmann H. (1987) Growth hormone (GH) response to GH-releasing hormone in depression. *J. Clin. Endocrinol. Metab.*, **65**: 1278–1281.
131. Risch S. (1991) Growth hormone-releasing factor and growth hormone. In *Neuropeptides and Psychiatric Disorders* (Ed. C. Nemeroff), pp. 93–108, American Psychiatric Press, Washington.
132. Krishnan K.R., Manepalli A.N., Ritchie J.C., Rayasam K., Melville M.L., Daughtry G., Thorner M.O., Rivier J.E., Vale W.W., Nemeroff C.B. (1988) Growth hormone-releasing factor stimulation test in depression. *Am. J. Psychiatry*, **145**: 90–92.

133. Skare S.S., Dysken M.W., Billington C.J. (1994) A review of GHRH stimulation test in psychiatry. *Biol. Psychiatry*, **36**: 249–265.
134. Gerner R.H., Yamada T. (1982) Altered neuropeptide concentrations in cerebrospinal fluid of psychiatric patients. *Brain Res.*, **238**: 298–302.
135. Agren H., Lundqvist G. (1984) Low levels of somatostatin in human CSF mark depressive episodes. *Psychoneuroendocrinology*, **9**: 233–248.
136. Bissette G., Widerlov E., Walleus H., Karlsson I., Eklund K., Forsman A., Nemeroff C.B. (1986) Alterations in cerebrospinal fluid concentrations of somatostatinlike immunoreactivity in neuropsychiatric disorders. *Arch. Gen. Psychiatry*, **43**: 1148–1151.
137. Molchan S.E., Hill J.L., Martinez R.A., Lawlor B.A., Mellow A.M., Rubinow D.R., Bissette G., Nemeroff C.B., Sunderland T. (1993) CSF somatostatin in Alzheimer's disease and major depression: relationship to hypothalamic–pituitary–adrenal axis and clinical measures. *Psychoneuroendocrinology*, **18**: 509–519.
138. Nemeroff C.B., Youngblood W.W., Manberg P.J., Prange A.J. Jr., Kizer J.S. (1983) Regional brain concentrations of neuropeptides in Huntington's chorea and schizophrenia. *Science*, **221**: 972–975.
139. Richardson U.I., Schonbrunn A. (1981) Inhibition of adrenocorticotropin secretion by somatostatin in pituitary cells in culture. *Endocrinology*, **108**: 281–290.
140. Heisler S., Reisine T.D., Hook V.Y., Axelrod J. (1982) Somatostatin inhibits multireceptor stimulation of cyclic AMP formation and corticotropin secretion in mouse pituitary tumor cells. *Proc. Natl. Acad. Sci. USA*, **79**: 6502–6506.
141. Brown M.R., Rivier C., Vale W. (1984) Central nervous system regulation of adrenocorticotropin secretion: role of somatostatins. *Endocrinology*, **114**: 1546–1549.

5

Neurophysiological Research in Psychiatry

John H. Gruzelier[1], Silvana Galderisi[2] and Werner Strik[3]

[1]*Department of Cognitive Neuroscience and Behaviour, Imperial College of Science, Technology and Medicine, St. Dunstan's Road, London W6 8RF, United Kingdom*
[2]*Department of Psychiatry, University of Naples SUN, Largo Madonna delle Grazie, 80138 Naples, Italy*
[3]*University Hospital of Clinical Psychiatry, Bollingen Str. 111, Berne 60, 3000 Switzerland*

INTRODUCTION

Mental activities, from simple sensory processing to high-order cognitive functions, are based on complex electrochemical neuronal activation patterns. This apparently trivial statement implies that the study of brain morphology and molecular biology will not be able to link the activity of the working brain with psychology and psychopathology until the dynamics and topological interactions of brain activity at the systems level are sufficiently understood. Since neurophysiological methods assess the summed electrical field potentials derived from postsynaptic dendritic currents of cortical neurons, they are able in principle to study the system physiology of the brain with a sufficiently high temporal resolution. Important insights into the time course of brain electrical activation during complex cognitive processes are possible. To give some examples, the time course of neuronal mass activation during conscious sensory discrimination, anticipation of movements even if only imagined, processing of semantic information, and decoding of human face expression has been reliably described. Multi-channel recordings have provided important information about the topography of brain electrical fields over time. However, attempts to relate the results of electrophysiological recordings to the topology of brain function have been hindered by the lack of reliable methods that provide an external validation of electrophysiological topographic findings.

Psychiatry as a Neuroscience. Edited by Juan José López-Ibor, Wolfgang Gaebel, Mario Maj and Norman Sartorius. © 2002 John Wiley & Sons Ltd.

In recent years, the upcoming techniques of functional imaging, in particular functional magnetic resonance imaging (fMRI), have contributed substantially to the validation of earlier electrophysiological results [1]. This has opened up a fascinating field which combines methods for integrative research utilizing the high time resolution of electroencephalography (EEG) and cortical event-related potentials (ERPs) and the high spatial resolution of functional imaging techniques. Not too surprisingly for contemporary neurophysiologists, and to the delayed gratification of many pioneers, several electrophysiological results that were plausible, but not proven due to the lack of adequate validation, have recently been confirmed by functional imaging. Examples include the preactivation of the motor cortex prior to a planned movement, the activation of modality-specific brain areas during mental imagery and the validation of source localization routines [2, 3]. Furthermore, exciting new discoveries relating fast-frequency EEG activity, in the form of gamma oscillations, to conscious experience, have contributed to a renaissance in EEG methodology, as have the methods of high-resolution EEG coherence demonstrating dynamic patterns of functional connectivity and disconnection [4, 5].

In clinical psychiatry, neurophysiological methods are still of limited impact compared with their importance for understanding physiological brain functions. EEG and ERPs are in general accepted only as a means of excluding "organic" brain pathology and for investigating sleep disorders; for psychiatric diseases an accepted indication is lacking. This is surprising, since robust results have been reported and independently confirmed in schizophrenia and depression demonstrating that late ERPs, for example, are related to subdiagnoses, risk factors, symptom dimensions and prognosis [6, 7]. So far, final validation of the parameters and their introduction into clinical practice has been held back by manifold problems. One is the apparent reluctance of research foundations to provide the necessary financial support for the last step needed to make basic research results available for clinical practice. Further limitations to progress in neurophysiology, as well as in many other disciplines of psychiatric research, derive from present psychiatric classification systems. In the case of schizophrenia, for example, although it is generally accepted that it is not one disease, empirical results that account for this are usually not adequately taken note of and further investigated.

Neurophysiology has recently gained new interest due to its extension into functional brain imaging, which allows validation of spatial information yielded previously. Now the combination of available techniques offers new perspectives for describing a neurophysiological syntax of higher brain functions that might improve our understanding of mechanisms underlying abnormal mental states and contribute to a revision of current psychopathological concepts and categories. Several encouraging results are available today, and this chapter will attempt a comprehensive overview of the state of the art.

RECORDING AND ANALYSIS OF BRAIN ELECTRICAL ACTIVITY

Electroencephalography

Since Hans Berger's discovery of the EEG, recording of the brain electrical activity from the scalp has been considered a window to mental processes. The EEG consists of the summed electrical field potentials generated by postsynaptic dendritic currents of cortical neurons [8–11]. The frequency and amplitude characteristics of the scalp EEG provide information on the underlying neural dynamics. They can be investigated with respect to different experimental conditions and/or diagnostic categories. The EEG is generally recorded from large arrays of electrodes; nowadays, 16–32 electrodes are used in most laboratories, while in more sophisticated research settings the number can be 124 or more [12]. The electrodes are placed over the scalp according to international systems [13, 14]. In the last ten years, the old EEG machines have been largely replaced by computer systems for the amplification, digitization, digital filtering, storing and quantitative analysis of multi-lead EEG, with several advantages [15]. Visual interpretation of the EEG has limited value in the study of neurocognitive functions, providing only a few parameters for assessment of the state of alertness and for the detection of epileptic or other abnormalities related to gross cerebral pathology [16, 17]. By contrast, quantitative analysis of EEG (qEEG) in the time, frequency and space domains has enormously enhanced the potential of the technique in the evaluation of brain functioning: changes in amplitude, frequency and/or topography, which cannot be resolved by the human eye, reflect changes in brain functions [12]. qEEG provides valuable information on the timing of neurocognitive events and brain functional connectivity, i.e. the functional coupling among different brain areas under various affective, motor and cognitive conditions [12, 18–20]. Two methods have been used in EEG quantification: time and frequency domain analysis.

In the time domain, the principal method is period analysis, which calculates the percentage of time spent in each frequency band, the average frequency, the frequency variability, as well as the amplitude and amplitude variability, for both the primary EEG wave and the first derivative [21].

In the frequency domain, qEEG parameters are most frequently derived from the spectral analysis of the EEG signal. This analysis calculates the power for all the frequency spectrum (total power) or for individual frequency bands (band power). By calculating the root mean square of the power, the total amplitude and the amplitude of each frequency band is obtained. The traditional four frequency bands—delta (up to 3.5 Hz), theta (3.5–7.5 Hz), alpha (7.5–13.5 Hz) and beta (13.5–30 Hz)—have been replaced by narrower frequency bands for which distinct functional correlates have been reported [22–26]. The analysis of frequencies above 30 Hz—the so-called gamma band—has started quite recently, after the discovery of its functional significance in experimental studies with intracerebral recordings [27–30]. As described in the next paragraph, the interpretation of the functional meaning of different EEG frequency bands has greatly changed in the last decades. In fact, while until the 1970s an excess of delta and theta activity in adults was considered as a sign of sleepiness or brain pathology, alpha rhythm as an index of an idling state of the brain, and the presence of beta activity was related to cognitive and sensory activation, in the last few decades several studies have demonstrated that all known EEG frequency bands may be involved in physiological brain states.

Coherent, rhythmic changes of electrical potentials in the high-frequency range (above 30 Hz, gamma band) have been demonstrated in distributed populations of neurons in response to sensory input [20, 27–30]. The demonstration of this "evoked" (stimulus-induced) gamma oscillatory activity in the mammalian brain was the first empirical validation of von der Malsburg's hypothesis that synchronization of neural groups (individually coding for different aspects of the sensory input) is the basic binding process in the central nervous system, yielding a unified percept [18, 30]. Recently, it has been hypothesized that other oscillatory rhythms are involved in cognitive processes requiring integration over large cortical distances (e.g. among areas of different sensory modalities) and in complex activities extending in time (such as working memory tasks) [25, 31, 32].

Task-related or event-related amplitude measures within a specific frequency band provide an estimate of synchronization of local sources. Event-related desynchronization (ERD), with positive values representing a reduction and negative values an increase in power with respect to a baseline reference interval, is a valuable example of this type of measure [33]. Some studies have also investigated the synchronization of the qEEG frequency with different rates of sensory stimulation in the gamma and alpha frequency ranges [34, 35]. Research focusing on oscillatory responses has changed the interpretation of the EEG rhythms. In particular, delta oscillation is believed to increase during the performance of tasks requiring internal concentration (i.e. subjects have to disregard external input); in these conditions, the increase is maximal over frontal regions [36, 37]. The activation of corticofugal pathways that inhibit thalamocortical neurons, producing a disconnection of the cortex from environmental stimuli, was hypothesized to mediate delta increase during internal concentration [37].

Recent findings seem to indicate an increase of delta for recalled versus non-recalled words [26]. Theta activity was shown to be involved in working memory functions and attention [22–26]. Alpha in the lower band (7.5–9.5 Hz) was demonstrated to index attentional processes, while in its higher band (9.5–13.5 Hz) it was implicated in memory functions [22, 24, 37–40]. Beta, like gamma activity, seems to have a role in the integration of sensory information to give a unified percept [41].

Coherence (i.e. the correlation coefficient among different recording sites within a frequency band) is a measure of the shared electrical activity among scalp sites and evaluates the functional interactions of brain areas on a large spatial scale [19, 26]. The coherence among distant recording sites separated by the rolandic fissure is termed "fascicle coherence" because it expresses the interactions along the superior longitudinal fasciculus, while coherence among post-rolandic sites is called "visual" because is restricted to areas connected by projections of the visual pathways [42]. Methodological problems in measurements and interpretation of coherence have been recently reviewed [19, 43] and the reader is referred to these papers for a comprehensive review of methodological issues.

The integration of highly specialized processes, involving spatially segregated areas of the neocortex, to form a coherent neural process underlying perception and cognition, cannot imply only a global synchronization of a large number of neural assemblies. It has been hypothesized that integration might be achieved by complex relationships among different brain areas, so that the neural dynamic of one population influences the dynamics of another population, not just inducing the same frequency (by synchronizing the other population), but constraining the frequency range that can be expressed by the second population. It has been shown that low-frequency oscillations in some brain regions might influence the high-frequency oscillatory response of distant areas [32, 44, 45]. According to some authors, the application of non-linear methods of analysis might be more appropriate than linear methods (such as power spectrum and coherence) to study this type of relationship among different brain regions and frequency bands [46, 47]. Dimensional complexity and a positive Lyapunov exponent are parameters derived from non-linear methods and provide an estimate of the coordination of brain processes by evaluating the number of independent processes which influence the behaviour of the whole system [46–48]. An analogous measure, omega complexity, based on linear analysis methodologies, has also been proposed [49]. Both the dimensional and the omega complexity have high values when many independent processes are active and poorly coordinated, possibly related to reduced functional connectivity. In fact, as shown by Friston [44] in a computer simulation, reduced connectivity among neural elements is reflected by an increase in the dimensional complexity of the electrical activity of the whole network. The Lyapunov exponent estimates the dependence of the system on its initial conditions and is thought to index system flexibility [50].

Computerized EEG topography (CET) or qEEG mapping has been developed for multi-lead qEEG data. The technique involves the construction of a two- or three-dimensional matrix for a topographic representation of qEEG parameters, such as instant amplitude and band power. Values of the matrix points not covered by the recording electrodes are calculated by interpolating the values from the nearest three or four recording electrodes. The introduction of colour-coded maps made the information more intelligible for non-neurophysiologists and led to renewed interest in these methods in the late 1980s and early 1990s. As for other imaging techniques, statistical probability mapping can also be implemented for comparisons between different subject populations or experimental conditions.

Without appropriate transformations of the qEEG parameters, the topographic information provided by the technique is critically dependent on the reference electrode used for EEG recording. Several transformations have been proposed to obtain reference-independent data, such as the average reference (subtraction of the mean of all electrode values from each electrode value) and Laplacian derivation (the second derivative in space of the potential field at each electrode) [51, 52]. Topography of the brain electrical fields changes over time. The field strength and its distribution is the summary result of the contemporaneous active neural source in the brain. Due to the limited spatial resolution and the so-called inverse solution problem (many different neural activation patterns can explain the same surface field) of electrophysiological recordings, there is no final proof for topographical interpretations in terms of activation of cortical areas. In spite of this general limitation, a parsimonious but valid statement is that a consistent change of the brain electrical field configuration must be due to a change in the relative contribution of distributed brain regions. In other words, while the same field can be generated by different neural activation patterns, different fields cannot be generated by the same activation pattern.

These facts are sufficient to give a physiological significance to field topography changes observed over time and have led to the development of a method for segmentation of the spontaneous EEG into topographically homogeneous periods. With this method [53] it has been demonstrated that the brain electrical fields are not continuously changing, but show epochs of topographic stability interrupted by rapid changes. Further, stable epochs are short (50–1000 milliseconds) compared to the changes in the EEG frequency content and are not merely an expression of the EEG carrier frequency. This has led to the introduction of the term "brain electrical microstates" for these topographically stable periods of the brain electrical fields, in distinction from the macrostates (more enduring frequency patterns) in which they are embedded [54].

The neurophysiological meaning of brain electrical microstates is being studied in terms of cognitive and psychopathological phenomena associated with particular brain electrical field configurations and their temporal characteristics. The particular temporal pattern of rapid changes and stability of variable duration has led to the hypothesis that these brain electrical microstates are related to basic mental operations. This is consistent with the fact that basic mental operations have a duration well within the range observed for brain electrical microstates, and implies that the stream of consciousness, though based on massive low-level parallel processing, results in a sequence of unique contents of mind that are represented by the instantaneous spatial activation patterns of the cerebral cortex. Further observations suggest that there may be a threshold of 100–150 milliseconds for a brain state to become a conscious content of mind [55]. Empirical studies have demonstrated that the brain electrical microstates identified with topographical segmentation of the EEG are related to conscious mind states. In particular, abstract thoughts have been associated with different brain electrical field configurations compared to visual mental representations [56]. Source localizations of these different fields showed a very convincing regional activation pattern involving the left frontal region during abstract thoughts (inner speech) and right parieto-occipital regions during visual mental sceneries [57]. On the basis of these results, the method appears suitable for identifying what Dietrich Lehmann calls the "atoms of thought".

A further important development in topographical analysis is the three-dimensional current source analysis of the brain electrical fields. Pascual-Marqui *et al.* have developed a method of low-resolution electromagnetic tomography (LORETA) that allows localization of the electrical sources of a surface field in the three-dimensional brain space [58]. In contrast to traditional dipole analysis, LORETA is based on the assumption that the scalp field is not generated by a single point source but rather by synchronous activation of neighbouring neurons. LORETA calculates the "smoothest" of all possible solutions by minimizing the total squared Laplacian derivation of source strengths and restricts the solution to brain regions contributing to the electrical scalp field. The method appears to be superior for the source localization of spontaneous EEG and for the cognitive components of the ERPs compared to traditional dipole analysis. It has been validated with concomitant EEG and fMRI recordings during epileptic discharges, with glucose metabolism in Alzheimer's disease (AD) [59] and with neuropsychological tests of frontal brain functions and face decoding [2, 60]. Combination with other functional imaging techniques allows validation of the method and has in several instances provided a fruitful integration between the high spatial resolution of functional imaging and insights obtained from the high time resolution of EEG and ERPs.

Event-Related Potentials

Another measure of electrocortical activity derived from EEG recordings is the ERP. This has been the psychophysiological parameter most widely investigated in psychopathology to date. ERPs are generated in response to specific stimuli and are depicted by positive (P) and negative (N) deflections typically averaged over a number of stimuli. They may be time-locked to the stimulus and termed "evoked", or may be "induced" by the stimulus, in which case the latency is more variable. ERPs have been classified into: (a) sensory potentials, which may occur in the various sensory modalities and include far-field very short latency auditory potentials whose deflections depict transmission through the auditory nerve and brain stem, (b) motor potentials, which precede and accompany motor movements, and (c) longer latency potentials, occurring after about 200 milliseconds and typically reflecting subjective responses, such as the P300, a widespread potential (with maximum positivity at centroparietal areas at about 300 milliseconds) related to novelty or expectancy, and the N400, associated with memory and semantic deviations as with unexpected endings of sentences. Such ERPs, occurring in the millisecond range, are contrasted with steady potential shifts, lasting over seconds, and including the contingent negative variation (CNV), which occurs during the waiting to respond following a warning signal, and the *bereitschaftspotential* or readiness potential, which accrues before the onset of a voluntary movement.

ERPs have been used to understand at what stage information processing may be dysfunctional, under what conditions, and, to a lesser extent, where in the brain the dysfunction may be located. Most sensory ERP components have an origin in or close to primary sensory cortex. In the auditory modality, ERPs depict a negative–positive N100–P200 complex generated in the auditory cortex of the temporal lobe. Monaural stimulation may produce a larger contralateral ERP, though there is not always an advantage for contralateral pathways. Visual ERPs typically are largest at the occipital pole and larger contralateral to the hemi-field of stimulation. Somatosensory potentials have been localized to post-central gyrus and to primary somatosensory cortex with larger contralateral responses to unilateral stimulation.

Attending to one ear and ignoring the other has revealed an N100 component that is related to attention [61]. If a deviant stimulus is presented in a stimulus train, a negative wave at about 200 milliseconds occurs, which is termed mismatch negativity (MMN). This is measured by subtracting standard from deviant stimuli; using magnetoencephalography (MEG), one generator has been localized to supratemporal auditory cortex. MMN has been attributed to an echoic memory process, for it occurs even if the subject is absorbed in another task and fails to register the auditory stimuli. Another

ERP component to an infrequent stimulus is the P300 response. This has been associated with a range of cognitive processes such as expectancy, decision making, relevance, information delivery and so on. As with all but early ERP components, multiple processes and generators are involved.

Neurochemical processes have been related to ERPs. Relations between stimulus intensity and the amplitude of ERP components at around 100 milliseconds, where specific and non-specific thalamocortical systems interact, involve serotonin [62]. ERP measures of sensory gating, whereby two stimuli are presented in succession to assess the influence of the first on the amplitude of the second, in the case of suppression of a P50 component have been related to α_7 nicotinic receptor sensitization under hippocampal and thalamic modulation [63].

PERIPHERAL MEASURES

Electrodermal Activity

Electrodermal activity, formerly called the galvanic skin response, has been one of the most widely utilized measures. This reflects eccrine sweat gland activity mediated by cholinergic activity and under sympathetic autonomic nervous system control. Top-down modulatory influences arise from the premotor and sensorimotor cortex, limbic structures, such as the amygdala, hippocampus, cingulate cortex, hypothalamus and the reticular formation. Electrodermal recording measures the resistance of the skin (or its reciprocal skin conductance) to a minute electrical current through bipolar placement of electrodes, typically placed on the phalanges of the fingers. Measures typically taken are phasic event-related responses, phasic non-specific responses and tonic levels. Non-specific responses may be called "spontaneous responses" and may have a physiological identity independent of cognitive influences.

There are striking individual differences in responsiveness or the lability of responding, as well as in habituation following the repetition of standard stimuli, which varies inversely with stress. A varying proportion of subjects also fail to show evoked responses to passive or non-signal stimuli. Electrodermal reactivity may be also used as an index of emotional arousal, and because it is unconfounded by parasympathetic influences, it is a useful measure of sympathetic reactivity.

Hemispheric influences have had important implications for psychopathology. The nature of lateralized influences has been controversial, and conceptualization has been prone to simplistic right-versus-left interpretations. Unsurprisingly, lateralized influences have been shown to depend (a) on the nature of the electrodermal measure, such as whether the response is a phasic evoked or non-specific response or is a tonic response, (b) the cognitive significance of the eliciting stimulus, such as whether it is verbal or non-verbal, or whether it involves motor preparation, and (c) whether the modulatory influences are predominantly cortical or subcortical. Most research in psychopathology has involved non-signal orienting responses, where subcortical limbic influences appear to predominate. Here, as with other functions, such as behavioural turning tendencies, influences are ipsilateral [64], as confirmed by intracranial stimulation studies in epileptic patients [65].

Cardiovascular Activity

Cardiovascular activity measures, including heart activity measured with the electrocardiogram and impedance cardiograph, blood pressure and blood volume, have also proved useful indicators of emotionality and stress. In addition, in view of significant interactions with somatic muscle activity and brain activity, heart rate recording has illuminated orienting versus defensive responding, signal detection and mental performance. The conventional measure is the electrocardiogram, while the impedance cardiograph provides information about the physical functioning of the heart such as cardiac output, stroke volume, ventricular ejection time, myocardial contractility and total peripheral resistance. Spectral analysis of the ECG allows delineation of sympathetic and parasympathetic influences. Electromyography (EMG) has been useful in evaluating effort and arousal processes, and more recently emotional processes through recording distinct muscle groups involved in facial displays of emotion. Pupillography may also assist in evaluating emotional valence and mental load.

Eye Movements–Startle Reflex–Pre-pulse Inhibition

Eye movements, recorded by the electro-oculogram (EOG), currently have widespread application in psychiatric research. Measured by electrodes placed horizontally or vertically surrounding the eye, they include saccadic movements from one fixation point to the next, smooth pursuit involving the tracking of a moving object together with assessment of intrusive saccades, the ability to inhibit saccades or to respond in a contrary direction (anti-saccades), blink rates and scan paths. Eye blink has also been used to index the startle response, especially the effect of a weak lead stimulus in modulating startle.

The acoustic startle reflex is thought to involve the auditory nerve, cochlear nucleus, lateral lemniscus, nucleus reticularis pontis caudalis and reticulospinal pathway to lower motor neurons. The inhibitory influences of a lead pre-pulse, usually in the form of a weak auditory stimulus termed "pre-pulse inhibition" (PPI), involves descending frontolimbic cortico-striato-pallido-pontine circuitry. The latter has been elucidated by means of pharmacological studies in animals, which have shown modulation by the hippocampal and medial prefrontal cortices and the basolateral amygdala. Disruption of PPI occurs with agonists of dopamine and serotonin and with glutamate/N-methyl-D-aspartate (NMDA) antagonists (see [66] for a review). Neurodevelopmental studies have shown that PPI is reduced by rearing rats in isolation, an effect reversed by typical and atypical antipsychotic drugs. Furthermore, in rats with neonatal neurotoxic lesions of the hippocampus, PPI is impaired after puberty, suggesting that early developmental lesions of the hippocampus create a vulnerability to hormonal influences on neuronal circuits that accompany puberty [67].

MAIN FINDINGS OF NEUROPHYSIOLOGICAL RESEARCH IN PSYCHIATRY

Schizophrenia

Quantitative EEG

The most frequently reported findings from qEEG studies in subjects with schizophrenia include an increase of slow (delta and theta) and fast (beta) activities, and a decrease in alpha power [68–79]. This pattern was initially attributed to the effects of neuroleptic treatment, since some drugs may induce a general slowing of EEG activity. However, this explanation has been ruled out by studies showing that slow wave activity is even more pronounced in untreated patients [74], and it is also present in children at genetic risk for schizophrenia [68]. Although some authors have found these abnormalities as a pattern, others have reported the presence of only some of them (e.g. increase of slow activities and decrease of alpha), or discrepant findings (increase of alpha or lack of differences) [73, 80, 81]. EEG characteristics of schizophrenic patients appear to be stable over time [82, 83]. The majority of studies carried out in subjects in their first episode of schizophrenia have confirmed the pattern of qEEG abnormalities described above [73, 75, 83–85]. However, discrepant findings have also been reported [86–88].

qEEG abnormalities cannot be considered pathognomonic characteristics of schizophrenia, since the degree of sensitivity and specificity is not adequate for diagnostic purposes. However, they have been regarded as: (a) markers of vulnerability to psychosis, (b) prognostic indicators of illness course, (c) tools for the identification of schizophrenia subtypes and

(d) correlates of psychopathological characteristics. The topography of the observed abnormalities has often stimulated hypotheses on pathophysiological mechanisms underlying the disorder.

qEEG Abnormalities and Vulnerability to Psychosis. In 1974, Itil *et al.* [89] reported preliminary findings of a study carried out in Copenhagen which included 71 children considered to be at high risk for schizophrenia (at least one parent suffering from schizophrenia) and 71 children of normal parents (controls). The high-risk group of children showed more slow delta waves (1.3–3.5 Hz), more fast beta activity (above 18 Hz), less alpha activity (10–13 Hz), higher average frequency and less average absolute amplitude than controls. Most significant differences were found over the right temporal and parietal leads. A similar pattern of EEG abnormalities had been found by the same research group in both adult subjects with schizophrenia and psychotic children in comparison with matched groups of healthy controls [68, 90].

Koukkou [91] proposed alpha power reactivity as a trait marker of schizophrenia. She found that before medication, while acutely psychotic patients showed a reduced reactivity of the alpha band power and frequency, the reactivity of the alpha frequency was restored to some extent in the remitted, non-psychotic state and after discontinuation of neuroleptic treatment for three months or more, but it was still reduced compared to normals. Koukkou interpreted the EEG reactivity as a sign of reorganization of working memory during the schizophrenic psychosis [86].

According to Clementz *et al.* [83] and Stassen *et al.* [92], EEG abnormalities observed in patients with schizophrenia do not reflect genetic vulnerability. Stassen *et al.* [92] have studied with repeated assessments 27 pairs of monozygotic (MZ) twins discordant and 13 pairs concordant for schizophrenia, 40 pairs of healthy MZ twins, and 91 healthy unrelated subjects. Healthy MZ twins appeared as similar to each other as the same person was to herself/himself over time. Concordance was much lower in twins concordant and discordant for schizophrenia. Increased theta and decreased alpha differentiated affected from non-affected co-twins, who were discriminated with 80% accuracy. The authors hypothesized that the "EEG abnormalities associated with schizophrenia, and manifested differently in MZ twins concordant for schizophrenia, reflect non-genetic, idiosyncratically different, pathologic developments of genetically identical brains".

qEEG Abnormalities as Prognostic Indices of Illness Course. In schizophrenia, besides the above-described pattern of EEG abnormalities characterized by an increase of slow (delta and theta) and fast (beta) activities and a decrease of alpha power, some authors have described the presence of a so-called "hypernormal" EEG, characterized by the prevalence of a highly stable and synchronized alpha rhythm. Such a pattern has been found in patients with an unfavourable response to treatment with standard neuroleptics [93, 94].

Galderisi *et al.* [95] investigated whether qEEG alterations before treatment could discriminate between subjects with and those without a subsequent favourable response to neuroleptic treatment. Although responders and non-responders showed significant group differences at baseline examination, the degree of overlap among individual values prevented a reliable assignment of subjects to either group; changes in the slow alpha band induced by a single dose of standard neuroleptic discriminated responders from non-responders with an overall accuracy of 89.3%. A significant increase of the slow alpha following neuroleptic treatment has been reported by other authors [68, 96–103]. It is also worth noting that in non-responders the administration of a single dose of a neuroleptic drug produced significant changes in the slow alpha band, which in most cases were the opposite of changes in responders. However, no significant qEEG change was observed after six weeks of treatment in non-responders, which might suggest that the observation reported by some authors that qEEG abnormalities in subjects with schizophrenia are stable traits, not influenced by drug treatment, applies to subjects with an unfavourable response to antipsychotic drugs [104].

qEEG as a Tool for the Identification of Schizophrenia Subtypes. Two strategies can be identified in the relevant literature: (a) subgroups are defined on the basis of clinical features and their EEG characteristics are compared; (b) subgroups are defined by either electrophysiological or other biological characteristics, such as qEEG, quantitative ERPs or lateral ventricular enlargement (LVE).

In studies carried out with the first strategy, patients have usually been dichotomized, for example, as paranoid versus non-paranoid (paranoid patients have higher amplitude for low and fast frequency rhythms), or positive versus negative schizophrenia (subjects with negative schizophrenia have more delta activity than those with the positive subtype of the syndrome) [105, 106]. Dichotomizing approaches to the psychopathology of schizophrenia, however, have been questioned, and the lack of stability of clinical subtypes represents a great limitation for research aimed at reducing the clinico-biological heterogeneity of the syndrome and fostering knowledge of its pathogenetic mechanisms.

A limited number of studies have employed the second research strategy. Karson *et al.* [72] reported that schizophrenic patients with reduced alpha frequency have significantly increased ventricle to brain ratios compared to other patients. The authors hypothesized that both LVE and reduced alpha frequency in subjects with schizophrenia might be related to neuropathological processes involving the thalamus. In a study by Kemali *et al.* [107], schizophrenic patients with LVE showed more alpha power and less beta relative activity than those without LVE. Gambini *et al.* [108] also found an increase of fast alpha (alpha-2) in patients with LVE.

The application of multivariate statistical methods allows control for the enormous amount of parameters provided by multi-channel recordings of the EEG (and its transformations into frequency bands). The most promising work in this direction was done by John and his group, who applied principal component analysis (PCA) to a huge resting-EEG database of controls and schizophrenic patients. They were able to identify patterns of EEG parameters that were related to schizophrenic subsyndromes and neuroleptic medication [87]. The system can be optimized to resemble psychiatric diagnosis and might be helpful for reorienting the diagnostic process while new insights on biologically defined schizophrenic subgroups are awaited.

In a recent study, Sponheim *et al.* [104] examined EEG power abnormalities, brain morphology, oculomotor functioning, electrodermal activity, and nailfold plexus visibility in 112 patients with schizophrenia (54 first-episode, 58 chronic), 78 with non-schizophrenic psychosis (33 with bipolar disorder, 29 with a major depressive disorder and 16 with other psychoses) and 107 non-psychiatric controls. Almost all patients were receiving medication. The two patient groups were subdivided in high and low "LFA" (augmented low frequencies, diminished alpha factor). In the group of patients with schizophrenia, those with high LFA exhibited more negative symptoms, a wider third ventricle, larger frontal horns of the lateral ventricles, and larger cortical sulci than those with low LFA; moreover, first-episode schizophrenic patients with high LFA showed worse oculomotor performance and chronic patients with high LFA had more deviant electrodermal activation. These associations were not observed in the group with non-schizophrenic psychosis. The authors concluded that the association between EEG power abnormalities on the one hand and negative symptoms, ventricular enlargement and oculomotor dysfunction on the other lends credence to recent hypotheses identifying thalamic and prefrontal cortical pathology in schizophrenia. Augmented low frequencies and reduced alpha are consistent with a dysfunction in thalamocortical circuits, particularly in medial dorsal prefrontal networks.

qEEG Correlates of Psychopathological Features of Schizophrenia. Studies of correlations between qEEG characteristics and psychopathological features represent an attempt to overcome limitations of clinical subgrouping. Relationships have been reported between increased low frequency activity and negative symptoms [75, 109, 110], as well as between decreased alpha activity and negative symptoms [111, 112]. In a study carried out in 37 DSM-III-R drug-free schizophrenic patients, a significant positive correlation between beta-2 relative power and disorganization was found. In the same group of subjects a positive correlation between disorganization and speed in the repetition of supraspan recurring spatial sequences was also observed, suggesting a disinhibition of the right hemisphere temporolimbic regions as a possible pathophysiological mechanism underlying disorganization [113]. In a group of 40 patients receiving medication, Harris et al. [114] reported significant positive correlations between psychomotor poverty and both delta and beta power, between disorganization and delta activity, and between reality distortion and alpha-2 power. Discrepancies in the results might be explained by the failure to deal with the issue of heterogeneity of negative symptoms, and/or to separate out the influence of possible confounding variables, such as drug treatment and duration of illness.

Topography of qEEG Abnormalities. The most controversial finding suggested by qEEG topographic studies has been the frontal localization of increased slow activity. According to some investigators, the increase of slow activities is confined to the frontal regions or, at least, is more pronounced in these regions [70, 115–117], while for others it is diffused to the whole scalp [72–74]. Karson et al. [71] demonstrated an important eye movement contribution to the predominance of delta over the anterior regions, showing that, after removal of EOG activity, the delta increase in schizophrenic subjects is widespread.

It has been proposed that frontal localization of increased delta activity may represent the electrophysiological correlate of hypofrontality reported by brain imaging studies examining metabolism or regional cerebral blood flow (rCBF). The few studies that have simultaneously investigated qEEG and PET have reported discrepant findings [117, 118]. Guich et al. [117] reported a negative correlation between positron emission tomography (PET) metabolism measured during continuous performance task (CPT) execution and frontal EEG delta power during the task. They interpreted these findings as evidence that the delta increase over frontal regions represents the electrophysiological correlate of decreased metabolism. However, Alper et al. [118] reported significant positive correlations between frontal PET metabolism and relative delta qEEG power at rest, as well as between subcortical metabolism and relative alpha power. According to these authors, both increased metabolism and delta activity should be regarded as correlates of cognitive activation, while increased subcortical metabolism along with increased alpha power are possible correlates of neuroleptic medication. The interpretation of Alper et al.'s findings is impeded by several methodological pitfalls, including the resting state, the small sample size, the unavailability of simultaneous recording in four out of nine subjects and the inclusion of medicated subjects. Increased delta relative power has also been regarded as a sign of cognitive activation by Guenther et al.

[119]. They found an increase of delta activity in healthy subjects during a motor task, and an extreme increase of delta activity over the frontal and central regions in type I schizophrenia, described by Crow [120] as characterized by positive symptoms, good response to neuroleptic treatment and dopaminergic hyperactivity. This was not found in subjects with type II schizophrenia.

The increase in beta activity in schizophrenia has been reported as more marked over the posterior quadrants of the scalp, either bilaterally [73] or with a left-sided prevalence [115, 121]. Karson *et al.* [72] found an increase of fast beta over all left hemisphere leads.

The LORETA analysis of the multi-channel resting EEG in acute and never-treated first-episode schizophrenics showed distinctive features for the different EEG frequencies. Three patterns of activity were described in these patients: (a) an anterior, bilateral, nearly symmetrical increase of delta activity; (b) an anterior-inferior deficit of theta frequencies along with an anterior-inferior left-sided deficit of alpha-1 and alpha-2 activity; and (c) a posterior-superior right-sided excess of beta-1, beta-2 and beta-3 frequency activity [122]. Deviations from normal brain activity were demonstrated by LORETA in patients along an anterior-left/posterior-right axis. The EEG features were specified not only as excess or deficit, but also as inhibitory, normal and excitatory. The patients showed a regionally discordant brain functional state, i.e. while prefrontal/frontal areas were inhibited, right parietal areas were simultaneously overexcited; left anterior, left temporal and left central areas, on the other hand, did not show the expected normal activity [122]. Interestingly enough, there are hints on dysfunctions involving the left–right hemispheric asymmetry, with overactivity in areas supposed to be active during mental imagery and underactivation of regions containing the specialized sensory and motor language processing areas.

More recently, several studies have investigated the qEEG oscillatory responses, coherence and complexity. The photic driving response (PDR) involves the synchronization of the EEG rhythm with the frequency (or its harmonics) of the photic stimulation. Studies investigating the PDR in drug-free or drug-naïve patients have found deficits in the frequency range of the alpha band (10–12 Hz) [35, 79, 123–125]. One study showed that the PDR was normalized by treatment with neuroleptic drugs in responders to these drugs [126]. A study investigating the PDR in patients with a major depressive episode showed increased synchronization in the alpha range for this diagnostic group with respect to both patients with schizophrenia and healthy controls [125]. The authors interpreted the findings as signs of dysfunctional thalamocortical circuits involved in alpha generation in schizophrenia and abnormal arousal functions in depression.

Elevated gamma oscillations have been reported to coincide with hallucinations in a patient when medicated and unmedicated [127]. Evoked gamma responses, i.e. gamma responses that are time- and phase-locked to the stimulus, were investigated by 20- to 40-Hz auditory stimulation in medicated patients with schizophrenia [34]. Results indicated a deficit of the 40-Hz response and an increased phase delay in patients with respect to healthy controls. A reduction in gamma activity was shown to mediate the sensory gating deficit measured by the P50 paradigm in schizophrenia [128]. On the whole, the 40-Hz abnormality found in patients with schizophrenia might index a basic dysfunction in perceptual processes requiring fast temporal integration, probably due to altered functional connectivity in the cortex. A recent study has investigated induced gamma power, i.e. a gamma response that is time-locked but not phase-locked to the stimulus, during a standard odd-ball auditory task in medicated patients with schizophrenia and matched healthy controls [129]. The gamma response for both target and standard tones, 200–600 milliseconds after stimulus onset, was reduced in patients compared to controls. The target gamma response was negatively correlated with the Positive and Negative Syndrome Scale (PANSS) total score in patients. Gordon *et al.* [130] reported further associations between gamma abnormalities and psychopathological dimensions of schizophrenia. Induced gamma amplitude for target stimuli correlated positively with reality distortion, indicating an automatic overprocessing of task-related information, and negatively with psychomotor poverty, possibly reflecting a shut-down of information processing. Induced gamma amplitude for non-target stimuli correlated negatively with disorganization, suggesting inadequate processing of task-irrelevant information. The interpretation of the findings remains speculative, since the functional role of induced gamma activity is poorly understood and more experimental work is needed to clarify it. The confounding role of drug treatment has not been adequately addressed in all the studies.

Coherence research in schizophrenia has yielded inconclusive results. There have been reports of either an increase of coherence in the delta, theta and beta bands [131–133] or a reduction in the same bands as well as in the alpha band [88, 134–137]. Discrepant findings might be related to differences in methodological approaches and patient medication status.

Research on non-linear dynamics of the EEG in schizophrenia has produced a more coherent picture of altered coordination of brain processes during both rest and cognition. In medicated patients at rest, with respect to controls, dimensional complexity was shown to be higher and to have an opposite distribution, with higher values over frontal than the central electrodes [138]. The findings were interpreted as expressing poor coordination of frontal activities in patients. First-episode drug-naïve patients with schizophrenia had higher values of dimensional complexity in the left temporo-parietal lead, but not in the parietal-occipital leads, than healthy controls, while this abnormality was not present in drug-free remitted schizophrenic patients and in neurotic subjects [86, 139]. More recently, dimensional complexity from both single- and multi-channel data, as well as the global and regional omega complexity, were assessed in a small group of first-episode drug-naïve patients with schizophrenia and healthy controls [140]. The results showed an increase of both the anterior regional omega and dimensional complexity, again favouring the hypothesis of loosened coordination of the active brain processes. The study also provided evidence that the abnormality was specific to the anterior regions of the scalp. Kirsch et al. [141] reported that, with respect to healthy controls, remitted, medicated patients with schizophrenia showed similar values of the dimensional complexity at baseline and while viewing an emotionally challenging movie. These findings are consistent with the hypothesis of Koukkou et al. [86, 139] that a loose coordination of brain processes is a state marker of acute psychosis. However, in the same study, higher values of complexity were found in patients with respect to controls during the execution of the CPT, due to the fact that in healthy controls a reduction of complexity values was observed during the task. The authors discussed these findings in terms of reduced adaptation of the information processing system to cognitive tasks in patients with schizophrenia. To our knowledge, only one study has evaluated the Lyapunov exponent in schizophrenia during wakefulness [50]. The results showed a decrease in the exponent in medicated schizophrenic versus healthy subjects in fronto-temporal areas, indicating reduced flexibility of neural networks in schizophrenia.

Event-Related Potentials

Evoked potential studies have provided extensive evidence of abnormalities at both early and later stages of information processing in schizophrenia [64]. Here the emphasis will be on earlier processing to complement the cognitive literature, which has in general focused on later stages of processing. Brain-stem auditory evoked potentials have revealed in some patients either permanent or transitory anomalies arising at different stages of transmission from the auditory pathways, through the brainstem to thalamic nuclei [142, 143]. Functional abnormalities have coincided with auditory hallucinations, as well as with negative symptoms, disappearing with clinical improvement [143]. Sensory evoked potential abnormalities have reflected both facilitatory (hyper-reactivity) and inhibitory (slower transmission and delayed recovery) processes, and in some instances these may coexist, as exemplified by shorter latencies together with attenuated amplitudes [144, 145]. There have commonly been syndrome differences, such as hypersensitivity and excitability to median nerve stimulation in chronic undifferentiated, chronic paranoid and schizoaffective schizophrenia, in contrast to acute and latent subtypes

[145]. Thought disorder in chronic schizophrenia has been associated with abnormally short auditory P50 latencies, while hallucinations have been associated with abnormally slow visual ERP recovery [146, 147]. In sum, deficits seem to be more consistent with a dysregulation of sensory input than with increased or decreased transmission. These abnormalities may be asymmetrical. Lateral asymmetry in the auditory modality in favour of the normal contralateral amplitude advantage was absent in more than half of schizophrenic patients [148], while in the visual modality the normal left hemisphere advantage was found to be reversed [149]. Disordered interhemispheric interactions have been supported by somatosensory ERPs to unilateral stimulation. There have been several reports of an apparent bilateral symmetry of amplitude instead of the normal larger contralateral response, and an abnormally short ipsilateral latency incompatible with the delay that should occur by virtue of callosal crossing (see [150] for review). While interpreted as evidence of structural abnormalities in the callosum, or in ipsilateral pathways, or both, the reduction of the abnormality with clinical improvement suggests a functional underpinning [151]. Andrews *et al.* [152] found that the abnormality was characteristic of patients with a withdrawn but not activated syndrome.

Anomalies of stimulus intensity control at around 100 milliseconds have been demonstrated in schizophrenia. It has been suggested that such anomalies are underpinned by irregularities of EEG desynchronization involving thalamocortical gating [64, 153]. In schizophrenia, an increase in potential with increasing intensity (augmenting) has been associated with paranoid and acute syndromes, whereas a decrease in potential with increasing intensity (reducing) has been associated with non-paranoid and chronic syndromes. The importance of a dimensional approach along with topography has been suggested by differential associations with activated, withdrawn and reality distortion syndromes [154, 155], whereas categorical approaches, such as comparisons between first-episode schizophrenic, schizophreniform, bipolar depressive and major depressive patients and first-degree relatives and controls, have been unsuccessful [156].

Abnormalities have been demonstrated in the maintenance of attention required in simple procedures of detecting target stimuli in a train of standard stimuli. Attenuation of the N100 has characterized undifferentiated/ disorganized schizophrenia, whereas later P200 and P300 components have been found to be attenuated in paranoid schizophrenia as well [157]. These reductions have also been found in obligate carriers, i.e. those parents who carry the genetic inheritance [158], but not in children at genetic risk [159], while patients with schizotypal personality disorders have shown results intermediate between those of schizophrenic patients and controls [160]. MMN has been found to be reduced in schizophrenia by a number of investigators [161, 162]. Similarly, the P300 component to odd-ball stimuli is commonly reduced in schizophrenia [163, 164]. Egan *et al.* [165] also found that positive correlations between the P300 and the earlier N200 distinguish schizophrenic patients from controls. The reduction of the P300 in schizophrenia was found to be associated with the negative symptoms [166–168] and a worse outcome [169]. However, there is as yet no clear symptom relation (see [64] for review).

Reports of lateral asymmetry in the P300 with left-hemisphere amplitude reductions and right lateralization of the P300 positivity were first provided by Morstyn *et al.* [170]. They were only described by groups using the P300 paradigm with silent counting and the auditory modality. Motor response and the visual stimulation do not appear to evoke asymmetries of the P300 in schizophrenia. A further source of inconsistencies is heterogeneity of the patient groups [171, 172]. The typical P300 asymmetries with left-hemisphere amplitude reductions were shown to be present only in chronic and subchronic schizophrenia [173], and to be associated with volume reductions of the left posterior-superior temporal lobe [164] and with deficits in a neuropsychological test of verbal, but not of visual, figure processing [168]. The latter findings were interpreted as an expression of deficits of left temporal functions in core schizophrenia, possibly related to the typical language-related symptoms such as incoherence and hallucinated speech.

Gruzelier *et al.* [172] found that the syndrome-asymmetry relations observed for P300 were also present at the earlier N100 and P200 components, supporting a generalized thalamo-cortical activation imbalance rather than a circumscribed memory deficit.

Recently, a patient group within the schizophrenia spectrum was identified as having increased P300 amplitudes, which have not been described for any other psychiatric diagnosis. The patients were classified according to the ICD-10 diagnosis of acute polymorphous psychosis, which is to be considered as a compromise among the European concepts of cycloid psychosis, bouffée délirante and acute reactive psychosis. The P300 amplitude increase in this group was accompanied by a symmetrical, i.e. normal, field configuration and is therefore specific for this diagnosis, distinguishing it from core schizophrenia on the one hand and from mania on the other [169]. The finding is in line with single photon emission tomography (SPECT) studies showing increased rCBF in cycloid psychosis and in differently defined groups of acute psychosis with emotional turmoil, and gives clues for a neurophysiological interpretation of these very dramatic clinical pictures with excellent prognosis in terms of generalized over-arousal (see [6] for review).

Evoked potential abnormalities in two-stimulus (S1, S2) paradigms have confirmed sensory gating abnormalities in schizophrenia. These have taken the form of a failure of the normal facilitation of S2 that occurs with intervals up to 100 milliseconds and a failure of suppression over longer intervals, from about 500 milliseconds to 2 seconds, intervals in which inhibitory effects mediated by thalamo-cortical and limbic pathways normally operate. Shagass [144] reported failure of facilitation in chronic schizophrenia as well as in bipolar and unipolar depression. Freedman *et al.* have pioneered research on the loss of suppression at longer intervals [174]. Not all investigators have been able to replicate the loss of P50 suppression in schizophrenia, and no symptom relationships have yet been agreed on. Possible reasons for this are that P50 suppression has been calculated as a ratio between S1 and S2, obscuring differential changes in response to the two stimuli, while averaging over trials obscures habituation and sensitization effects. The latter are important, because the loss of P50 suppression in schizophrenia has been attributed to desensitization of the α_7 nicotinic receptor. In keeping with these surmises, abnormalities in response to S1 have been associated with positive symptoms of schizophrenia [175] and the unreality dimension of schizotypy [176], while abnormal differential habituation to the two stimuli has also been associated with "unreality" [176]. A loss of suppression has been associated only with disorganized and undifferentiated schizophrenia [177, 178]. Consistent with P50 anomalies in psychometrically defined schizotypy, a loss of P50 suppression has been found in about 50% of patient relatives, suggesting a genetic influence [179]. From a study of obligate carriers, Freedman *et al.* have concluded that the gating deficit may predispose to schizophrenia, but additional hippocampal pathology may be necessary for the psychosis to develop [180]. Hippocampal volume may be one such factor, since in a sibling study, while schizophrenic and non-schizophrenic siblings shared the P50 gating deficit, hippocampal volumes were reduced only in the siblings with schizophrenia [181]. Furthermore, Waldo *et al.* [181] reported that while P50 suppression failure coexisted with N100 diminution in schizophrenic patients, in those relatives with the P50 suppression impairment, N100 amplitudes were larger than normal, which was interpreted as a compensatory mechanism. The α_7 receptor, sensitization of which is thought to underpin P50 suppression, is expressed in cortical neurons as part of the response to afferent innervation, engendering functional connection between thalamic and basal forebrain cholinergic afferents. While widely distributed in the brain, it is found in the CA3 region of the hippocampus and in the reticular nucleus of the thalamus. In this regard, Clementz *et al.* [128] have shown that the P50 may be a subcomponent of the fast transient gamma band response emanating from thalamic mechanisms, while Erwin *et al.* [175] found it mirrored in the P100 recovery cycle of similar origin.

Peripheral Measures

Sensory gating has also been examined in schizophrenia with the startle blink to a loud noise and the inhibitory influences of a lead pre-pulse, usually in the form of a weak auditory stimulus, PPI [182]. Applications to individuals with schizophrenia spectrum disorders have shown that PPI is diminished in schizophrenia [182] and in schizotypal patients having both positive and negative symptoms [183]. At the same time, there have been negative reports in schizophrenia [184] and in psychometrically defined schizotypy [185]. Interest in PPI has led to examination of the habituation of the startle response; deficits in the two have been found to be correlated, suggesting a shared central mechanism [186]. In many but not all schizophrenic patients, habituation of startle is retarded [187–189]. The PPI deficit has been associated with thought disorder and is impaired in patients with Wisconsin Card Sorting deficits. In chronic patients, PPI suppression has been associated with distractibility on the CPT and lateralized inattention on the Posner task (see [64] for review). While recent-onset schizophrenic patients who were relatively asymptomatic failed to demonstrate PPI in the conventional passive attention paradigm, they did manifest a deficit in conditions where they attended to the pre-pulse [184]. This was a condition requiring greater involvement of descending forebrain influences and controlled rather than automatic processes.

Eye movement recording has disclosed deviant smooth pursuit eye tracking with intrusive saccadic eye movements [190]. This has been promoted as a genetic marker of schizophrenia, with evidence of deviant tracking in family members [191]. Siever et al. [192] identified the same abnormality in college students with a schizotypal personality diagnosis. Evidence of a functional basis to the deficit follows the demonstration in recent-onset schizophrenia of improvement by attentional manipulations, suggesting an association with diminished voluntary attention [193], in keeping with frontal involvement in smooth pursuit tracking [194].

Electrodermal recording in schizophrenia identified two patient subgroups, one with heightened responsivity and delayed or irregular habituation to the repetition of passive orienting stimuli, while the other failed to respond [195]. Non-responsiveness, the focus of initial enquiry encouraged by deficit models of schizophrenia, has in fact remained enigmatic and is in all probability heterogeneous in causation [196]. Greater clarity has followed investigation on heightened responsiveness, and, contrary to the expectations of many, in a recent review Dawson and Schell [197] concluded that, with few exceptions, it is heightened responsiveness that has proved to be the sign of poor symptomatic prognosis and poor social and occupational outcome. This is in keeping with stress–diathesis models of schizophrenia, given associations between delayed habituation of responses and stress. Similarly, in schizotypy, a review of the literature suggested that responsiveness, particularly irregular responding including sensitization, rather than non-responding, may prove to be the hallmark, and may accompany disorganization [198].

Classifying patients on the basis of lateral asymmetry in electrodermal orienting response amplitude has delineated contrasting activated and withdrawn syndromes in schizophrenia [199]. Activated patients have greater right-hemispheric activation and withdrawn patients greater left-hemispheric activation. A wide range of psychophysiological and neurocognitive evidence has been seen to support this finding [153, 200]. This has led to a syndrome asymmetry model, whereby cardinal aspects of positive and negative symptoms arise from imbalances in lateralized thalamo-cortical arousal systems, and symptom expression is in keeping with theories of approach/withdrawal, thought to involve left and right hemisphere activation respectively [172, 196, 200]. In schizophrenia, eye movement recording of spontaneous lateral deviations from a central fixation showed opposite rightward versus leftward deviations in excited versus socially withdrawn patients, while eye movements during a letter matrix visual search task depicted serial (left hemisphere) versus gestalt (right hemisphere) scan paths respectively [201, 202]. Eye movement recording in socially withdrawn patients during visual retention of complex figures showed evidence of relative neglect of the right side of space in memory performance, which was corroborated by fewer rightward eye movements [203]. Motor neuron excitability, measured with the Hoffman reflex, which has been associated with cognitive asymmetries in schizophrenia, revealed in unmedicated patients an association between withdrawal–retardation and a dominance of right-hemisphere influences, while the opposite asymmetry was associated with agitation [204, 205]. Opposite cognitive asymmetries have been found to distinguish high versus low heart rate variability subgroups of schizophrenic and schizoaffective patients, characterized respectively by excitement and withdrawal [206]. P300 asymmetries recorded from posterior temporal placements in activated and withdrawn patients provided a test of the model [172], while there has been replication of electrodermal findings through opposite asymmetries in withdrawn schizophrenic patients [207] and positive schizotypy [208].

The functional nature of hemispheric imbalance in schizophrenia and schizophrenia spectrum disorders is indicated by evidence of reversals in asymmetry with changes in symptom profile, clinical recovery and neuroleptic treatment (see [153] for review). It is proposed that the asymmetries arise from influences of genes, hormones and early experience, including stressors, on lateralization of thalamo-cortical non-specific arousal systems, which precede language development and underpin approach/withdrawal behaviour, manifested in temperament, personality and clinical syndromes.

Affective Disorders

Quantitative EEG

Increases of alpha [209–211] and/or beta [211–213] activity have frequently been reported in subjects with depressive disorders compared with healthy controls. Increased slow-wave activity, generally observed in subjects with dementia, has been found in elderly depressed patients by some authors, though to a lesser degree [210, 214, 215]. Studies investigating early- and late-onset depressed patients failed to find differences between the two groups, but reported a relationship between increased delta-wave activity and poor performance on several neurocognitive tests in patients with late-onset depression [216, 217].

According to some authors, alpha power is greater over the left than the right frontal regions in currently or previously depressed patients [218, 219] and in subclinically depressed students [209, 220], while the opposite asymmetry pattern (alpha power higher over the right than over the left) has been found for the parietal regions in currently or previously depressed subjects [218, 220]. As alpha power suppression has been interpreted as reflecting cortical activation, the frontal asymmetry pattern might be due to decreased left frontal activation and would be associated with a deficit in approach-related behaviours [221]. The parietal asymmetry pattern might instead be associated with cognitive deficits suggesting right posterior dysfunction in depression [220, 222]. The parietal asymmetry remains a controversial finding, since it has not been found by some authors in either depressed students or subjects with major depression [209, 219]. Bruder *et al.* [223] demonstrated that the presence of anxiety in the clinical picture influences the laterality pattern observed over the posterior regions. Non-anxious depressed patients showed more alpha activity (less activation) over the right than over the left posterior leads, whereas anxious depressed patients showed the opposite pattern.

Mania has been neglected in qEEG studies, probably because of the difficulty of obtaining cooperation from these patients, especially when unmedicated. Shagass *et al.* [224] found that patients with mania have higher EEG frequencies and greater variability than those with depression. Small *et al.* [225] recorded qEEG in 37 patients who were able to cooperate after a drug-free period and again on completion of a period of pharmacotherapy. At baseline, non-responders to pharmacotherapy had more fast theta activity (6–8 Hz) than responders all over the scalp. After treatment, non-responders had more delta and theta over frontal and temporal regions, as well as more beta-1 activity over left temporal leads. In bipolar subjects left-hemisphere abnormalities have been reported, akin to those in schizophrenia [226, 228].

The study of brain electrical microstates has shown a significantly increased topographical variability in depressive patients, i.e. the spatial changes of the fields were more frequent per time unit and had a greater magnitude than in healthy controls. The spatial configuration of the microstates, however, did not differ between patients and controls. On the basis of previous results in healthy volunteers during spontaneous cognition and in other patient groups, the findings were explained by formal alterations of the cognition stream in depression rather than by functional over-recruitment/under-representation of specific brain areas as described in schizophrenic patients. Automatic and schematic processing as well as attention deficits have been described in depressive patients and might account for the finding of less sustained brain electrical microstates [228].

Event-Related Potentials

ERPs are impaired during severe depressive episodes. The most consistent finding is amplitude reductions of the P300 component. The reductions have been found to be less pronounced than in schizophrenia and disappear after the remission of the depressive disorder [229]. They are to be considered, therefore, as a state marker of depression. The clinical benefit of the parameter is probably quite limited, since it is suspected to be an expression of a motivational deficit, and, owing to the presence of P300 amplitude reductions in many psychiatric conditions, no actual contribution for differential diagnosis may be expected.

Surprisingly, P300 studies on manic patients have been published only recently. The first study showed a normal global field strength with slightly reduced amplitudes at central electrode sites combined with a distinctive topographical pattern with relative amplitude reductions in frontal areas. This leads to a shift towards posterior regions of the P300 positivity. By analogy with recent findings of the P300 features in a Go–NoGo paradigm, the result was interpreted as a sign of reduced inhibitory frontal control in mania instead of general cerebral overactivity [230]. This result was confirmed by an independent group with the same interpretation [231]. Further support for this interesting neurophysiological interpretation of manic psychopathology (disinhibition instead of overexcitation) came from a recent PET study showing a reduction of frontal activity in mania [232].

The early P50, considered to be an expression of sensory gating, is altered in acute mania: the normal P50 amplitude reduction after repetition of the stimulus is missing during the acute episode. However, this feature returns to normality after remission of the disorder. The acute finding is not distinguishable from the one described in schizophrenia. The CNV tends to be reduced in depressive patients. This amplitude reduction correlates negatively with the severity of depression [233]. However, a subgroup of depressive patients with increased dopamine reactivity in the apomorphine test had increased instead of reduced CNV amplitudes [234].

ERPs have been widely investigated in relation to depression. As yet, however, there is no diagnostic specificity [235]. A common finding has been longer P300 latency, with further prolongation of latency accompanying cognitive deterioration as also found in Alzheimer's disease [236, 237]. Comparisons of elderly patients with unipolar affective disorder have indicated that late-onset patients showed more evidence of structural changes on MRI than did early-onset cases, whereas impairments in ERPs and cognitive functions were independent of both age at onset and structural changes, and, importantly, persisted after recovery from depression [217].

Topographical considerations are important but little explored and may distinguish bipolar disorder from schizophrenia [238, 239]. Buchsbaum *et al.* [240] examined a bipolar patient through five regular and rapid switches from mania to depression, finding that changes in the P200 amplitude were synchronous with the switches, decreasing at the vertex and increasing occipitally with mania. Altered stimulus dependency relations, revealed with the P100, preceded the switch from depression to mania by 8–10 days.

Peripheral Measures

Abnormal eye tracking has been found in bipolar patients [190, 241, 242]. While Holzman *et al.* [190] considered that in bipolar patients this might be an artefact of lithium treatment, in a careful study of patients on and off medication Gooding *et al.* [242] have ruled out this possibility. Levy *et al.* [243] in a study of first-degree relatives, found that, whereas in schizophrenia smooth pursuit abnormalities were in evidence in family members, they were no more prevalent in the relatives of patients with unipolar and bipolar affective disorders than in normal individuals without a family history of major psychoses.

Affective disorders have been examined for dysregulated electrodermal activity. Whereas one hypothesis has been that mania and depression may be characterized by opposite extremes of activity, this does not appear to be the case. On the whole, low responsiveness has been representative of both unipolar and bipolar affective disorders. Electrodermal non-responding has been reported in as high a proportion of acutely ill manic as in schizophrenic patients [244], and in endogenous depression [245]. Electrodermal activity was found to be uniformly lower in both passive, non-signal conditions and task conditions in remitted unipolar and bipolar patients compared with controls [246]. Furthermore, in a comparison of depressive subtypes, unipolar and bipolar patients could not be distinguished, nor could responders to the dexamethasone suppression test, though a symptom profile of psychomotor retardation was found to be associated with lower tonic activity in both unipolar and bipolar patients [247]. Bilateral recording has been informative. In order to determine whether non-responsiveness was a trait marker for depression, electrodermal activity was recorded in children of bipolar parents in response to non-signal orienting tones and during reaction time and mental arithmetic tasks [248]. Only during tasks were the children at genetic risk distinguished from controls, when in fact they displayed evidence of hyper-responsiveness, particularly in left-hand responses, and this coincided with higher self-rated depression. Larger left- than right-hand responses to non-signal stimuli had earlier been reported in endogenous depression [249, 250]. This was subsequently reported in college students described as subsyndromal and at risk for bipolar disorder [251], in whom there was also a bias towards leftward conjugate eye movements in response to cognitive problems. Together the laterality measures provided evidence of right-hemispheric hyperexcitability. However, in contradiction to these studies, Iacono and Tuason [246] were unable to detect consistent lateral asymmetries in electrodermal activity in unipolar and bipolar patients.

Anxiety Disorders

Quantitative EEG

Early qEEG studies carried out in patients with obsessive-compulsive disorder (OCD) have reported either no difference or a reduced absolute power for all investigated frequency bands, with respect to healthy controls [212, 252]. However, these studies were carried out in patients on medication and in whom depressive comorbidity was not controlled for. In a study of non-depressed, drug-free OCD patients, compared with healthy controls, a reduction of delta, beta-1 and beta-2 absolute and relative power was reported, as well as an increase of alpha relative power [253]. The same study found higher hemispheric asymmetry indices $(L - R/L + R)$ for all frequency bands in OCD patients. The higher asymmetry index for beta-2 power was associated with worse performance on a visuospatial task and better execution of the logical memory scale, indicating greater left than right hemisphere activation in OCD patients. Discrepant results were reported [254]. Non-depressed, drug-free OCD patients showed an increase of power in delta, theta and beta bands over anterior regions compared to healthy controls. Four of these patients who were investigated after six weeks of treatment with fluoxetine or clomipramine showed a reduction of delta and theta power from baseline. The same patients showed a reduction after treatment of frontal and caudate blood flow as assessed by SPECT. The authors interpreted the increase of slow activity at baseline as a correlate of frontal hyperactivity shown by the SPECT evaluation.

Apart from several methodological factors, such as differences in the calculation of power measures and the definition of frequency bands, discrepancies in the results of the qEEG studies in OCD patients might be due to a biological heterogeneity of the disorder, as suggested by some authors [255]. In fact, OCD patients with an excess of frontal theta before treatment were shown to be non-responders to serotonin reuptake inhibitors, while patients with an excess of alpha power were responders. No replication of these data has been published to date and, therefore, they should be considered as preliminary.

Relations between qEEG abnormalities and OCD symptoms have mostly been neglected. A recent study reported a reduction of slow alpha band absolute and relative power in drug-free non-depressed OCD subjects, as compared with healthy controls, which correlated with slowness on executive tests [256]. Since slow alpha desynchronization is related to increased attentional allocation, and neuropsychological slowness on executive tasks might suggest a hyperactivity of the supervisory attentional system, the results of this study are in line with brain imaging evidence of increased activation of circuits involved in attention and executive control in OCD patients. The only study investigating qEEG changes induced by symptom provocation in OCD patients [257] found a decrease of alpha power with respect to baseline over anterior regions during live exposure to feared contaminants. The authors considered their findings in line with functional brain imaging evidence of increased activation of anterior regions during symptom provocation in OCD patients [258–260].

Patients with panic disorder (PD) have shown increased absolute delta, theta and alpha power and reduced beta relative power when compared with healthy controls [261]. In the same study, subjective ratings of anxiety during the EEG recording correlated positively with relative beta power, while anticipatory anxiety correlated inversely with both delta and theta absolute power. Reduced alpha power in the right frontal region, with a frontal brain asymmetry favouring right hemisphere activation, was found at rest and during the presentation of both negative and positive emotional stimuli in drug-free patients with PD [262]. The same asymmetry was absent during the presentation of neutral stimuli. The frontal asymmetry index correlated with state anxiety scores. The findings were interpreted as a sign of increased activation of the avoidance–withdrawal right hemisphere system in PD. An activation of right prefrontal brain regions has also been found in subjects with social phobia when anticipating a public speech [263].

Event-Related Potentials

ERP studies in patients with OCD have consistently found reduced latencies of N200 and P300 with respect to healthy controls, for both auditory and visual stimuli [264–266]. Findings concerning the amplitude of the same ERP components in patients compared with healthy controls were inconsistent [264, 265, 267, 268].

Studies that have examined the difference wave between ERP waveforms elicited by salient and unattended stimuli reported an increase of the so-called processing negativities (such as the mismatch negativity) for both early and late phases in OCD patients versus healthy controls [268]. The reduced latencies of the late ERP components, the lack of latency increase of the same components for difficult versus easy tasks and the increased amplitude of the processing negativities led to the conclusion that OCD patients might present an overfocused attention to salient stimuli [268]. A recent study reported that the "error-related negativity" (a negative ERP component occurring at the moment of an error during cognitive tasks, reflecting monitoring of actions and involving the activity of the cingulate cortex) is increased in patients with OCD versus healthy controls [269]. The amplitude of the component correlated with symptom severity. This study also analysed, by dipole modelling, the source of the activity enhancement in OCD patients, reporting a medial frontal locus possibly involving the anterior cingulate cortex.

Abnormalities of early processing have been implicated in PD through ERP recording. Iwanami *et al.* [270] recorded the P300 in a conventional two-tone odd-ball task. While there was no difference in the P300 in the comparison with controls, patients with PD showed elevated N100 components to both standard and target stimuli and elevated N200 amplitudes to target stimuli. Neither panic nor anticipatory anxiety seem to affect P300. Grillon and Ameli [271] found that in normal subjects the anticipation of electric shocks had no effect on P300. Slow cortical potential recording in PD patients has shown that body-related words produced enhanced positive potentials, a reduction of which over more than a year correlated with symptom improvement on an anxiety scale [272].

ERP brain electrical microstates have recently been investigated in patients with PD [273]. Results showed deviations of microstate topography in PD patients versus healthy subjects, during both early and late processing phases. In particular, the first microstate topographic descriptor showed a rightward shift, while that of the fourth microstate, corresponding to the ERP late positive complex (LPC), presented a leftward shift. The findings indicated overactivation of the right-hemisphere circuits involved in early visual processing, and hypoactivation of the right-hemisphere networks involved in the generation of the LPC. The topographic abnormalities of the LPC microstate were associated with worse performance on a test exploring temporo-hippocampal functioning and with a higher number of panic attacks, suggesting a pathogenetic role of the temporo-hippocampal dysfunction in PD.

Preattentive processing in the form of auditory memory has been implicated in post-traumatic stress disorder (PTSD) [274]. An augmented MMN wave was found in PTSD, compared with controls, and was associated with sexual assault. Importantly, the amplitude of MMN correlated positively with a PTSD symptom scale. Similarly, symptom subgroups have been revealed that correlate with auditory ERP patterns of augmenting and reducing in children with and without PTSD who have suffered physical and/or sexual abuse [275]. Those with PTSD were characterized by an augmenting pattern in the P200-N200 component, while the same pattern was also associated with a high number of re-experiencing trauma-related symptoms, whether or not there was PTSD. Independent of PTSD, arousal symptoms, including startle and hypervigilance, were associated with a reducing pattern.

Peripheral Measures

Measurement of electrodermal activity has revealed some parallels with findings in affective disorders, particularly with regard to nosological categories and lateral asymmetry. On the whole, there has been little success in using electrodermal activity or other autonomic indices for the purposes of differential diagnosis amongst anxiety disorders, but there have been symptom relations, especially when hemispheric influences were taken into account. In general, anxiety has been associated with an over-reactive pattern in normal subjects [276], and some clear differences have been shown when patients are compared with controls, such as elevated electrodermal levels and a high incidence of non-specific responses in anxiety neurotics and patients with agitated depression [277].

Distinguishing amongst patient diagnoses has been more challenging. With a stepwise regression analysis, Rabavilas [278] failed in an attempt to use electrodermal orienting and habituation to distinguish patients with generalized anxiety, phobia, obsessive-compulsive, dysthymic and conversion disorders. Argyle [279] compared PD patients with and without major depression with regard to differences in tonic skin conductance levels. There was some evidence of lower tonic levels in panic associated with depression, and the wide variance in those without depression was suggestive of a different aetiology of panic associated with depression compared with primary depression. Kopp et al. [280] compared PD patients with and without agoraphobia with regard to relations between electrodermal lability and the suppression of cortisol with dexamethasone. Higher electrodermal lability and slower habituation was associated with higher basal cortisol, whereas those who were rapid habituators showed lower basal cortisol and cortisol suppression. These two patterns of results, which were suggestive of different patterns of hypothalamic–pituitary–adrenal dysregulation, could not be discriminated on the basis of psychiatric classification.

Consideration of lateral asymmetry may prove useful, as it has been in schizophrenia and affective disorders in delineating syndrome relations. In students, while high anxiety was associated with slow habituation of electrodermal responses, lateral asymmetry was related to degree of anxiety and gave clues to differences in the quality of anxiety [281]. Students with greater left-hemispheric excitability were characterized by cognitive aspects of anxiety such as apprehension–worrying, frustration–tension and suspicion, whereas those with greater right-hemispheric excitability were characterized more by non-specific features such as emotional instability and lack of self-control. Kopp and Gruzelier [282] and Kopp [283] subdivided DSM-III anxiety disorders (generalized anxiety, panic and panic with agoraphobia) according to electrodermal lability. Both lability and lateral asymmetries in specific electrodermal responses distinguished generalized anxiety patients from panic patients: higher on the left hand of the panic patients, who were the most labile, and higher on the right hand of the generalized anxiety patients, who were at an intermediate level of lability between controls and panic patients. In sum, the results were in keeping with hemispheric specialization; generalized, non-verbal, non-specific anxiety associated with the right hemisphere, and specific, apprehensive, verbalizable anxiety associated with the left hemisphere.

Germane to this, Papousek and Schulter [284] found that relations between extremes of normal affect and electrodermal reactivity were clarified by taking into account the topography of hemispheric influences measured with the EEG and quality of affect in terms of anxiety and depression. A positive relation between anxiety and higher electrodermal responsiveness was associated with greater right-hemispheric activation in orbitofrontal cortex, whereas depression was positively associated with higher electrodermal responsiveness when there was greater left than right hemispheric activation in dorsolateral prefrontal cortex.

Psychophysiological recording with measures including electrodermal responsiveness, heart rate, blood pressure, skin temperature and EMG responses, eye blink and eye fixation has provided insights into the nature of dysfunctional processing. Phobic patients have on the whole been characterized by exaggerated responses to phobic stimuli. Roth et al. [285] reported higher tonic levels of skin conductance and heart rate among panic patients with agoraphobia than in healthy controls. Segerstrom et al. [286] demonstrated that worriers showed larger electrodermal and heart rate responses to phobic than to neutral stimuli, and this was coupled with an attenuation of the normal circadian increase in natural killer cell activity. Hamm et al. [287] found that animal and mutilation phobics showed abnormal eye blink facilitation that was specific to slides depicting their feared objects, as has been demonstrated in patients with simple and social phobias, PD and PTSD when imagining or viewing threatening pictures [288]. Exaggerated autonomic responses in patients with PTSD have been found on a par with responses in panic patients [289]. At the same time there is general agreement that responses in PTSD are greater to trauma-related stimuli than to neutral stimuli [290, 291], to startling stimuli compared with neutral stimuli [292–295] and to reminders of other stressors [296]; moreover, individuals with PTSD seem to be more autonomically conditionable [297]. Prospective studies of trauma victims have shown that slower electrodermal habituation and increased heart rate and EMG responses to startle stimuli develop along with PTSD in the months following a trauma. Theoretically, this links PTSD with progressive neuronal sensitization. Process considerations have also revealed psychophysiologically validated subgroups. Women who scored high on a peritraumatic dissociation index showed suppression of electrodermal and heart rate responses compared with low-scoring women. Dissociation between cognitive and emotional factors was also suggested by a discrepancy between self-reports of distress and objective laboratory stress indicators [298].

Ohman and Soares [299] using backward masking have demonstrated larger skin conductance responses to masked phobic stimuli compared with neutral stimuli. This provided evidence that unconscious preattentive perceptual analysis occurred in snake and spider phobics. One possibility was that nonconscious fear alerts cognitive systems that initiate scanning of the environment, kindling the expectancy that untoward events will occur. Accordingly, phobic behaviour may represent a response to unrecognized external and internal cues which produce oversensitization to potentially threatening stimuli.

Psychological interventions such as relaxation training have been effective in reducing electrodermal and heart rate reactivity in snake phobics subjected to controlled in vivo exposure. This was observed in a lowering of tonic arousal throughout the course of exposure, rather than in an attenuation of specific phasic responses [300]. Biofeedback procedures have also been successful. Canter et al. [301] compared biofeedback with progressive muscle relaxation in patients with anxiety neurosis with and without panic. Biofeedback produced a greater reduction in muscle tension and relief from anxiety in the majority of patients. Weinman et al. [302] found beneficial effects for biofeedback combined with relaxation training in anxiety patients with recent stressful life events, when compared with patients without recent life events. Levels of anxiety, depression and muscle tension were reduced effectively. Most impressively, gains were demonstrated through biofeedback in chronic anxiety disorders refractory to treatment. Following 2–12 weeks of training, sleep improved in 87% of cases, anxiety was reduced in 40% and there was a reduction in frequency and intensity of headaches among headache sufferers [303].

Dementia

Quantitative EEG

An increase of slow delta and theta activity and a reduction of alpha activity are the most frequently reported qEEG abnormalities in patients with AD, during both early and late stages of the illness [304–309]. However, some observations suggest that the early stages are characterized by a reduction in beta power and an increase in theta power [305, 306, 310, 311], while the later ones are characterized by a progressive decrease in alpha and an increase in delta [312–315]. Alpha and beta equivalent dipoles (representing the centre of gravity of the electrical activity) have been shown to shift towards anterior regions in mild AD stages, and the amount of the anterior shift correlated with the degree of cognitive impairment [316]. A correlation has been repeatedly reported between the slowing of the mean frequency and the severity of the cognitive deficit as assessed by the Mini-Mental State Examination [210, 317]. Follow-up investigations have documented an absence of qEEG abnormalities during the early stages in subjects who at initial evaluation had a Global Deterioration Scale (GDS) of 2 or 3 (corresponding to a mild impairment) and did not show any cognitive deterioration two to three years later. These findings suggest that the qEEG might be useful in the identification of patients with non-progressive cognitive decline [306, 313, 318, 319]. In line with these observations, a recent study showed that subjects with mild cognitive impairment (MCI) who progressed to probable AD, after a mean follow-up of 21 months, had more theta, less alpha and a lower mean alpha frequency, compared with non-progressive MCI subjects [320]. The baseline qEEG alone correctly classified 82% of the subjects in non-progressive and progressive MCI subgroups. Results from this study also showed an increase of theta and a reduction of both beta amplitude and beta mean frequency at follow-up only in progressive MCI subjects. In a slightly larger group of MCI subjects, it has been shown that progressive MCI subjects had less alpha relative and absolute power, less fast beta absolute power and more theta relative power than non-progressive MCI subjects, together with a more anterior location of the alpha, theta and fast beta equivalent dipoles [321]. Baseline relative theta and alpha power correctly classified 87% of the cases in both the progressive and the non-progressive group.

Some authors have hypothesized that qEEG changes observed in AD patients are the expression of the cholinergic deficit found in these subjects [319, 322]. This hypothesis is in line with the observations that the administration of anticholinergic drugs to healthy subjects induces an increase in delta and very fast beta and a reduction in alpha activity [322, 323]. Animal studies have also shown that an increase of delta is observed after deafferentation of the cortex by lesions of the cholinergic pathways or by lesions of the hemispheric white matter [17, 324]. Nootropic and cholinergic drugs commonly used in the treatment of dementia, after both acute and short-term administration, have induced qEEG changes with respect to the pre-drug condition, including a reduction of slow and an increase of alpha activity [322, 325–329]. No study, however, has examined the long-term effects of the treatment with the same drugs on qEEG characteristics.

Findings similar to those reported in AD patients were observed in patients with vascular dementia [309, 330–332]; however, some authors reported that in the latter the reduction of alpha and the increase of slow activity is less pronounced than in patients with AD [333].

A reduction of the coherence in alpha and beta bands was repeatedly shown in patients with AD versus healthy controls [42, 334–337]. A reduction of the long-range coherence in the 14- to 18-Hz band was more often observed in AD patients, while a reduction of the local coherence in posterior areas (visual coherence) was reported in vascular dementia [42, 335, 338–340]. A reduction of the dimensional complexity has also been observed in AD patients and seems to be related to the severity of the cognitive decline [341].

The space-oriented segmentation of the resting EEG into brain electrical microstates in mild and moderate dementia of the Alzheimer type yielded a significant anteriorization of the centres of gravity of the microstate fields, an increase of the microstates' spatial variability and a reduced duration of sustained microstates. These differences were statistically more robust than the typical changes in the frequency domain (diffuse slowing) and were significantly correlated with the cognitive decline. It was concluded that the adaptive spatial segmentation into microstates is a method to extract meaningful EEG parameters for the early diagnosis and staging of AD [342]. The results, including the correlation with clinical severity, were confirmed in an independent sample of Swedish patients [343]. Further confirmation comes from a study involving the fast Fourier transform approximation method, which allows the calculation of intracerebral model sources of individual frequency bands. A more anterior location of the alpha-1 sources was found, supporting the previous results obtained with other methods; in addition, a more superficial location of all frequency band sources was observed [344]. This latter result can be explained either by a more superficial brain electrical generator or, more plausibly, by less widespread cortical activation due to reduced activity in occipital and temporo-parietal regions.

Interesting results were reported regarding the correlation between the location of the intracerebral electrical EEG sources and cerebral glucose metabolism (GluM) evaluated by PET. It has been shown that healthy subjects have similar metabolic and neuroelectric spatial patterns. In healthy controls and patients with different degrees of cognitive decay, the localization of intracerebral EEG generators correlated with the spatial distribution of GluM. These results convincingly demonstrate that the EEG sources provide spatial information about brain function that is consistent with degree of glucose consumption [59].

Event-Related Potentials

In dementia with primary degeneration of the association areas, there are no impairments of the early components of the evoked potentials unless there is a concomitant pathological process impairing subcortical signal conduction or important degeneration of the primary sensory cortex areas. Late ERPs, on the other hand, are often impaired from the early stages of the disease. As a typical finding, P300 amplitudes are reduced and latencies are increased. Amplitude reductions are not specific and cannot be reliably used for diagnosis or staging. Although a P300 latency increase is also found in schizophrenia and other psychoses, in these clinical conditions it is inconsistent and possibly an effect of medication [230]. In dementia, the finding is consistent and considered to be characteristic of the cognitive decline.

In a meta-analysis of latency increases, the sensitivity varied between 13% and 80%, and the specificity even reached 90% compared to other general psychiatric patients [345]. The sensitivity was best in studies on severely demented patients, though in these groups, obviously, the diagnostic contribution of ERPs will be minimal. A field of particular interest, however, is the differential diagnosis of early AD from depressive pseudo-dementia. Here the latency increase is a very promising marker, since it is not a typical finding in depression. However, validation of the parameter as a supplementary tool for differential diagnosis between these clinical conditions has not yet been performed. According to present knowledge, in the later stages of dementia ERPs are not expected to be clinically useful because of their limited contribution to diagnosis and, most importantly, because patients' attentional deficits mean that they are unable to perform the task that would evoke the potential.

CONCLUSIONS

When the psychiatrist Hans Berger discovered the EEG, he was hopeful of depicting physiological and pathological mental processes. In his diary he wrote more than 70 years ago: "May I succeed in finding a sort of mirror of brain function—the *elektrenkephalogram*". During the intervening period, the techniques for recording and, especially, analysing brain electrical activity have undergone constant progress, such that clinicians and researchers can now assess brain function with unique time resolution and the possibility of topographic and even tomographic imaging of the brain electrical fields and sources.

Compared to other imaging methods, the analysis of brain electrical activity still suffers from relatively poor spatial resolution. Combining it with other methods in the field of nuclear medicine and neuroradiology that have high spatial resolution, such as PET and fMRI, makes it possible to look at normal and pathological brain function with both high spatial and high temporal resolution. However, it should be borne in mind that the recording of brain electrical activity not only measures the quantity of neuronal activity, but can also assess neuronal synchronization within brain areas and, with the appropriate tools, between neuronal assemblies. This ability is unique to analysis of brain electrical activity and not available with other imaging techniques. Since normal functioning of the brain is certainly dependent on synchronous activity between functional areas, the analysis of the brain electrical activity has an exceptional standing and future outlook among imaging techniques. For a long time this ability of the EEG was not focused on; the reasons could in part be restrictions in methods of analysis (for instance, the standard method of assessing synchronicity between areas was coherence between surface channels, which is inappropriate) and limitations in the number of recording electrodes. Since the symptoms of mental diseases depend not just on "more" or "less" activity in circumscribed brain regions, but rather on disruption of physiological networks, the removal of these limitations in the analysis of brain electrical activity opens up new frontiers for the understanding of pathological brain function in mental diseases.

For psychiatrists, recent developments have shown solid areas of possible clinical utility, but have also opened new exciting perspectives for improved understanding of the neurophysiological mechanisms underlying psychosis [6]. We hope that this development will contribute to approaching another dream of Hans Berger: to formulate something he liked to call a "physiological psychology", although he was aware of being far from being able to describe human psychology in terms of neurophysiological mechanisms and events. Today, as 80 years ago, this appears a necessary step to escape from the centenary impasse of the psychiatry of psychoses, which has been criticized in many statements from researchers and clinicians. Psychiatric symptoms are defined as disorders of behaviour and subjective experience, but they still are weighted and bundled (in terms of syndromes) mainly on the basis of their social implications, together with their course and sensitivity to specific treatments, rather than on underlying dysfunctions of highest-order brain functions. Classification systems, like that of Carl Wernicke, tried to rely on such hypothetical dysfunctions, but became unpopular due to their theoretical superstructure, which could not be proven, thus giving rise to unresolvable controversies. With the new insights into brain functions offered by the combination of powerful functional neuroimaging methods, this old idea has gained a new and more realistic optimism.

REFERENCES

1. Dierks T., Linden D.E., Jandl M., Formisano E., Goebel R., Lanfermann H., Singer W. (1999) Activation of Heschl's gyrus during auditory hallucinations. *Neuron*, **22**: 615–621.

2. Strik W.K., Fallgatter A.J., Brandeis D., Pascual-Marqui R.D. (1998) Three-dimensional tomography of event-related potentials during response inhibition: evidence for phasic frontal lobe activation. *Electroencephalogr. Clin. Neurophysiol.*, **108**: 406–413.

3. Federspiel A., Müller T.J., Fallgatter A.J., Strik W.K. (1999) The response of the human brain to a continuous performance test as measured with fMRI. *Neuroimage*, **9**: 744.

4. Gruzelier J.H. (1996) New advances in EEG and cognition. *Int. J. Psychophysiol.*, **24**: 1–5.

5. Hermann C.S. (2000) Gamma activity in the human EEG. *Int. J. Psychophysiol.*, **38**: vii–viii.

6. Strik W.K. (2000) Anxiety as a primary symptom in cycloid psychosis. *CNS Spectrums*, **5**: 47–51.

7. Strik W.K. (1999) Psychiatrische neurophysiologie. In *Psychiatrie der Gegenwart*, 4th ed. (Eds H. Helmchen, F.A. Henn, H. Lauter, N. Sartorius), pp. 251–272, Springer, Berlin.

8. Cooper R., Winter A.L., Crow H.J., Walter W. (1965) Comparison of subcortical, cortical and scalp activity using chronically indwelling electrodes in man. *Electroencephalogr. Clin. Neurophysiol.*, **18**: 217–228.

9. Speckmann E.J., Elger C.E. (1987) Introduction to the neurophysiological basis of EEG and DC potentials. In *Electroencephalography. Basic Principles, Clinical Applications and Related Fields* (Eds E. Niedermeyer, F. Lopes Da Silva), pp. 1–14, Urban & Schwarzenberg, Munich.

10. Lopes Da Silva F. (1991) Neural mechanisms underlying brain waves: from neural membranes to networks. *Electroencephalogr. Clin. Neurophysiol.*, **79**: 81–93.

11. Nunez P.L. (1995) *Neocortical Dynamics and EEG Rhythms*, Oxford University Press, New York.

12. Gevins A. (1998) The future of electroencephalography in assessing neurocognitive functioning. *Electroencephalogr. Clin. Neurophysiol.*, **106**: 165–172.

13. Jasper H.H. (1958) The ten–twenty electrode system of the International Federation. *Electroencephalogr. Clin. Neurophysiol.*, **10**: 370–375.

14. Nuwer M.R., Lehmann D., Lopes Da Silva F., Matsuoka S., Sutherling W., Vibert J.F. (1994) IFCN guidelines for topographic and frequency analysis of EEGs and EPs. Report of an IFCN committee. *Electroencephalogr. Clin. Neurophysiol.*, **91**: 1–5.

15. Van Cott A., Brenner R.P. (1998) Technical advantages of digital EEG. *J. Clin. Neurophysiol.*, **15**: 464–475.

16. Niedermeyer E. (1987) The normal EEG of the waking adult. In *Electroencephalography. Basic Principles, Clinical Applications and Related Fields* (Eds E. Niedermeyer, F. Lopes Da Silva), pp. 97–117, Urban & Schwarzenberg, Munich.

17. Schaul N. (1990) Pathogenesis and significance of abnormal nonepileptiform rhythms in the EEG. *J. Clin. Neurophysiol.*, **7**: 229–248.

18. Singer W., Gray C.M. (1995) Visual feature integration and the temporal correlation hypothesis. *Annu. Rev. Neurosci.*, **18**: 555–586.

19. Nunez P.L., Silberstein R.B., Shi Z., Carpenter M.R., Srinivasan R., Tucker D.M., Doran S.M., Cadush P.J., Wijesinghe R.S. (1999) EEG coherency, II: experimental comparison of multiple measures. *Clin. Neurophysiol.*, **110**: 469–486.

20. Sannita W.G. (2000) Stimulus-specific oscillatory responses of the brain: a time/frequency-related coding process. *Clin. Neurophysiol.*, **111**: 565–583.

21. Frost J.D. (1987) Mimetic techniques. In *Methods of Analysis of Brain Electrical and Magnetic Signals. Handbook of Electroencephalography and Clinical Neurophysiology*, revised series, Vol. 1 (Eds A.S. Gevins, A. Remond), pp. 195–209, Elsevier, Amsterdam.

22. Klimesch W., Schimke H., Schwaiger J. (1994) Episodic and semantic memory: an analysis in the EEG-theta and alpha band. *Electroencephalogr. Clin. Neurophysiol.*, **91**: 428–441.

23. Klimesch W., Doppelmayr M., Schimke H., Ripper B. (1997) Theta synchronization and alpha desynchronization in a memory task. *Psychophysiology*, **34**: 169–176.

24. Klimesch W. (1999) EEG alpha and theta oscillations reflect cognitive and memory performance: a review and analysis. *Brain Res. Rev.*, **29**: 169–195.

25. Karacas S., Erzengin O.U., Basar E. (2000) A new strategy involving multiple cognitive paradigms demonstrates that ERP components are determined by the superposition of oscillatory responses. *Clin. Neurophysiol.*, **111**: 1719–1732.

26. Weiss S., Rappelsberger P. (2000) Long-range EEG synchronization during word encoding correlates with successful memory performance. *Brain Res. Cogn. Brain Res.*, **9**: 299–312.

27. Freeman W.J., Skarda C.A. (1985) Spatial EEG patterns, non-linear dynamics and perception: the neo-sherringtonian view. *Brain Res. Rev.*, **10**: 147–175.

28. Gray C.M., Singer W. (1989) Stimulus-specific neuronal oscillations in orientation columns of cat visual cortex. *Proc. Natl. Acad. Sci. USA*, **86**: 1698–1702.

29. Gray C.M., Engel K., König P., Singer W. (1990) Stimulus-dependent neuronal oscillations in cat visual cortex: receptive field properties and feature dependence. *Eur. J. Neurosci.*, **2**: 607–619.

30. Engel A.K., König P., Kreiter A., Schillen T.B., Singer W. (1992) Temporal coding in the visual cortex: new vistas on integration in the nervous system. *Trends Neurosci.*, **15**: 218–226.

31. Dinse H.R., Kruger K., Akhavan A.C., Spengler F., Schoner G., Schreiner C.E. (1997) Low-frequency oscillations of visual, auditory and somatosensory cortical neurons evoked by sensory stimulation. *Int. J. Psychophysiol.*, **26**: 205–227.

32. Sewards T.V., Sewards M.A. (1999) Alpha-band oscillations in visual cortex: part of the neural correlate of visual awareness? *Int. J. Psychophysiol.*, **32**: 35–45.

33. Pfurtscheller G. (1977) Graphical display and statistical evaluation of event-related desynchronization (ERD). *Electroencephalogr. Clin. Neurophysiol.*, **43**: 757–760.

34. Kwon J.S., O'Donnel B.F., Wallenstein G.V., Greene R.W., Hirayasu Y., Nestor P.G., Hasselmo M.E., Potts G.F., Shenton M.E., McCarley R.W. (1999) Gamma frequency-range abnormalities to auditory stimulation in schizophrenia. *Arch. Gen. Psychiatry*, **56**: 1001–1005.

35. Jin Y., Castellanos A., Solis E.R., Potkin S.G. (2000) EEG resonant responses in schizophrenia: a photic driving study with improved harmonic resolution. *Schizophr. Res.*, **44**: 213–220.

36. Fernández T., Harmony T., Rodríguez M., Reyes A., Marosi E., Bernal J. (1993) Test-retest reliability of EEG spectral parameters during cognitive tasks. I. Absolute and relative power. *Int. J. Neurosci.*, **68**: 255–261.

37. Fernández T., Harmony T., Rodríguez M., Bernal J., Silva J., Reyes A., Marosi E. (1995) EEG activation patterns during the performance of tasks involving different components of mental calculation. *Electroencephalogr. Clin. Neurophysiol.*, **94**: 175–182.
38. Klimesch W., Schimke H., Ladurner G., Pfurtscheller G. (1990) Alpha frequency and memory performance. *J. Psychophysiol.*, **4**: 381–390.
39. Klimesch W., Schimke H., Schwaiger J., Doppelmayer M., Ripper B., Pfurtscheller G. (1996) Event-related desynchronization (ERD) and the Dm-effect: does alpha desynchronization during encoding predict later recall performance? *Int. J. Psychophysiol.*, **24**: 47–60.
40. Stam C.J. (2000) Brain dynamics in theta and alpha frequency bands and working memory performance in humans. *Neurosci. Lett.*, **286**: 115–118.
41. von Stein A., Sarnthein J. (2000) Different frequencies for different scales of cortical integration: from local gamma to long range alpha/theta synchronization. *Int. J. Psychophysiol.*, **38**: 301–313.
42. Leuchter A.F., Newton T.F., Cook I.A., Walter D.O., Rosenberg-Thompson S., Lachenbruch P.A. (1992) Changes in brain functional connectivity in Alzheimer-type and multi-infarct dementia. *Brain*, **115**: 1543–1561.
43. Nunez P.L., Srinivasan R., Westdorp A.F., Wijesinghe R.S., Tucker D.M., Silberstein R.B., Cadusch P.J. (1997) EEG coherency. I: Statistics, reference electrode, volume conduction, Laplacians, cortical imaging, and interpretation at multiple scales. *Electroencephalogr. Clin. Neurophysiol.*, **103**: 499–515.
44. Friston K.J. (1996) Statistical parametric mapping and other analyses of functional imaging data. In *Brain Mapping: the Methods* (Eds A.W. Toga, J.C. Mazziotta), pp. 363–386, Academic Press, San Diego.
45. Schanze T., Eckhorn R. (1997) Phase correlation of cortical rhythms at different frequencies: higher order spectral analysis of microelectrode recordings from cat and monkey visual cortex. *Int. J. Psychophysiol.*, **26**: 171–189.
46. Grassberger P., Procaccia I. (1983) Measuring the strangeness of strange attractors. *Physica*, **9**: 189–208.
47. Pritchard W.S., Duke D.W. (1992) Dimensional analysis of no-task human EEG using the Grassberger–Procaccia method. *Psychophysiology*, **29**: 182–192.
48. Wackermann J., Lehmann D., Dvorak I., Michel C.M. (1993) Global dimensional complexity of multi-channel EEG indicates change of human brain functional state after a single dose of a nootropic drug. *Electroencephalogr. Clin. Neurophysiol.*, **86**: 193–198.
49. Wackermann J. (1996) Beyond mapping: estimating complexity of multichannel EEG recordings. *Acta. Neurobiol. Exp.*, **56**: 197–208.
50. Kim D.-J., Jeong J., Chae J.-H., Park S., Kim S.Y., Go H.J., Paik I.-H., Kim K.-S., Choi B. (2000) An estimation of the first positive Lyapunov exponent of the EEG in patients with schizophrenia. *Psychiatry Res.*, **98**: 177–189.
51. Lehmann D. (1987) Principles of spatial analysis. In *Methods of Analysis of Brain Electrical and Magnetic Signals. Handbook of Electroencephalography and Clinical Neurophysiology*, Vol. 1 (Eds A.S. Gevins, A. Remond), pp. 309–354, Elsevier, Amsterdam.
52. Nunez P.L., Pilgreen K.L. (1991) The spline-Laplacian in clinical neurophysiology: a method to improve EEG spatial resolution. *J. Clin. Neurophysiol.*, **8**: 397–413.
53. Lehmann D. (1984) EEG assessment of brain activity: spatial aspects, segmentation and imaging. *Int. J. Psychophysiol.*, **1**: 267–276.

54. Lehmann D., Ozaki H., Pal I. (1987) EEG alpha map series: brain microstates by space-oriented adaptive segmentation. *Electroencephalogr. Clin. Neurophysiol.*, **67**: 271–288.
55. Newell A. (1992) Precis of unified theories of cognition. *Behav. Brain Sci.*, **15**: 425–492.
56. Lehmann D., Strik W.K., Henggeler B., Koenig T., Koukkou M. (1998) Brain electric microstates and momentary conscious mind states as building blocks of spontaneous thinking: I. Visual imagery and abstract thoughts. *Int. J. Psychophysiol.*, **29**: 1–11.
57. Lehmann D. (2001) Hirnarbeit–Wacharbeit–Traumarbeit: mikrozustände als atome des denkens. In *Psychoanalyse im Dialog der Wissenschaften*, Vol. 1 (Ed. P. Giampieri-Deutsch), Kohlhammer, Stuttgart (in press).
58. Pascual-Marqui R.D., Michel C.M., Lehmann D. (1984) Low resolution electromagnetic tomography: a new method for localizing electrical activity in the brain. *Int. J. Psychophysiol.*, **18**: 49–65.
59. Dierks T., Jelic V., Pascual-Marqui R.D., Wahlund L., Julin P., Linden D.E., Maurer K., Winblad B., Nordberg A. (2000) Spatial pattern of cerebral glucose metabolism (PET) correlates with localization of intracerebral EEG-generators in Alzheimer's disease. *Clin. Neurophysiol.*, **111**: 1817–1824.
60. Mueller T.J., Federspiel A., Dierks T. (2001) Activation in landmarks and faces: a LORETA-ERP study. *Brain Topogr.* (in press).
61. Nataanan R. (1992) *Attention and Brain Function*, Erlbaum, London.
62. Spoont M.R. (1992) Modulatory role of serotonin in neural information processing: implications of human psychopathology. *Psychol. Bull.*, **112**: 330–350.
63. Griffith J.M., O'Neill J.E., Petty F., Garver D., Young D., Freedman R. (1998) Nicotine receptor desensitisation and sensory gating deficits in schizophrenia. *Biol. Psychiatry*, **44**: 98–106.
64. Gruzelier J. (1999) A review of the implications of early sensory processing and subcortical involvement for cognitive dysfunction in schizophrenia. In *Review of Psychiatry, 25* (Ed. C. Tamminga), pp. 29–76, American Psychiatric Association, Washington.
65. Mangina C.A., Beuzeron-Mangina J.H. (1996) Electrical stimulation of the human brain and bilateral electrodermal activity. *Int. J. Psychophysiol.*, **22**: 1–8.
66. Swerdlow N.R., Geyer M.A. (1998) Using an animal model of deficient sensorimotor gating to study the pathophysiology and new treatments of schizophrenia. *Schizophr. Bull.*, **24**: 285–301.
67. Lipska B.K., Swerdlow N.R., Geyer M.A., Jaskiw G.E., Braff D.L., Weinberger D.R. (1995) Neonatal excitotoxic hippocampal damage in rats causes postpubertal changes in prepulse inhibition of startle and its disruption by apomorphine. *Psychopharmacology*, **122**: 35–43.
68. Itil T.M. (1977) Qualitative and quantitative EEG findings in schizophrenia. *Schizophr. Bull.*, **3**: 61–79.
69. Buchsbaum M.S., Rigal F., Coppola R., Cappelletti J., King A.C., Johnson J. (1982) A new system for gray-level surface distribution maps of electrical activity. *Electroencephalogr. Clin. Neurophysiol.*, **53**: 237–242.
70. Morihisa J.M., Duffy F.H., Wyatt R.J. (1983) Brain electrical activity mapping (BEAM) in schizophrenic patients. *Arch. Gen. Psychiatry*, **40**: 719–728.
71. Karson C.N., Coppola R., Morihisa J.M., Weinberger D.R. (1987) Computed electroencephalographic activity mapping in schizophrenia: the resting state reconsidered. *Arch. Gen. Psychiatry*, **44**: 514–517.

72. Karson C.N., Coppola R., Daniel D.G. (1988) Alpha frequency in schizophrenia: an association with enlarged cerebral ventricles. *Am. J. Psychiatry*, **145**: 861–864.
73. Miyauchi T., Tanaka K., Hagimoto H., Miura T., Kishimoto H., Matsushita M. (1990) Computerized EEG in schizophrenic patients. *Biol. Psychiatry*, **28**: 488–494.
74. Galderisi S., Mucci A., Mignone M.L., Maj M., Kemali D. (1992) CEEG mapping in drug-free schizophrenics: differences from healthy subjects and changes induced by haloperidol treatment. *Schizophr. Res.*, **6**: 15–24.
75. Gattaz W.F., Mayer S., Ziegler P., Platz M., Gasser T. (1992) Hypofrontality on topographic EEG in schizophrenia. *Eur. Arch. Psychiatry Clin. Neurosci.*, **241**: 328–332.
76. Kemali D., Galderisi S., Maj M., Mucci A., Di Gregorio M., Bucci P. (1992) Computerized EEG topography findings in schizophrenic patients before and after haloperidol treatment. *Int. J. Psychophysiol.*, **13**: 283–290.
77. Sponheim S.R., Clementz B.A., Iacono W.G., Beiser M. (1994) Resting EEG in first-episode and chronic schizophrenia. *Psychophysiology*, **31**: 37–43.
78. Takeuchi K., Takigawa M., Fukuzako H., Hokazono Y., Hirakawa K., Fukuzako T., Ueyama K., Fujimoto T., Matsumoto K. (1994) Correlation of third ventricular enlargement and EEG slow wave activity in schizophrenic patients. *Psychiatry Res.*, **55**: 1–11.
79. Wada Y., Takizawa Y., Kitazawa S., Zheng-Yan J., Yamaguchi N. (1994) Quantitative EEG analysis at rest and during photic stimulation in drug-naive patients with first-episode paranoid schizophrenia. *Eur. Arch. Psychiatry Clin. Neurosci.*, **244**: 247–251.
80. Omori M., Koshino Y., Murata I., Nishio M., Sakamoto K., Isaki K. (1995) Quantitative EEG in never-treated schizophrenic patients. *Biol. Psychiatry*, **38**: 305–309.
81. Wada Y., Takizawa Y., Yamaguchi N. (1995) Abnormal photic driving responses in never-medicated schizophrenia patients. *Schizophr. Bull.*, **21**: 111–115.
82. Itil T.M., Saletu B., Davis S., Allen M. (1974) Stability studies in schizophrenics and normals using computer-analyzed EEG. *Biol. Psychiatry*, **8**: 321–335.
83. Clementz B.A., Sponheim S.R., Iacono W.G., Beiser M. (1994) Resting EEG in first-episode schizophrenia patients, bipolar psychosis patients, and their first-degree relatives. *Psychophysiology*, **31**: 486–494.
84. Mucci A., Galderisi S., Catapano F., Fabrazzo M., Maj M. (1996) Correlati neurofisiologici della risposta clinica ai neurolettici tipici in pazienti schizofrenici al primo episodio di malattia. *Riv. Riabil. Psichiatr. Psicosoc.*, **2**: 105–115.
85. Galderisi S., Mucci A., Bucci P., Maj M. (1997) Quantitative EEG reactivity to neuroleptic challenge in first-episode and chronic schizophrenia. *Biol. Psychiatry*, **42**: 64S.
86. Koukkou M., Lehmann D., Federspiel A., Merlo M.C.G. (1995) EEG reactivity and EEG activity in never-treated acute schizophrenics, measured with spectral parameters and dimensional complexity. *J. Neural Transm.*, **99**: 89–102.
87. John E.R., Prichep L.S., Alper K.R., Mas F.G., Cancro R., Easton P., Sverdlov L. (1994) Quantitative electrophysiological characteristics and subtyping of schizophrenia. *Biol. Psychiatry*, **36**: 801–826.
88. Tauscher J., Fischer P., Neumeister A., Rappelsberger P., Kasper S. (1998) Low frontal electroencephalographic coherence in neuroleptic-free schizophrenic patients. *Biol. Psychiatry*, **44**: 438–447.

89. Itil T.M., Hsu W., Saletu B., Mednick S. (1974) Computer EEG and auditory evoked potential investigations in children at high risk for schizophrenia. *Am. J. Psychiatry*, **8**: 892–900.
90. Itil T.M., Simeon J., Coffin C. (1976) Qualitative and quantitative EEG in psychotic children. *Dis. Nerv. Syst.*, **37**: 247–252.
91. Koukkou M. (1997) Models of the workings of the human brain and the search for the pathogenesis of schizophrenia. *Hellenic Med. J.*, **1**: 21–25.
92. Stassen H.H., Coppola R., Gottesman I.I., Torrey E.F. Kuny S., Rickler K.C., Hell D. (1999) EEG differences in monozygotic twins discordant and concordant for schizophrenia. *Psychophysiology*, **36**: 109–117.
93. Itil T.M., Shapiro D.M., Schneider S.J., Francis I.B. (1981) Computerized EEG as a predictor of drug response in treatment resistant schizophrenics. *J. Nerv. Ment. Dis.*, **169**: 629–637.
94. Czobor P., Volavka J. (1991) Pretreatment EEG predicts short-term response to haloperidol treatment. *Biol. Psychiatry*, **30**: 927–942.
95. Galderisi S., Maj M., Mucci A., Bucci P., Kemali D. (1994) QEEG alpha-1 changes after a single dose of high-potency neuroleptics as a predictor of short-term response to treatment in schizophrenic patients. *Biol. Psychiatry*, **35**: 367–374.
96. Itil T.M. (1974) Computerized EEG findings in schizophrenia and effects of neuroleptic drugs. In *Biological Mechanisms of Schizophrenia and Schizophrenia-like Psychoses* (Eds H. Mitsuda, T. Fukuda), pp. 196–207, Igaka Shoin, Tokyo.
97. Saito M. (1978) CEEG study on patients under the psychiatric drug treatment: the correlation between EEG alteration and clinical evolution. In *Biological Psychiatry Today* (Eds J. Obiols, C. Ballùs, E. Gonzales Monclùs, J. Pujol), pp. 1036–1311, Elsevier, Amsterdam.
98. Herrmann W.M., Schaerer E. (1982) Pharmaco-EEG: computer EEG analysis to describe the projection of drug effects on a functional cerebral level in humans. In *Handbook of Electroencephalography and Clinical Neurophysiology*, Vol. 2 (Eds F.H. Lopes da Silva, W. Storm van Leeuwen, A. Rémond), pp. 385–445, Elsevier, Amsterdam.
99. Ulrich G., Müller-Oerlinghausen B., Gaebel W. (1986) Changes in the topographical distribution of absolute alpha-power in the resting EEG of schizophrenic in-patients under neuroleptic medication. *Pharmacopsychiatry*, **19**: 220–221.
100. Galderisi S., Mucci A., Di Gregorio M.R., Bucci P., Maj M., Kemali D. (1990) C-EEG brain mapping in DSM III schizophrenics after acute and chronic haloperidol treatment. *Eur. Neuropsychopharmacol.*, **1**: 51–54.
101. Saletu B., Kufferle B., Grunberger J., Foldes P., Topitz A., Anderer P. (1994) Clinical, EEG mapping and psychometric studies in negative schizophrenia: comparative trials with amisulpride and fluphenazine. *Neuropsychobiology*, **29**: 125–135.
102. Schellenberg R., Milch W., Schwarz A., Schober F., Dimpfel W. (1994) Quantitative EEG and BPRS data following haldol-decanoate administration in schizophrenics. *Int. Clin. Psychopharmacol.*, **9**: 17–24.
103. Moore N.C., Tucker K.A., Brin F.B., Merai P., Shillcutt S.D., Coburn K.L. (1997) Positive symptoms of schizophrenia: response to haloperidol and remoxipride is associated with increased alpha EEG activity. *Hum. Psychopharmacol.*, **12**: 75–80.

104. Sponheim S.R., Clementz B.A., Iacono W.G., Beiser M. (2000) Clinical and biological concomitants of resting state EEG power abnormalities in schizophrenia. *Biol. Psychiatry*, **48**: 1088–1097.

105. Saletu B., Kufferle B., Anderer P., Grunberger J., Steinberger K. (1990) EEG-brain mapping in schizophrenics with predominantly positive and negative symptoms. Comparative studies with remoxipride/haloperidol. *Eur. Neuropsychopharmacol.*, **1**: 27–36.

106. Begic D., Hotujac L., Jokic-Begic N. (2000) Quantitative EEG in "positive" and "negative" schizophrenia. *Acta Psychiatr. Scand.*, **101**: 307–311.

107. Kemali D., Maj M., Galderisi S., Salvati A., Starace F., Valente A., Pirozzi R. (1987) Clinical, biological, and neuropsychological features associated with lateral ventricular enlargement in DSM-III schizophrenic disorder. *Psychiatry Res.*, **21**: 137–149.

108. Gambini O., Colombo C., Macciardi F., Locatelli M., Calabrese G., Sacchetti E., Scarone S. (1990) EEG power spectrum profile and structural CNS characteristics in schizophrenia. *Biol. Psychiatry*, **27**: 1331–1334.

109. Fenton G.W., Fenwick P.B.C., Dollimore J., Dunn T.L., Hirsch S.R. (1980) EEG spectral analysis in schizophrenia. *Br. J. Psychiatry*, **136**: 445–455.

110. Omori M., Koshino Y., Murata T., Murata I., Horie T., Isaki K. (1992) Quantitative EEG of elderly schizophrenic patients. *Jpn. J. Psychiatry Neurol.*, **46**: 681–692.

111. Merrin E.L., Floyd T.C. (1992) Negative symptoms and EEG alpha activity in schizophrenic patients. *Schizophr. Res.*, **8**: 11–20.

112. Merrin E.L., Floyd T.C. (1996) Negative symptoms and EEG alpha in schizophrenia: a replication. *Schizophr. Res.*, **19**: 151–161.

113. Galderisi S., Mucci A., Catapano F., Colucci D'Amato A., Maj M. (1995) Neuropsychological and QEEG mapping correlates of psychopathological dimensions in drug-free schizophrenic patients. In *Critical Issues in the Treatment of Schizophrenia* (Eds N. Brunello, G. Racagni, S.Z. Langer, J. Mendlewicz), pp. 44–47, Karger, Basel.

114. Harris A.W.F., Williams L., Gordon E., Bahramali H., Slewa-Younan S. (1999) Different psychopathological models and quantified EEG in schizophrenia. *Psychol. Med.*, **29**: 1175–1181.

115. Morstyn P., Duffy F.H., McCarley R.W. (1983) Altered topography of EEG spectral content in schizophrenia. *Electroencephalogr. Clin. Neurophysiol.*, **56**: 263–271.

116. Guenther W., Steinberg R., Petsch R., Streck P., Kugler J. (1989) EEG mapping in psychiatry: studies on type I/II schizophrenia using motor activation. In *Topographic Brain Mapping of EEG and Evoked Potentials* (Ed. K. Maurer), pp. 438–450, Springer-Verlag, Berlin.

117. Guich S.M., Buchsbaum M.S., Burgwald L., Wu J., Haier R., Asarnow R., Nuechterlein K., Potkin S. (1989) Effect of attention on frontal distribution of delta activity and cerebral metabolic rate in schizophrenia. *Schizophr. Res.*, **2**: 439–448.

118. Alper K., Günther W., Pritchep L.S., John E.R., Brodie J. (1998) Correlation of qEEG with PET in schizophrenia. *Neuropsychobiology*, **38**: 50–56.

119. Guenther W., Davous P., Godet J.-L., Guillibert E., Breitling D., Rondot P. (1988) Bilateral brain dysfunction during motor activation in type II schizophrenia measured by EEG mapping. *Biol. Psychiatry*, **23**: 295–311.

120. Crow T.J. (1980) Molecular pathology of schizophrenia: more than one disease process? *Br. Med. J.*, **280**: 66–68.

121. Morihisa J.M. (1986) Electrophysiological evidence implicating frontal lobe dysfunction in schizophrenia. *Psychopharmacol. Bull.*, **22**: 885–889.
122. Pascual-Marqui R.D., Lehmann D., Koenig T., Kochi K., Merlo M.C., Hell D. (1999) Low resolution brain electromagnetic tomography (LORETA) functional imaging in acute, neuroleptic-naive, first-episode, productive schizophrenics. *Psychiatry Res.*, **90**: 169–179.
123. Rice D.M., Potkin S.G., Jin Y., Isenhart R., Heh C.W., Sramek J., Costa J., Sandman C.A. (1989) EEG alpha photic driving abnormalities in chronic schizophrenia. *Psychiatry Res.*, **30**: 313–324.
124. Jin Y., Potkin S.G., Rice D., Sramek J., Costa J., Isenhart R., Heh C., Sandman C.A. (1990) Abnormal EEG response to photic stimulation in schizophrenic patients. *Schizophr. Bull.*, **16**: 627–634.
125. Jin Y., Potkin S.G., Sandman C.A., Bunney W.E. (1997) Electroencephalographic photic driving in patients with schizophrenia and depression. *Biol. Psychiatry*, **41**: 496–499.
126. Jin Y., Potkin S.G., Sandman C. (1995) Clozapine increases EEG photic driving in clinical responders. *Schizophr. Bull.*, **21**: 263–268.
127. Baldeweg T., Spence S., Hirsch S.R., Gruzelier J. (1998) Gamma-band electroencephalographic oscillations in a patient with somatic hallucinations. *Lancet*, **352**: 620–621.
128. Clementz B.A., Blumenfeld L.D., Cobb S. (1997) The gamma band response may account for poor P50 suppression in schizophrenia. *Neuroreport*, **8**: 3889–3893.
129. Haig A.R., Gordon E., De Pascalis V., Meares R.A., Bahramali H., Harris A. (2000) Gamma activity in schizophrenia: evidence of impaired network binding? *Clin. Neurophysiol.*, **111**: 1461–1468.
130. Gordon E., Williams L., Haig A.R., Wright J., Meares R.A. (2001) Symptom profile and "gamma" processing in schizophrenia. *Cognitive Neuropsychiatry*, **6**: 7–19.
131. Merrin E.L., Floyd T.C., Fein G. (1989) EEG coherence in unmedicated schizophrenic patients. *Biol. Psychiatry*, **25**: 60–66.
132. Pockberger H., Thau K., Lovrek A., Petshe H., Pappelsberger P. (1989) Coherence mapping reveals differences in the EEG between psychiatric patients and healthy persons. In *Topographic Brain Mapping of EEG and Evoked Potentials* (Ed. K. Maurer), pp. 451–457, Springer, Heidelberg.
133. Nagase Y., Okubo Y., Matsuura M., Kojima T. Toru M. (1992) EEG coherence in unmedicated schizophrenic patients: topographical study of predominantly never medicated cases. *Biol. Psychiatry*, **32**: 1028–1034.
134. Hoffman R.E., Buchsbaum M.S., Escobar M.D., Makuch R.W., Nuechterlein K.H., Guich S.M. (1991) EEG coherence of prefrontal areas in normal and schizophrenic males during perceptual activation. *J. Neuropsychiatry Clin. Neurosci.*, **3**: 169–175.
135. Michelogiannis S., Paritsis N., Trikas P. (1991) EEG coherence during hemispheric activation in schizophrenics. *Eur. Arch. Psychiatry Clin. Neurosci.*, **241**: 31–34.
136. Morrison-Stewart S.L., Williamson P.C., Cornig W.C., Kutcher S.P., Merskey H. (1991) Coherence on electroencephalography and aberrant function organisation of the brain in schizophrenic patients during activation tasks. *Br. J. Psychiatry*, **159**: 636–644.

137. Morrison-Stewart S.L., Velikonja D., Corning W.C., Williamson P. (1996) Aberrant interhemispheric alpha coherence on electroencephalography in schizophrenic patients during activation tasks. *Psychol. Med.*, **26**: 605–612.
138. Elbert T., Lutzenberger W., Rockstroh B., Berg P., Cohen R. (1992) Physical aspects of the EEG in schizophrenics. *Biol. Psychiatry*, **32**: 595–606.
139. Koukkou M., Lehmann D., Wackermann J., Dvorak I., Henggeler B. (1993) Dimensional complexity of EEG brain mechanisms in untreated schizophrenia. *Biol. Psychiatry*, **33**: 397–407.
140. Saito N., Kuginuki T., Yagyu T., Kinoshita T., Koenig T., Pascual-Marqui R.D., Kochi K., Wackermann J., Lehmann D. (1998) Global, regional, and local measures of complexity of multichannel electroencephalography in acute, neuroleptic-naive, first-break schizophrenics. *Biol. Psychiatry*, **43**: 794–802.
141. Kirsch P., Besthorn C., Klein S., Rindfleisch J., Olbrich R. (2000) The dimensional complexity of the EEG during cognitive tasks reflects the impaired information processing in schizophrenic patients. *Int. J. Psychophysiol.*, **36**: 237–246.
142. Buchsbaum M.S., Mirsky A.F., DeLisi LE., Morihisa J., Karson C.N., Mendelson W.B., King A.C., Johnson J., Kessler R. (1984) The Genain quadruplets: electrophysiological, positron emission, and X-ray tomographic studies. *Psychiatry Res.*, **13**: 95–108.
143. Igata M., Ohta M., Hayashida Y., Abe K. (1994) Missing peaks in auditory brainstem responses and negative symptoms in schizophrenia. *Jpn. J. Psychiatry Neurol.*, **48**: 571–578.
144. Shagass C. (1977) Early evoked potentials. *Schizophr. Bull.*, **3**: 80–92.
145. Shagass C., Roemer R.A., Straumanis J.J., Amadeo M. (1979) Temporal variability of somatosensory, visual, and auditory evoked potentials in schizophrenia. *Arch. Gen. Psychiatry*, **36**: 1341–1351.
146. Saletu B., Itil T.M., Saletu M. (1971) Auditory evoked response, EEG, and thought process in schizophrenics. *Am. J. Psychiatry*, **128**: 336–344.
147. Ishikawa K. (1968) Studies on the visual evoked responses to paired light flashes in schizophrenics. *Kurume Med. J.*, **15**: 153–167.
148. Connolly J.F., Manchanda R., Gruzelier J.H. (1985) Pathway and hemispheric differences in the event-related potential (ERP) to monaural stimulation: a comparison of schizophrenic patients with normal controls. *Biol. Psychiatry*, **20**: 293–303.
149. Jutai J., Gruzelier J.H., Connolly J. (1984) Schizophrenia and spectral analysis of the visual evoked potential. *Br. J. Psychiatry*, **145**: 496–501.
150. Gruzelier J. (1996) Lateralised dysfunction is necessary but not sufficient to account for neuropsychological deficits in schizophrenia. In *Schizophrenia: A Neuropsychological Perspective* (Eds C. Pantelis, H. Nelson, H. Barnes), pp. 125–160, Wiley, New York.
151. Tress K.H., Kugler B.T., Caudrey D.J. (1979) Interhemispheric integration in schizophrenia. In *Hemisphere Asymmetries of Function* (Eds J.H. Gruzelier, P. Flor-Henry), pp. 449–462, Elsevier, Amsterdam.
152. Andrews H.B., House A.O., Cooper J.E., Barber C. (1986) The prediction of abnormal evoked potentials in schizophrenic patients by means of symptom pattern. *Br. J. Psychiatry*, **149**: 46–50.
153. Gruzelier J. (1999) Functional neuro-psychophysiological asymmetry in schizophrenia: a review and reorientation. *Schizophr. Bull.*, **25**: 91–120.

154. Connolly J.F., Gruzelier J.H, Manchanda R. (1983) Visual evoked potentials in schizophrenia: intensity effects and hemispheric asymmetry. *Br. J. Psychiatry*, **153**: 153–155.
155. Gruzelier J., Jutai J., Connolly J. (1993) Cerebral asymmetry in EEG spectra in unmedicated schizophrenic patients: relationships with active and withdrawn syndromes. *Int. J. Psychophysiol.*, **15**: 239–246.
156. Katsanis J., Iacono W.G., Beiser M. (1996) Visual event-related potentials in first-episode psychotic patients and their relatives. *Psychophysiology*, **33**: 207–217.
157. Boutros N., Nasrallah H., Leighty R. (1997) Auditory evoked potentials, clinical versus research applications. *Psychiatry Res.*, **24**: 183–195.
158. Frangou S., Sharma T., Alarcon G., Sigmudsson T., Takei N., Binnie C., Murray R.M. (1997) The Maudsley Family Study, II: Endogenous event-related potentials in familial schizophrenia. *Schizophr. Res.*, **23**: 45–53.
159. Friedman D., Cornblatt B., Vaughan H. Jr., Erlenmeyer-Kimling L. (1988) Auditory event-related potentials in children at risk for schizophrenia: the complete initial sample. *Psychiatry Res.*, **26**: 203–221.
160. Trestman R.L., Horvath T., Kalus O., Peterson A.E., Coccaro E., Mitropoulou V., Apter S., Davidson M., Siever L.J. (1996) Event-related potentials in schizotypal personality disorder. *J. Neuropsychiatry Clin. Neurosci.*, **8**: 33–40.
161. Shelley A.M., Ward P.B., Catts S.V., Michie P.T., Andrews S., McConaghy N. (1991) Mismatch negativity: an index of a preattentive processing deficit in schizophrenia. *Biol. Psychiatry*, **30**: 1059–1062.
162. Javitt D.C., Doneshka P., Zylberman I., Ritter W., Vaughn H.G. Jr. (1993) Impairment of early cortical processing in schizophrenia: an event-related potential confirmation study. *Biol. Psychiatry*, **33**: 513–519.
163. Pfefferbaum A., Roth W.T., Kopell B.S. (1979) State-trait considerations of event-related potential markers of psychopathology. *Psychopharmacol. Bull.*, **15**: 36–39.
164. McCarley R.W., Shenton M.E., O'Donnell B.F., Faux S.F., Kikinis R., Nestor P.G., Jolesz F.A. (1993) Auditory P300 abnormalities and left posterior superior temporal gyrus volume reduction in schizophrenia. *Arch. Gen. Psychiatry*, **50**: 190–197.
165. Egan M.F., Duncan C.C., Suddath R.L., Kirch D.G., Mirsky A.F., Wyatt R.J. (1994) Event-related potential abnormalities correlate with structural brain alterations and clinical features in patients with chronic schizophrenia. *Schizophr. Res.*, **11**: 259–271.
166. Galderisi S., Maj M., Mucci A., Monteleone P., Kemali D. (1988) Lateralization patterns of verbal stimuli processing assessed by reaction time and event-related potentials in schizophrenic patients. *Int. J. Psychophysiol.*, **6**: 167–176.
167. Strik W.K., Dierks T., Franzek E., Stöber G., Maurer K. (1994) P300 in schizophrenia: interactions between amplitudes and topography. *Biol. Psychiatry*, **35**: 850–856.
168. Heidrich A., Strik W.K. (1997) Auditory P300 topography and neuropsychological test performance: evidence for left hemisphere dysfunction in schizophrenia. *Biol. Psychiatry*, **41**: 327–335.
169. Strik W.K., Fallgatter A.J., Stöber G., Franzek E., Beckmann H. (1996) The predictive value of auditory P300 on the course of schizophrenia. *J. Neural Transm.*, **103**: 1351–1359.
170. Morstyn R., Duffy F.H., McCarley R.W. (1983) Altered P300 topography in schizophrenia. *Arch. Gen. Psychiatry*, **40**: 729–734.

171. Strik W.K., Dierks T., Franzek E., Maurer K., Beckmann H. (1993) Differences in P300 amplitude and topography between cycloid psychosis and schizophrenia in Leonhard's classification. *Acta Psychiatr. Scand.*, **87**: 179–183.
172. Gruzelier J., Kaiser J., Richardson A., Liddiard D., Cheema S., Puri B., McEvedy C. (1999) Opposite patterns of P300 asymmetry in schizophrenia are syndrome related. *Int. J. Psychophysiol.*, **34**: 276–282.
173. Strik W.K., Dierks T., Franzek E., Stöber G., Maurer K. (1994) P300 asymmetries in schizophrenia revisited with reference-independent methods. *Psychiatry Res. Neuroimaging*, **55**: 153–166.
174. Freedman R. (2001) Genetic risk for schizophrenia and biological mechanisms. *Schizophr. Res.* (in press).
175. Erwin R.J., Mawhinney-Hee M., Gur R.C. (1991) Midlatency auditory evoked responses in schizophrenia. *Biol. Psychiatry*, **30**: 430–442.
176. Croft R.J., Lee A., Bertolo J., Gruzelier J.H. (2001) Associations of P50 suppression and habituation with perceptual and cognitive features of "unreality" in schizotypy. *Biol. Psychiatry* (in press).
177. Boutros N.N., Zouridakis G., Overall J. (1991) Replication and extension of P50 findings in schizophrenia. *Clin. Electroencephalogr.*, **22**: 40–45.
178. Boutros N., Zouridakis G., Rustin T., Peabody C., Warner D. (1993) The P50 component of the auditory evoked potential and subtypes of schizophrenia. *Psychiatry Res.*, **47**: 243–254.
179. Siegel C., Waldo M., Mizner G., Adler L.E., Freedman R. (1984) Deficits in sensory gating in schizophrenic patients and their relatives. Evidence obtained with auditory evoked responses. *Arch. Gen. Psychiatry*, **41**: 607–612.
180. Harris J.G., Adler L.E., Young D.A., Cullum C.M., Rilling L.M., Cicerello A., Intemann P.M., Freedman R. (1996) Neuropsychological dysfunction in parents of schizophrenics. *Schizophr. Res.*, **20**: 253–260.
181. Waldo M.C., Adler L.E., Freedman R. (1988) Defects in auditory sensory gating and their apparent compensation in relatives of schizophrenics. *Schizophr. Res.*, **1**: 19–24.
182. Braff D.L. (2001) Advances in translationsal research in schizophrenia. *Schizophr. Res.* (in press).
183. Cadenhead K.S., Geyer M.A., Braff D.L. (1993) Impaired startle prepulse inhibition and habituation in patients with schizotypal personality disorder. *Am. J. Psychiatry*, **150**: 1862–1867.
184. Dawson M.E., Hazlett E.A., Filion D.L. (1993) Attention and schizophrenia: impaired modulation of the startle reflex. *J. Abnorm. Psychol.*, **102**: 633–641.
185. Cadenhead K.S., Perry W., Braff D.L. (1996) The relationship of information-processing deficits and clinical symptoms in schizoptypal personality disorder. *Biol. Psychiatry*, **40**: 853–858.
186. Schwarzkopf S.B., Lamberti J.S., Smith D.A. (1993) Concurrent assessment of acoustic startle and auditory P50 evoked potential measures of sensory inhibition. *Biol. Psychiatry*, **33**: 815–828.
187. Geyer M.A., Braff D.L. (1982) Habituation of the blink reflex in normals and schizophrenic patients. *Psychophysiology*, **19**: 1–6.
188. Bolino F., Manna V., Di Cicco L., Di Michele V., Daneluzzo E., Rossi A., Casacchia M. (1992) Startle reflex habituation in functional psychoses: a controlled study. *Neurosci. Lett.*, **145**: 126–128.
189. Braff D.L., Saccuzzo D.P., Geyer M.A. (1991) Information processing dysfunctions in schizophrenia; studies of visual backward masking, sensorimotor gating, and habituation. In *Handbook of Schizophrenia: Neuropsychology, Psycho-*

physiology and Information Processing (Eds S.R. Steinhauer, J.H. Gruzelier, J. Zubin), pp. 303–334, Elsevier, Amsterdam.

190. Holzman P.S., O'Brian C., Waternaux C. (1991) Effects of lithium treatment on eye movements. *Biol. Psychiatry*, **29**: 1001–1015.

191. Iacono W.G. (1988) Eye movement abnormalities in schizophrenic and affective disorders. In *Neuropsychology of Eye Movements* (Eds C.W. Johnston, F.J. Pirozzolo), pp. 115–146, Erlbaum, Hillsdale.

192. Siever L.J., Coursey R.D., Alterman I.S., Buchsbaum M.S., Murphy D.L. (1984) Impaired smooth pursuit eye movement: vulnerability marker of schizotypal personality disorder in a normal volunteer population. *Am. J. Psychiatry*, **141**: 1560–1566.

193. Yee C.M., Nuechterlein K.H., Dawson M.E. (1998) A longitudinal analysis of eye tracking dysfunction and attention in recent onset schizophrenia. *Psychophysiology*, **35**: 443–451.

194. Lewin S. (1984) Frontal lobe dysfunction in schizophrenia: I: Eye movement impairments. *J. Psychiatr. Res.*, **18**: 27–55.

195. Gruzelier J.H., Venables P.H. (1972) Skin conductance orienting activity in a heterogeneous sample of schizophrenics: possible evidence of limbic dysfunction. *J. Nerv. Ment. Dis.*, **155**: 277–287.

196. Gruzelier J.H. (2001) A Janusian perspective on the nature, development and structure of schizophrenia and schizotypy. *Schizophr. Res.* (in press).

197. Dawson M.E., Schell A.M. (2001) What does electrodermal activity tell us about prognosis in the schizophrenia spectrum? *Schizophr. Res.* (in press).

198. Gruzelier J., Raine A. (1994) Schizophrenia, schizotypal personality, syndromes, cerebral lateralisation and electrodermal activity. *Int. J. Psychophysiol.*, **16**: 1–16.

199. Gruzelier J.H., Manchanda R. (1982) The syndrome of schizophrenia: relations between electrodermal response lateral asymmetries and clinical ratings. *Br. J. Psychiatry*, **141**: 488–495.

200. Gruzelier J.H. (2001) Functional lateral asymmetries and interhemispheric connectivity in the schizophrenic spectrum. Submitted for publication.

201. Gaebel W., Ulrich G., Frick K. (1986) Eye movement research with schizophrenic patients and normal controls using corneal reflection pupil centre measurements. *Eur. Arch. Psychiatry Neurol. Sci.*, **235**: 243–254.

202. Gaebel W., Ulrich G., Frick K. (1987) Visuomotor performance of schizophrenic patients and normal controls in a picture viewing task. *Biol. Psychiatry*, **22**: 1227–1237.

203. Kawazoe S., Fujiwara M., Tsuru N. (1987) Eye movements and the Benton Visual Retention Test in schizophrenics. In *Cerebral Dynamics, Laterality and Psychopathology* (Eds R. Takahashi, P. Flor-Henry, J. Gruzelier, S. Niwa), pp. 157–172, Elsevier, Amsterdam.

204. Goode D.J., Glenn S., Manning A.A., Middleton J.F. (1980) Lateral asymmetry of the Hoffman reflex: relation to cortical laterality. *J. Neurol. Neurosurg. Psychiatry*, **43**: 831–840.

205. Goode D.J., Manning A.A., Middleton J.F. (1981) Cortical laterality and asymmetry of the Hoffmann reflex in psychiatric patients. *Biol. Psychiatry*, **16**: 1137–1145.

206. Malaspina D., Bruder G., Dalack G.W., Storer S., van Kammen M., Amador X., Glassman A., Gorman J. (1997) Diminished cardiac vagal tone in schizophrenia: associations to brain laterality and age of onset. *Biol. Psychiatry*, **41**: 612–717.

207. Gruzelier J., Davis S. (1995) Social and physical anhedonia in relation to cerebral laterality and electrodermal habituation in unmedicated psychotic patients. *Psychiatry Res.*, **56**: 163–172.
208. Mason O., Claridge G., Clark K. (1997) Electrodermal relationships with personality measures of psychosis-proneness in psychotic and normal subjects. *Int. J. Psychophysiol.*, **27**: 137–146.
209. Schaffer C.E., Davidson R.J., Saron C. (1983) Frontal and parietal electroencephalogram asymmetry in depressed and nondepressed subjects. *Biol. Psychiatry*, **18**: 753–762.
210. Brenner R.P., Ulrich R.F., Spiker D.G., Sclabassi R.J., Reynolds C.F., Marin R.S., Boller F. (1986) Computerized EEG spectral analysis in elderly normal, demented and depressed subjects. *Electroencephalogr. Clin. Neurophysiol.*, **64**: 483–492.
211. John E.R., Prichep L.S., Fridman J., Easton P. (1988) Neurometrics: computer-assisted differential diagnosis of brain dysfunctions. *Science*, **239**: 162–169.
212. Flor-Henry P., Koles Z.J., Howarth B.G., Burton L. (1979) Neurophysiological studies of schizophrenia, mania and depression. In *Hemisphere Asymmetries of Function and Psychopathology* (Eds J. Gruzelier, P. Flor-Henry), pp. 189–221, Elsevier, Amsterdam.
213. Knott V.J., Lapierre Y.D. (1987) Computerized EEG correlates of depression and antidepressant treatment. *Prog. Neuropsychopharmacol. Biol. Psychiatry*, **11**: 213–221.
214. Nyström C., Matousek M., Hällström T. (1986) Relationships between EEG and clinical characteristics in major depressive disorder. *Acta Psychiatr. Scand.*, **73**: 390–394.
215. Have G., Kolbeinsson H., Petursson H. (1991) Dementia and depression in old age: psychophysiological aspects. *Acta Psychiatr. Scand.*, **83**: 329–333.
216. Visser S.L., Van Tilburg W., Hooijer C., Jonker C., De Rijke W. (1985) Visual evoked potentials (VEPs) in senile disorders in the elderly; comparison with EEG parameters. *Electroencephalogr. Clin. Neurophysiol.*, **60**: 115–121.
217. Dahabra S., Ashton C.H., Bahrainian M., Britton P.G., Ferrier I.N., McAllister V.A., Marsh V.R., Moore P.B. (1998) Structural and functional abnormalities in elderly patients clinically recovered from early- and late-onset depression. *Biol. Psychiatry*, **44**: 34–46.
218. Henriques J.B., Davidson R.J. (1990) Regional brain electrical asymmetries discriminate between previously depressed and healthy control subjects. *J. Abnorm. Psychol.*, **99**: 22–31.
219. Henriques J.B., Davidson R.J. (1991) Left frontal hypoactivation in depression. *J. Abnorm. Psychol.*, **100**: 535–545.
220. Davidson R.J., Chapman J.P., Chapman L.J. (1987) Task dependent EEG asymmetry discriminates between depressed and nondepressed subjects. *Psychophysiology*, **24**: 585.
221. Davidson R.J. (1992) Anterior cerebral asymmetry and the nature of emotion. *Brain Cogn.*, **20**: 125–151.
222. Tucker D.M., Stenslie C.E., Roth R.S., Shearer S.L. (1981) Right frontal activation and right hemisphere performance: decrement during a depressed mood. *Arch. Gen. Psychiatry*, **38**: 169–174.
223. Bruder G.E., Fong R., Tenke C.E., Leite P., Towey J.P., Stewart J.E., McGrath P.J., Quitkin F.M. (1997) Regional brain asymmetries in major depression with or without an anxiety disorder: a quantitative electroencephalographic study. *Biol. Psychiatry*, **41**: 939–948.

224. Shagass C., Roemer R.A., Straumanis J.J., Josiassen R.C. (1984) Psychiatric diagnostic discriminations with combinations of quantitative EEG variables. *Br. J. Psychiatry*, **144**: 581–592.
225. Small J.G., Milstein V., Malloy F.W., Medlock C.E., Klapper M.H. (1999) Clinical and quantitative EEG studies of mania. *J. Affect. Disord.*, **53**: 217–224.
226. Davidson R.J. (1987) Cerebral asymmetry and the nature of emotion: implications for the study of individual differences and psychopathology. In *Cerebral Dynamics, Laterality and Psychopathology* (Eds R. Takahashi, P. Flor-Henry, J. Gruzelier, S. Niwa), pp. 71–83, Elsevier, Amsterdam.
227. Flor-Henry P. (1987) Cerebral dynamics, laterality and psychopathology: a commentary. In *Cerebral Dynamics, Laterality and Psychopathology* (Eds R. Takahashi, P. Flor-Henry, J. Gruzelier, S. Niwa), pp. 3–21, Elsevier, Amsterdam.
228. Strik W.K., Dierks T., Becker T., Lehmann D. (1995) Larger topographical variance and decreased duration of brain electric microstates in depression. *J. Neural Transm. Gen. Sect.*, **99**: 213–222.
229. Picton T.W. (1992) The P300 wave of the human event-related potential. *J. Clin. Neurophysiol.*, **9**: 456–479.
230. Strik W.K., Ruchsow M., Abele S., Fallgatter A.J., Mueller T. (1998) Distinct neurophysiological mechanisms for manic and cycloid psychoses: evidence from a P300 study on manic patients. *Acta Psychiatr. Scand.*, **98**: 459–466.
231. Salisbury D.F., Shenton M.E., McCarley R.W. (1999) P300 topography differs in schizophrenia and manic psychosis. *Biol. Psychiatry*, **45**: 98–106.
232. Blumberg H.P., Stern E., Martinez D., Ricketts S., de Asis J., White T., Epstein J., McBride P.A., Eidelberg D., Kocsis J.H. *et al.* (2000) Increased anterior cingulate and caudate activity in bipolar mania. *Biol. Psychiatry*, **48**: 1045–1052.
233. Ashton H., Golding J.F., Marsh V.R., Thompson J.W., Hassanyeh F., Tyrer S.P. (1988) Cortical evoked potentials and clinical rating scales as measures of depressive illness. *Psychol. Med.*, **18**: 305–307.
234. Timsit-Berthier M. (1986) Contingent negative variation (CNV) in psychiatry. In *Cerebral Psychophysiology: Studies in Event-Related Potentials* (Eds W.C. McCallum, R. Zappoli, F. Denoth), pp. 429–438, Elsevier, Amsterdam.
235. Mialet J.P., Pope H.G., Yurgelun-Todd D. (1996) Impaired attention in depressive states: a non-specific deficit? *Psychol. Med.*, **26**: 1009–1020.
236. Vandoolaeghe E., van Hunsel F., Nuyten D., Maes M. (1998) Auditory event related potentials in major depression: prolonged P300 latency and increased P200 amplitude. *J. Affect. Disord.*, **48**: 105–113.
237. Charles G., Hansenne M. (1992) P300 slow potential. Clinical interest in 3 mental diseases and neurobiology: a review. *Encephale*, **18**: 225–236.
238. Shagass C., Roemer R.A. (1992) Evoked potential topography in major depression. I. Comparisons with nonpatients and schizophrenics. *Int. J. Psychophysiol.*, **13**: 241–254.
239. Shagass C., Roemer R.A. (1992) Evoked potential topography in major depression. II. Comparisons between subgroups. *Int. J. Psychophysiol.*, **13**: 255–261.
240. Buchsbaum M.S., Post R.M., Bunney W.E. Jr. (1977) Average evoked responses in a rapidly cycling manic-depressive patient. *Biol. Psychiatry*, **12**: 83–99.
241. Iacono W.G., Peloquin L.J., Lumry A.E., Valentine R.H., Tuason V.B. (1982) Eye tracking in patients with unipolar and bipolar affective disorders in remission. *J. Abnorm. Psychol.*, **91**: 35–44.

242. Gooding D.C., Iacono W.G., Katsanis J., Beiser M., Grove W.M. (1993) The association between lithium carbonate and smooth pursuit eye tracking among first-episode patients with psychotic affective disorders. *Psychophysiology*, **30**: 3–9.

243. Levy D.L., Yasillo N.J., Dorus E., Shaughnessy R., Gibbons R.D., Peterson J., Janicak P.G., Gaviria M., Davis J.M. (1983) Relatives of unipolar and bipolar patients have normal pursuit. *Psychiatry Res.*, **10**: 285–293.

244. Schnur D.B., Smith S., Smith A., Marte V., Horwitz E., Sackeim H.A., Mukherjee S., Bernstein A.S. (1999) The orienting response in schizophrenia and mania. *Psychiatry Res.*, **88**: 41–54.

245. Wolfersdorf M., Straub R., Barg T., Keller F. (1996) Depression and electrodermal response measures in a habituation experiment. Results from over 400 depressed inpatients. *Fortschr. Neurol. Psychiatrie*, **64**: 105–109.

246. Iacono W.G., Tuason V.B. (1983) Bilateral electrodermal asymmetry in euthymic patients with unipolar and bipolar affective disorders. *Biol. Psychiatry*, **18**: 303–315.

247. Williams K.M., Iacono W.G., Remick R.A. (1985) Electrodermal activity among subtypes of depression. *Biol. Psychiatry*, **20**: 158–162.

248. Zahn T.P., Nurnberger J.I. Jr., Berrettini W.H. (1989) Electrodermal activity in young adults at genetic risk for affective disorder. *Arch. Gen. Psychiatry*, **46**: 1120–1124.

249. Gruzelier J.H., Venables P.H. (1974) Bimodality and lateral asymmetry of skin conductance orienting activity in schizophrenics: replication and evidence of lateral asymmetry in patients with depression and disorders of personality. *Biol. Psychiatry*, **8**: 55–73.

250. Myslobodsky M.S., Horesh N. (1988) Bilateral electrodermal activity in depressive patients. *Biol. Psychol.*, **6**: 111–120.

251. Lenhart R.E., Katkin E.S. (1986) Psychophysiological evidence for cerebral laterality effects in a high-risk sample of students with subsyndromal bipolar depressive disorder. *Am. J. Psychiatry*, **143**: 602–607.

252. Khanna S. (1988) Obsessive-compulsive disorder: is there a frontal lobe dysfunction? *Biol. Psychiatry*, **24**: 602–613.

253. Kuskowski M.A., Malone S.M., Kim S.W., Dysken M.W., Okaya A.J., Christensen K.J. (1993) Quantitative EEG in obsessive-compulsive disorder. *Biol. Psychiatry*, **33**: 423–430.

254. Molina V., Montz R., Pérez-Castejòn M.J., Carreras J.L., Calcedo A., Rubia F.J. (1995) Cerebral perfusion, electrical activity and effects of serotonergic treatment in obsessive-compulsive disorder. A preliminary study. *Neuropsychobiology*, **32**: 139–148.

255. Prichep L.S., Mas F., Hollander E., Liebowitz M., John E.R., Almas M., DeCaria C.M., Levine R. (1993) Quantitative electroencephalographic subtyping of obsessive-compulsive disorder. *Psychiatry Res. Neuroimaging*, **50**: 25–32.

256. Volpe U., Mucci A., Bernardo A., Caputo F.M., Galderisi S. (2000) Executive hypercontrol in obsessive-compulsive disorder: neuropsychophysiological measures. *Giorn. Ital. Psicopat.*, **6**: 353–358.

257. Blair Simpson H., Tenke C.E., Towey J.B., Liebowitz M.R., Bruder G.E. (2000) Symptom provocation alters behavioral ratings and brain electrical activity in obsessive-compulsive disorder: a preliminary study. *Psychiatry Res.*, **95**: 149–155.

258. McGuire P.K., Bench C.J., Frith C.D., Marks I.M., Frackowiak R.S.J., Dolan R.J. (1994) Functional anatomy of obsessive-compulsive phenomena. *Br. J. Psychiatry*, **164**: 459–468.

259. Rauch S.L., Jenike M.A., Alpert N.M., Baer L., Breiter H.C.R., Savage C.R., Fischman A.J. (1994) Regional cerebral blood flow measured during symptom provocation in obsessive-compulsive disorder using oxygen 15-labeled carbon dioxide and positron emission tomography. *Arch. Gen. Psychiatry*, **51**: 62–70.

260. Breiter H.C., Rauch S.L., Kwong K.K., Baxter J.R., Weisskoff R.M., Kennedy D.N., Kendrick A.D., Davis T.L., Jiang A., Cohen M.S. *et al.* (1996) Functional magnetic resonance imaging of symptom provocation in obsessive-compulsive disorder. *Arch. Gen. Psychiatry*, **53**: 595–606.

261. Knott V.J., Bakish D., Lusk S., Barkely J., Perugini M. (1996) Quantitative EEG correlates of panic disorder. *Psychiatry Res. Neuroimaging*, **68**: 31–39.

262. Wiedemann G., Pauli P., Dengler W., Lutzenberger W., Birbaumer N., Buchkremer G. (1999) Frontal brain asymmetry as a biological substrate of emotions in patients with panic disorders. *Arch. Gen. Psychiatry*, **56**: 78–84.

263. Davidson R.J., Marshall J.R., Tomarken A.J., Henriques J.B. (2000) While a phobic waits: regional brain electrical and autonomic activity in social phobics during anticipation of public speaking. *Biol. Psychiatry*, **47**: 85–95.

264. Beech H.R., Ciesielski K.T., Gordon P.K. (1983) Further observations of evoked potentials in obsessional patients. *Br. J. Psychiatry*, **142**: 605–609.

265. Malloy P., Rasmussen S., Braden W., Haier R.J. (1989) Topographic evoked potential mapping in obsessive-compulsive disorder: evidence of frontal lobe dysfunction. *Psychiatry Res.*, **28**: 63–71.

266. Towey J., Bruder G., Hollander E., Friedman D., Erhan H., Liebowitz M., Sutton S. (1990) Endogenous event-related potentials in obsessive-compulsive disorder. *Biol. Psychiatry*, **28**: 92–98.

267. Savage C.R., Weilburg J.B., Duffy F.H., Baer L., Shera D.M., Jenike M.A. (1994) Low-level sensory processing in obsessive-compulsive disorder: an evoked potential study. *Biol. Psychiatry*, **35**: 247–252.

268. Towey J., Bruder G., Tenke C., Leite P., DeCaria C., Friedman D., Hollander E. (1993) Event-related potential and clinical correlates of neurodysfunction in obsessive-compulsive disorder. *Psychiatry Res.*, **49**: 167–181.

269. Gehring W.J., Himle J., Nisenson L.G. (2000) Action-monitoring dysfunction in obsessive-compulsive disorder. *Psychol. Sci.*, **11**: 1–6.

270. Iwanami A., Isono H., Okajima Y., Kamijima K. (1997) Auditory event-related potentials in panic disorder. *Eur. Arch. Psychiatry Clin. Neurosci.*, **247**: 107–711.

271. Grillon C., Ameli R. (1994) P300 assessment of anxiety effects on processing novel stimuli. *Int. J. Psychophysiol.*, **17**: 205–217.

272. Dengler W., Wiedemann G., Pauli P. (1999) Associations between cortical slow potentials and clinical rating scales in panic disorder: a 1.5-year follow-up study. *Eur. Psychiatry*, **14**: 399–404.

273. Galderisi S., Bucci P., Mucci A., Bernardo A., Koenig T., Maj M. (2001) Brain electrical microstates in subjects with panic disorder. *Brain Res. Bull.*, **54**: 427–435.

274. Morgan C.A. III, Grillon C. (1999) Abnormal mismatch negativity in women with sexual assault-related posttraumatic stress disorder. *Biol. Psychiatry*, **45**: 827–32.

275. McPherson W.B., Newton J.E., Ackerman P., Oglesby D.M., Dykman R.A. (1997) An event-related brain potential investigation of PTSD and PTSD symptoms in abused children. *Integr. Physiol. Behav. Sci.*, **32**: 31–42.

276. Gruzelier J.H., Phelan M. (1991) Laterality-reversal in a lexical divided visual field task under stress. *Int. J. Psychophysiol.*, **11**: 267–276.
277. Lader M., Noble P. (1975) The affective disorders. In *Research in Psychophysiology* (Eds P.H. Venables, M.J. Christie), pp. 14–44, Wiley, New York.
278. Rabavilas A.D. (1989) Clinical significance of the electrodermal habituation rate in anxiety disorders. *Neuropsychobiology*, **22**: 68–71.
279. Argyle N. (1991) Skin conductance levels in panic disorder and depression. *J. Nerv. Ment. Dis.*, **179**: 563–566.
280. Kopp M.S., Arato M., Magyar I., Buza K. (1989) Basal adrenocortical activity and DST in electrodermally differentiated subgroups of panic patients. *Int. J. Psychophysiol.*, **7**: 77–83.
281. Gruzelier J.H. (1989) Lateralisation and central mechanisms in clinical psychophysiology. In *Handbook of Clinical Psychophysiology* (Ed. G. Turpin), pp. 135–174, Wiley, Chichester.
282. Kopp M., Gruzelier J.H. (1988) Electrodermally differentiated subgroups of anxiety patients and controls. II. Auditory, somatosensory and pain thresholds, agoraphobic fear, depression and cerebral laterality. *Int. J. Psychophysiol.*, **7**: 65–76.
283. Kopp M.S. (1989) Psychophysiological characteristics of anxiety patients and controls. *Psychother. Psychosom.*, **52**: 74–79.
284. Papousek I., Schulter G. (2001) Associations between EEG asymmetry and electrodermal lability in low vs. high depressive anxious normal individuals. *Int. J. Psychophysiol.*, **41**: 105–118.
285. Roth W.T., Telch M.J., Taylor C.B., Sachitano J.A., Gallen C.C., Kopell M.L., McClenahan K.L., Agras W.S., Pfefferbaum A. (1986) Autonomic characteristics of agoraphobia with panic attacks. *Biol. Psychiatry*, **21**: 1133–1154.
286. Segerstrom S.C., Glover D.A., Craske M.G., Fahey J.L. (1999) Worry affects the immune response to phobic fear. *Brain Behav. Immun.*, **13**: 80–92.
287. Hamm A.O., Cuthbert B.N., Globisch J., Vaitl D. (1997) Fear and strartle reflex: blink modulation and autonomic response patterns in animal and mutilation fear subjects. *Psychophysiology*, **34**: 97–107.
288. Filion D.L., Dawson M.E., Schell A.M. (1998) The psychological significance of human startle eyeblink modification: a review. *Biol. Psychol.*, **47**: 1–43.
289. Shalev A.Y., Bloch M., Peri T., Bonne O. (1998) Alprazolam reduces response to loud tones in panic disorder but not in posttraumatic stress disorder. *Biol. Psychiatry*, **44**: 64–68.
290. Blanchard E.B., Kolb L.C., Pallmeyer T.P., Gerardi R.J. (1982) A psychophysiological study of post-traumatic stress disorder in Vietnam veterans. *Psychiatr. Q.*, **54**: 220–229.
291. Casada J.H., Amdur R., Larsen R., Liberzon I. (1998) Psychophysiologic responsivity in posttraumatic stress disorder: generalized hyperresponsiveness versus trauma specificity. *Biol. Psychiatry*, **44**: 1037–1044.
292. Orr S.P., Lasko N.B., Shalev A.Y., Pitman R.K. (1995) Physiologic responses to loud tones in Vietnam veterans with posttraumatic stress disorder. *J. Abnorm. Psychol.*, **104**: 75–82.
293. Orr S.P., Lasko N.B., Metzger L.J., Pitman R.K. (1997) Physiologic responses to non-startling tones in Vietnam veterans with post-traumatic stress disorder. *Psychiatry Res.*, **73**: 103–107.
294. Orr S.P., Solomon Z., Peri T., Pitman R.K., Shalev A.Y. (1997) Physiologic responses to loud tones in Israeli veterans of the 1973 Yom Kippur War. *Biol. Psychiatry*, **41**: 319–326.

295. Shalev A.Y., Peri T., Gelpin E., Orr S.P., Pitman R.K. (1997) Psychophysiologic assessment of mental imagery of stressful events in Israeli civilian posttraumatic stress disorder patients. *Compr. Psychiatry*, **38**: 269–273.
296. Shalev A.Y., Peri T., Orr S.P., Bonne O., Pitman R.K. (1997) Auditory startle responses in help-seeking trauma survivors. *Psychiatry Res.*, **69**: 1–7.
297. Orr S.P., Metzger L.J., Lasko N.B., Macklin M.L., Peri T., Pitman R.K. (2000) De novo conditioning in trauma-exposed individuals with and without posttraumatic stress disorder. *J. Abnorm. Psychol.*, **109**: 290–298.
298. Griffin M.G., Resick P.A., Mechanic M.B. (1997) Objective assessment of peritraumatic dissociation: psychophysiological indicators. *Am. J. Psychiatry*, **154**: 1081–1088.
299. Ohman A., Soares J.J. (1994) "Unconscious anxiety": phobic responses to masked stimuli. *J. Abnorm. Psychol.*, **103**: 231–240.
300. McGlynn F.D., Moore P.M., Lawyer S., Karg R. (1999) Relaxation training inhibits fear and arousal during in vivo exposure to phobia-cue stimuli. *J. Behav. Ther. Exp. Psychiatry*, **30**: 155–168.
301. Canter A., Kondo C.Y., Knott J.R. (1975) A comparison of EMG feedback and progressive muscle relaxation training in anxiety neurosis. *Br. J. Psychiatry*, **127**: 470–477.
302. Weinman M.L., Semchuk K.M., Gaebe G., Mathew R.J. (1983) The effect of stressful life events on EMG biofeedback and relaxation training in the treatment of anxiety. *Biofeedback and Self Regulation*, **8**: 191–205.
303. Raskin M., Johnson G., Rondestvedt J.W. (1973) Chronic anxiety treated by feedback-induced muscle relaxation. *Arch. Gen. Psychiatry*, **28**: 263–267.
304. Soininen H., Partanen V.J., Helkala E.L. Riekkinen P.J. (1982) EEG findings in senile dementia and normal aging. *Acta Neurol. Scand.*, **65**: 59–70.
305. Coben L.A., Danziger W.L., Berg L. (1983) Frequency analysis of the resting awake EEG in mild senile dementia of Alzheimer type. *Electroencephalogr. Clin. Neurophysiol.*, **55**: 372–380.
306. Coben L.A., Danziger W., Storandt M. (1985) A longitudinal EEG study of mild senile dementia of Alzheimer type: changes at 1 year and at 2.5 years. *Electroencephalogr. Clin. Neurophysiol.*, **61**: 101–112.
307. Giannitrapani D., Collins J., Vassiliadis D. (1991) The EEG spectra of Alzheimer's disease. *Int. J. Psychophysiol.*, **10**: 259–269.
308. Szelies B., Gron D., Herholz K., Kassler J., Wullen T., Heiss W.-D. (1992) Quantitative EEG mapping and PET in Alzheimer's disease. *J. Neurol. Sci.*, **110**: 46–56.
309. Szelies B., Mielke R., Herholz K., Heiss W.-D. (1994) Quantitative topographical EEG compared to FDG PET for classification of vascular and degenerative dementia. *Electroencephalogr. Clin. Neurophysiol.*, **91**: 131–139.
310. Dierks T., Perisic I., Frolich L., Ihl R., Maurer K. (1991) Topography of the quantitative electroencephalogram in dementia of the Alzheimer type: relation to severity of dementia. *Psychiatry Res.*, **40**: 181–194.
311. Jelic V., Shigeta M., Julin P., Almkvist O., Winblad B., Wahlund L.O. (1996) Quantitative electroencephalography power and coherence in Alzheimer's disease and mild cognitive impairment. *Dementia*, **7**: 314–323.
312. Penttilä M., Partanen J.V., Soininen H., Riekkinen P.J. (1985) Quantitative analysis of occipital EEG in different stages of Alzheimer's disease. *Electroencephalogr. Clin. Neurophysiol.*, **60**: 1–6.

313. Soininen H., Partanen V.J., Laulumaa V., Pääkkönen A., Helkala E.-L., Riekkinen P.J. (1991) Serial EEG in Alzheimer's disease: 3 year follow-up and clinical outcome. *Electroencephalogr. Clin. Neurophysiol.*, **79**: 342–348.

314. Schreiter-Gasser U.S., Gasser T., Ziegler P. (1994) Quantitative EEG analysis in early onset Alzheimer's disease: correlations with severity, clinical characteristics, visual EEG and CCT. *Electroencephalogr. Clin. Neurophysiol.*, **90**: 267–272.

315. Elmståhl S., Rosén I., Gullberg B. (1994) Quantitative EEG in elderly patients with Alzheimer's disease and healthy controls. *Dementia*, **5**: 119–124.

316. Dierks T., Ihl R., Frolich L., Maurer K. (1993) Dementia of the Alzheimer type: effects on the spontaneous EEG described by dipole sources. *Psychiatry Res.*, **50**: 151–162.

317. Primavera A., Novello P., Finocchi C., Canevari E., Corsello L. (1990) Correlation between Mini-Mental State Examination and quantitative electroencephalography in senile dementia of Alzheimer type. *Neuropsychobiology*, **23**: 74–78.

318. Soininen H., Partanen V.J., Laulumaa V., Helkala E.L., Laakso M., Riekkinen P.J. (1989) Longitudinal EEG spectral analysis in early stage of Alzheimer's disease. *Electroencephalogr. Clin. Neurophysiol.*, **79**: 290–297.

319. Helkala E.L., Laulumaa V., Soininen H., Partanen J., Riekkinen P. (1991) Different pattern of cognitive decline related to normal or deteriorating EEG in a 3 year follow-up of patients with Alzheimer's disease. *Neurology*, **41**: 528–532.

320. Jelic V., Johansson S.-E., Almkvist O., Shigeta M., Julin P., Nordberg A., Winblad B., Wahlund L.-O. (2000) Quantitative electroencephalography in mild cognitive impairment: longitudinal changes and possible prediction of Alzheimer's disease. *Neurobiol. Aging*, **21**: 533–540.

321. Huang C., Wahlund L.-O., Dierks T., Julin P., Winblad B., Jelic V. (2000) Discrimination of Alzheimer's disease and mild cognitive impairment by equivalent EEG sources: a cross-sectional and longitudinal study. *Clin. Neurophysiol.*, **111**: 1961–1967.

322. Itil T.M., Menon G.N., Songar A., Itil K.Z. (1986) CNS pharmacology and clinical therapeutic effects of oxiracetam. *Clin. Neuropharmacol.*, **9**(Suppl. 3): 70–72.

323. Itil T.M. (1966) Anticholinergic drug-induced delirium: experimental modification, quantitative EEG and behavioral correlations. *J. Nerv. Ment. Dis.*, **143**: 492–507.

324. Steriade M., Gloor P., Llinas R.R., Lopes da Silva F.H., Mesulam M.M. (1990) Basic mechanisms of cerebral rhythmic activities. *Electroencephalogr. Clin. Neurophysiol.*, **76**: 481–508.

325. Itil T.M., Murkherjee S., Dayican G., Shapiro D.M., Freedman A.M., Borgen L.A. (1983) Pramiracetam, a new nootropic: a controlled quantitative pharmaco-electroencephalographic study. *Psychopharmacol. Bull.*, **19**: 709–716.

326. Herrmann W.M., Kern U., Rohmel J. (1986) On the effects of pyritinol on functional deficits of patients with organic mental disorders. *Pharmacopsychiatry*, **19**: 378–385.

327. Saletu B., Anderer P., Kinsperger K., Grunberger J. (1987) Topographic brain mapping of EEG in neuropsychopharmacology, part II. Clinical applications (pharmaco EEG imaging). *Methods Find. Exp. Clin. Pharmacol.*, **9**: 385–408.

328. Saletu B., Grünberger J., Anderer P. (1990) Pharmaco-EEG and brain mapping in cognitive enhancing drugs. *Clin. Neuropharmacol.*, **13** (suppl. 2): 575–576.

329. Saletu B., Anderer P., Fischhof P.K., Lorenz H., Barousch R., Böhmer F. (1992) EEG mapping and psychopharmacological studies with denbufylline in SDAT and MID. *Biol. Psychiatry*, **32**: 668–681.

330. Erkinjuntti T., Larsen T., Sulkava R., Ketonen L., Laaksonen R., Palo J. (1988) EEG in the differential diagnosis between Alzheimer's disease and vascular dementia. *Acta Neurol. Scand.*, **77**: 36–43.

331. Martin-Loeches M., Gil P., Jimenez F., Exposito F.J., Miguel F., Cacabelos R., Rubia F.J. (1991) Topographic maps of brain electrical activity in primary degenerative dementia of the Alzheimer type and multiinfarct dementia. *Biol. Psychiatry*, **29**: 211–223.

332. Maurer K., Dierks T. (1992) Functional imaging procedures in dementias: mapping of EEG and evoked potentials. *Acta Neurol. Scand.*, **139**: 40–46.

333. Sloan E.P., Fenton G.W. (1993) EEG power spectra and cognitive change in geriatric psychiatry: a longitudinal study. *Electroencephalogr. Clin. Neurophysiol.*, **86**: 361–367.

334. Besthorn C., Förstl H., Geiger-Kabisch C., Sattel H., Gasser T., Schreiter-Gasser U. (1994) EEG coherence in Alzheimer disease. *Electroencephalogr. Clin. Neurophysiol.*, **90**: 242–245.

335. Dunkin J.J., Leuchter A.F., Newton T.F., Cook J.A. (1994) Reduced EEG coherence in dementia: state or trait marker? *Biol. Psychiatry*, **35**: 870–879.

336. Sloan E.P., Fenton G.W., Kennedy N.S.J., MacLennan J.M. (1994) Neurophysiology and SPECT cerebral blood flow patterns in dementia. *Electroencephalogr. Clin. Neurophysiol.*, **91**: 163–170.

337. Locatelli T., Cursi M., Liberati D., Franceschi M., Comi G. (1998) EEG coherence in Alzheimer's disease. *Electroencephalogr. Clin. Neuropsysiol.*, **106**: 229–237.

338. O'Connor K., Shaw J., Ongley C. (1979) The EEG and differential diagnosis in psycho-geriatrics. *Br. J. Psychiatry*, **135**: 156–162.

339. Leuchter A.F., Spar J.E., Walter D.O., Weiner H. (1987) Electroencephalographic spectra and coherence in the diagnosis of Alzheimer's-type and multi-infarct dementia. *Arch. Gen. Psychiatry*, **44**: 993–998.

340. Leocani L., Comi G. (1999) EEG coherence in pathological conditions. *J. Clin. Neurophysiol.*, **16**: 548–555.

341. Woyshville M.J., Calabrese J.R. (1994) Quantification of occipital EEG changes in Alzheimer's disease utilizing a new metric: the fractal dimension. *Biol. Psychiatry*, **35**: 381–387.

342. Strik W.K., Chiaramonti R., Muscas G.C., Paganini M., Mueller T.J., Fallgatter A.J., Versari A., Zappoli R. (1997) Decreased EEG microstate duration and anteriorisation of the brain electric fields in mild and moderate dementia of the Alzheimer type. *Psychiatry Res.*, **75**: 183–191.

343. Dierks T., Jelic V., Julin P., Maurer K., Wahlund L.O., Almkvist O., Strik W.K. (1997) EEG microstates in mild memory impairment and Alzheimer's disease: possible association with disturbed information processing. *J. Neural Transm.*, **104**: 483–495.

344. Fornara C., Cursi M., Roveri L., Minicucci F., Locatelli T., Comi G. (1998) FFT approximation in Alzheimer's disease. *Ital. J. Neurol. Sci.*, **19**: 211–216.

345. Goodin D.S. (1990) Clinical utility of long latency "cognitive" event-related potentials (P3): the pros. *Electroencephalogr. Clin. Neurophysiol.*, **76**: 2–5.

6

Neuropsychological Research in Psychiatry

Karen Ritchie[1] and Marcus Richards[2]

[1]INSERM EPI 9930-Epidemiology of Nervous System Disorders, CRLC Val d'Aurelle,
326 rue des Apothicaires, 34298 Montpellier Cedex 5, France
[2]MRC National Survey of Health and Development, University College Medical School,
1–19 Torrington Place, London WC1E 6BT, United Kingdom

INTRODUCTION

Contemporary neuropsychological assessment is essentially a refinement of the neurological examination focusing on integrative central nervous system (CNS) functioning. It may be defined as the observation of an individual's behaviour in relation to a standardized stimulus selected for its likelihood of provoking an abnormal response in the presence of damage or dysfunction of specific neuroanatomical structures. Its theoretical basis derives from the quite separate academic traditions of cognitive psychology and behavioural neurology, their integration providing both a quantitative and qualitative approach to the understanding of the neuroanatomical substrates of cognition and to the detection of pathology.

Cognitive psychology is principally concerned with the development of theories of normal information processing and the development of standardized measures of mental processes. One source is psychometrics and the factor analytical school, but more recent influences come from information theory, linguistics and the genetic epistemology of Piaget and his followers. It is essentially a quantitative approach based on an underlying assumption of the normal distribution of human abilities, and thus generates testing procedures that are dimensional rather than categorical, implicitly requiring the determination of a cut-off point for "abnormality". Such a cut-off point is based on improbability (deviation from a statistical mean) rather than reference to a clinical syndrome. Behavioural neurology, on the other hand, derives from the classification of normal and abnormal responses to

Psychiatry as a Neuroscience. Edited by Juan José López-Ibor, Wolfgang Gaebel, Mario Maj and Norman Sartorius. © 2002 John Wiley & Sons Ltd.

cognitive stimuli, in the tradition of Luria, by reference to pathological behaviours not seen in healthy individuals.

On the basis of information processing models of normal cognition and observations of deviant behaviour resulting from localized CNS trauma, it has been possible for neuropsychologists to construct and validate quantitative measures of cognitive dysfunction that may be related to underlying neurophysiological changes. In conjunction with qualitative observations of behaviour occurring in the course of test performance, it has been possible to develop diagnostic indicators for a wide range of neurological disorders. More recently, the development of functional imaging has permitted neuropsychologists to explore directly the relationships between cognitive models and their anatomical location in cortical and subcortical structures and subsequently to use these observations to develop more precise neuropathological screening techniques. For a recent review of developments in functional imaging the reader is referred to Cabeza and Nyberg [1].

INTEGRATION OF NEUROPSYCHOLOGY INTO PSYCHIATRIC RESEARCH

Although both psychiatry and neuropsychology are concerned with the identification of abnormal behavioural patterns, historically there has been surprisingly little interaction between the two disciplines. The development of neuropsychology under the influence of pioneers such as Luria, Reitan, Halstead and Rey began in the 1950s and 1960s at a time when academic psychiatry was moving away from biological theories towards social and psychoanalytical models of mental functioning. While in psychiatry unconscious conflicts and social pressures were given priority over the CNS as causes of morbidity, neurobiologists had begun to question the notion of equipotentiality which had assumed that higher mental functions were diffusely represented throughout the cortex. Thus the way was opened for the integration of early models of information processing derived from experimental research in cognitive psychology. Clinical neurology also provided the cases of highly localized cerebral lesions with their associated cognitive impairments, which became the foundation of neuropsychological theories of disassociation. Neuropsychology thus limited its range of interest primarily to the exploration of neurological disorders.

By the 1980s, coherent theories of localization in cognitive functioning validated by neuroimaging had been largely accepted within neurology. In parallel, the development of efficient psychopharmacological treatment of many major mental disorders led to renewed interest in the neurobiology of these disorders and the neuroanatomical correlates of their associated cognitive disturbances. Cognitive dysfunction was also recognized within psychiatry as a major cause of disability. In a therapeutic setting increasingly inclined towards the rapid social reintegration of individuals with mental illness, the causes of poor judgement, mental slowing and memory disorder and other cognitive disorders interfering with the performance of everyday activities became of interest to clinical psychiatrists and psychopharmacologists. As a result, there has been a gradual increase of interest in the neuropsychology of mental disorders in recent years.

The traditional differentiation of "disorders of mind" as opposed to "disorders of body" which has segregated psychiatry from the neurosciences is disappearing. Increasing acceptance that functions of the mind occur within the CNS has opened up exploration into the biological components of mental activity. Conversely, the potential ability of mental activity to produce changes in neural organization and even gene expression (epigenetic regulation) has stimulated clinical interest in the biological implications of psychotherapy. The association of neuropsychology with psychiatry is, however, relatively recent. Thus, the present overview is principally confined to knowledge gained over the past decade.

APPLICATION OF NEUROPSYCHOLOGICAL METHODS TO RESEARCH AND CLINICAL PRACTICE

Neuropsychology has been applied to the area of mental health with three principal objectives: the identification of underlying neuropathology for research purposes; differential diagnosis of specific psychiatric syndromes; and the monitoring of cognitive changes in the course of treatment to assess modifications in cognitive ability, neurotoxic effects and learning. Attempts to identify, measure and localize cognitive disorders occurring in psychiatric syndromes have largely concerned developmental neuropsychiatric disorders, depression, schizophrenia, obsessive-compulsive disorder, neurodegenerative diseases of ageing and, to a lesser extent, traumatic stress disorders. These conditions will be the principal focus of this review.

Developmental Neuropsychiatric Disorders

This section does not aim to present a comprehensive overview of the neuropsychology of childhood mental disorders. Rather, two important neuropsychiatric disorders illustrate the diversity of this field.

Autism

Autism involves disturbance of reciprocal social interaction, disturbance of communication, including expressive and receptive language, and extreme behavioural restriction [2]. Although autism is frequently associated with mental retardation [3], a more specific pattern of cognitive deficit was proposed by Hermelin and O'Connor [4], characterized by difficulty in perceiving order and meaning in events [5]. Broadly consistent with this are observations which have demonstrated that autism is a frontal lobe disturbance with involvement of the amygdala [6, 7], neuropsychological evidence of impaired executive function [8, 9], and the proposal that autistic children lack a "theory of mind", i.e. ability to understand the thinking of others from the social context [10].

Attention Deficit Hyperactivity Disorder

Imaging studies have shown that some frontal and basal ganglia regions are smaller in children with attention deficit hyperactivity disorder (ADHD) than in controls, consistent with neuropsychological evidence of impaired executive function (see [11] for a review). Although poor performance of hyperactive children on neuropsychological tests of attention has been reported [12], other work has focused on response initiation and inhibition. The rate of inhibition failure in a "go–no go" task was high in ADHD [13], a finding which is consistent with the construct of impulsiveness, i.e. reduced ability or willingness to inhibit inappropriate actions and to wait for a delayed consequence [12]. However, subsequent work suggests that the response style in children with ADHD may be inefficient (slow and inaccurate) rather than impulsive (fast and inaccurate) [11, 14, 15].

Depression

Neuropsychological deficits are now recognized to be a common and significant feature of depressive disorder, resembling the profile of cognitive deficiencies seen in traumatic brain injury [16]. Attentional, executive and secondary memory functioning are the areas principally affected [17–21]. Two different patterns of attentional deficit have been described in depression: distractor inhibition, and deficits in the processing of resources, that is, the central executive component of working memory [22]. Memory disorder in depression is principally due to a retrieval rather than encoding deficit [23], but has not been consistently reported, perhaps because testing is often limited to verbal or visual stimuli, and there is some evidence to suggest the deficit may in some cases be related to dysfunction in a single hemisphere [17, 24].

The association of neuropsychological tests with neuroimaging (positron emission tomography, PET, and magnetic resonance imaging, MRI) indicate dysfunction of frontostriatal circuits, the mediotemporal lobe, hippocampus and cingulate as the principal underlying neuroanatomical correlates of cognitive impairment in depression [16, 19, 25–27]. Abnormal responses to negative feedback are observed in depressed patients compared to normal subjects and those with other forms of psychopathology, which may in part explain the link between mood and cognition [27]. At a biological level, this link has been attributed to interactions between the serotonergic system and the hypothalamic–pituitary–adrenal axis [28, 29].

Not all depressed subjects show the same patterns of neuropsychological deficits, suggesting either a dominant role of moderating variables [19] or the existence of subtypes of depressive disorder. Different patterns of neuropsychological deficit have been identified, for example for major depression with and without psychotic features, the former showing significantly greater impairment in attention, psychomotor speed, response inhibition and verbal rather than visual secondary memory [25, 30, 31]. There is also some evidence to suggest the possibility of a late-onset form of depression linked to cerebrovascular pathology evidenced as white matter lesions on T2-weighted MRI scans. These are associated with a separate pattern of cognitive deficits, characterized by significantly poorer performance on frontal executive, language and secondary verbal memory tasks [32]. However, unrecognized subclinical dementia may be a confounding factor in identifying a specific pattern of neuropsychological deficit in this group.

Neuropsychological tests have also been used in the differential diagnosis of unipolar depression and chronic fatigue syndrome [33], and to measure treatment effects with electroconvulsive therapy [34, 35], transcranial magnetic stimulation [36] and pharmacological intervention [37, 38].

Studies of bipolar depression have been less common. Clinical studies suggest that memory functioning in mania is usually intact and that the principal area of cognitive disorder is in executive function, notably impaired judgement. Functional imaging using PET and verbal fluency tests shows rostral and orbitofrontal cortex activation during manic episodes [39], with poorer performance on neuropsychological tests being associated with small prefrontal and hippocampal volume [40, 41].

Schizophrenia

Neuropsychological impairment is virtually universal in schizophrenia, and is usually evident early in the disorder. Overall, schizophrenic patients perform worse than subjects with psychotic affective disorders [42], notably on tests of attention. Compared to normal control subjects, they are seen to have specific difficulties in the complex integration of stimuli, conceptual shifting, response initiation and inhibition, verbal fluency, ability to imitate, and encoding and retrieval in secondary verbal memory [24, 43–46]. Attention and memory disorders in childhood have been further demonstrated to be significant predictors of schizophrenia in mid-adulthood [47], suggesting that the cognitive deficits precede the onset of clinical symptoms. Attentional deficits and retroactive inhibition are also observed more frequently in otherwise symptom-free relatives of persons with schizophrenia [43, 48].

Cognitive functioning in schizophrenia is seen to be further impaired in the presence of obsessive-compulsive disorder [49, 50], particularly in frontal lobe executive functions, raising the possibility that this group may constitute a separate subtype of schizophrenia. The co-occurrence of depression also alters the cognitive profile in schizophrenia, leading to significantly greater impairment in attention [51]. On the other hand, paranoid schizophrenia has been associated with less cognitive impairment than other forms of the disorder, although these findings have not been consistently supported [52].

Several attempts have been made to relate specific cognitive disorders to symptomatology in schizophrenia. Referring to the three-factor model of symptom complexes of hallucinations/delusions, disorganization of behaviour and thought, and negative symptoms, a number of studies have reported specific patterns of deficit. Psychotic symptoms appear to be unrelated to cognitive deficits, whereas disorganized thoughts and behaviour appear to be associated with lower IQ, and negative symptoms to problems of verbal and visual memory, verbal fluency and visual–motor sequencing [53, 54]. Deficits in verbal fluency have also been observed in conjunction with negative symptoms [55]. The Continuous Performance and Wisconsin Card Sorting Tests (both tests of frontal functioning) have been described as putative indicators for the predisposition to develop negative symptoms [56].

Abnormality on the Wisconsin test is the most commonly reported deficit in schizophrenia, and has been assumed to reflect dorsolateral prefrontal cortex dysfunction [57, 58]. Functional imaging and morphometric studies point, however, to more widespread neuropathology, such that the cognitive deficits seen in schizophrenia are now considered to be the result of dysfunction in cortico-subcortical connectivity with a neurotransmitter imbalance in the thalamic-prefrontal motor cortex and basal ganglia [59].

Obsessive-Compulsive Disorder

Once considered to be related to unresolved internal conflict, obsessive-compulsive disorder (OCD) is now regarded as a model of neuropsychiatric disorder, with complex information processing deficits which go beyond the effects of any associated mood disturbance. Low overall performance on cognitive tests has also been found to be significantly associated with the presence of neurological soft signs [60]. At the neuropsychological and physiological level, OCD in fact shares many of the features of Tourette's syndrome: lack of laterality, bilateral or left frontal lobe dysfunction, shortened rapid eye movement (REM) sleep latency and abnormal glucose metabolism in the caudate nucleus [61]. Studies of children with OCD indicate no impairment differences on neuropsychological testing [62], suggesting that information processing circuits may not be disturbed in very early stages of the illness. It is perhaps difficult, however, to determine the extent of damage in children, given that such studies are carried out before full maturation of the frontal cortex, and in the face of the high neuronal plasticity present in younger brains.

The neuropsychological disturbances of OCD are principally characterized by a frontal lobe syndrome with accompanying difficulties in motor initiation, shifting and frequent perseverative errors [63–65], a profile commonly observed in lesions of the orbitofrontal cortex. A case study described by Simpson and Baldwin [66] of sudden-onset OCD with frontal lobe signs showed in fact low activation in the left orbitofrontal region on single photon emission computed tomography (SPECT). Spatial recognition and spatial working memory deficits consistent with frontostriatal dysfunction have also been consistently observed [65, 67]. Clinical observations of qualitative aspects of test performance by Veale *et al.* [68] also point to frontostriatal involvement, namely distractability in the face of competing stimuli, excessive monitoring and rigidity in tasks requiring change of set. The authors refer to this pattern of behaviours as dysfunction of the "supervising attentional system". Supporting evidence for anatomical localization has come from clinical follow-up studies of subjects undergoing ventromedial frontal leucotomy, subjects with frontostriatal lesions showing the most striking improvement [69].

Visual and praxic memory deficits have been linked by Tallis [65] to checking behaviour, but a subsequent study found a relationship only with symptom severity and not with checking [70]. Motor slowing has also been observed in some studies [37], which has been limited to psychomotor tasks involving the fronto-subcortical system and thus cannot be simply attributed to interference due to thought intrusion. Disassociation on neuropsychological testing has been found between the orbitofrontal deficits observed in OCD and the dorsolateral functions observed in schizophrenia, the dorsolateral prefrontal cortex being apparently spared in OCD [57].

Dementia

Cognitive impairment is observed in a range of neurodegenerative diseases, and neuropsychological assessment is routinely used to document this impairment in detail. However, the rapid growth of the world's elderly population has brought a focusing on dementia as a major public health burden, leading to a massive research effort to understand its aetiology and to generate effective therapies. One particular contribution made by neuropsychology has been to the discussion of whether the multiple diseases encompassed by the term "dementia" are discrete or overlapping entities. An older distinction was made between cognitive function in the "cortical" dementia of Alzheimer's disease (AD) and that in "subcortical" dementia, such as occurs in progressive supranuclear palsy [71]. More recently, Spinnler and Della Sala [72] have proposed an alternative dichotomy of instrumental cortical (retrorolandic) dementias (e.g. AD) and dysexecutive cortical (prefrontal) dementias with (e.g. Huntington's chorea) or without (e.g. Pick's disease) subcortical damage.

A more difficult issue has been the distinction between AD and vascular dementia. Again, there has been considerable debate over whether these are distinct diseases or variant consequences of common risk factors [73], or whether vascular dementia is in fact of valid nosological status [74]. To some extent, however, neuropsychological research has identified a distinct cognitive profile in this disease. This is suggestive of predominantly subcortical damage, and is characterized by cognitive slowing and disorders of retrieval and attention [75] and executive impairment [76], with relative sparing of cortical functions such as those underlying aphasia, apraxia and agnosia [77]. However, comorbidity in vascular disease complicates the attempt to separate neuropsychological features of vascular dementia, neurodegenerative dementias and other pathologies [77].

Finally, neuropsychology has been influential in defining the nature of mild cognitive decline in ageing. To a large extent this relates to normal ageing and is therefore beyond the scope of the present chapter. However, neuropsychology has played a role in the prediction of dementia [e.g. 78–80], as well as an essential part in the formulation of research criteria for subclinical states such as age-associated memory impairment [81] and ageing-associated cognitive decline [82, 83].

Stress Disorders

Stress disorder is characterized by sleep disturbance, emotional numbing and symptoms of autonomic instability, depression and cognitive disorder. There has been some interest in recent years in the cognitive consequences of exposure to stress. This area has received less attention, however, than other psychiatric syndromes, despite a high prevalence in the general population of 0.5% for men and 1.2% for women [84]. This is perhaps because the affective component is initially the principal presenting cause of disability.

In the longer term, however, cognitive disorder may seriously impair reintegration into working life.

Clinical observations of cognitive impairment following adverse life events have been paralleled by biological observations that exposure to severe stress, notably maternal separation in childhood and combat-related post-traumatic stress disorder, leads to increases in glucocorticoids, hippocampal damage and subsequently disorders of memory [85, 86]. An 8% reduction in right hippocampal volume has, for example, been observed in war veterans with stress disorder [85]. Two principal areas of cognitive functioning appear to be affected in stress disorders: attention and organization of sequential stimuli, and secondary declarative memory. As subjects experiencing severe stress have also usually been exposed to physical trauma such as head injury, and are also at high risk for drug and alcohol dependency, it is often difficult for the neuropsychologist to attribute test performance difficulties specifically to psychological stress-related changes in the CNS. Hickling *et al.* [87] have, however, demonstrated that subjects with post-traumatic stress syndrome following motor vehicle accidents have impairment of secondary declarative memory independently of physical injury. Beckham *et al.* [88] have found, for example, significant difficulties on tests of working memory central executive functioning in Vietnam veterans, controlling for drug effects and comorbid conditions.

CONCLUSIONS

It may be concluded from the above review of selected pathologies that neuropsychology has made some significant contributions to the understanding of the anatomical correlates of mental disorders. Such procedures cannot, however, be used on their own as diagnostic tools. This is because of the inherent nature of neuropsychological testing, which is based on observations of the behavioural correlates of localized lesions rather than direct biological markers. That is, from a known pathology it may be possible to specify on which cognitive tests a patient is likely to perform poorly, but it is more difficult to do the reverse, i.e. to predict with any great precision from test results the specific anatomical site of an underlying lesion.

Although specific neuropsychological tests may be recommended for the exploration of a particular brain region or a specific cognitive function, they often implicate multiple functions and anatomical sites. For example, the Wisconsin Card Sorting Test and the Verbal Fluency Test are known to be poorly performed by subjects with frontal lobe disorders, but functional imaging has demonstrated that performance on these tests involves not only prefrontal areas but also the right side of the cerebellum, with significant decremental responses over a large area of the posterior cortex [89, 90].

Within a research framework, neuropsychological tests are best used to describe the consequences of pathology rather than its origins, unless used in the context of functional imaging.

With regard to therapy, the role of neuropsychology has mainly been limited so far to the monitoring of treatment effects and the identification of impairment in specific cognitive systems for the targeting of cognitive therapy. Kandel [91] has indicated a possible future role for neuropsychology in validating clinical concepts from psychoanalysis and thus fulfilling the earlier prediction by Freud [92] that "all of our provisional ideas in psychology will presumably one day be based on an organic substructure". The rapid development of the neurosciences at present renders much of psychoanalytic theory obsolete. However, as Kandel has pointed out, there may continue to be an important role for psychoanalysis at a broader conceptual level. The integration of observations from psychoanalysis with cognitive models may permit the extension of neurocognitive research beyond the exploration of specific clinical syndromes to the scientific observation of complex areas of human mental functioning such as unconscious mental processes and motivation.

The unconscious mind is a central element of psychoanalytic theory and many clinical examples have been cited of the manner in which it may both protect the individual in situations of poorly apprehended danger, and interfere with everyday functioning. Within neuropsychology there is now increasing evidence of the existence of both conscious and unconscious information processing systems. Implicit or unconscious learning is now believed to constitute a more primitive intellectual process governed by neural systems other than the limbic structures associated with the explicit or conscious treatment of information [93, 94]. The more recent association of neuropsychological assessment with cerebral imaging techniques has led to the identification of separate loci for implicit and explicit processing [95], with PET studies implicating the left prefrontal cortex in conceptual priming [96, 97] and a structural–perceptual memory system located in the right occipital cortex being related to perceptual priming [97].

In conclusion, neuropsychological tests have many advantages over the clinical mental status examination. They are standardized, so that norms can be established and the extent of individual variation and change across time estimated with some precision. They also extend the present state examination beyond the identification of underlying pathology to an appreciation of the real-life consequences the pathology is likely to have for the individual. Reviewing the contribution of neuropsychology to clinical psychiatry, Lishman [98] concludes that the psychiatrist has tended to underestimate the organic component of psychiatric syndromes, whereas the neuropsychologist has tended to overestimate it. This comment underlines the importance of placing neuropsychology within a broader clinical context.

Neuropsychological test results cannot be interpreted in isolation, but must be seen against general clinical impressions and more precise biological investigations.

REFERENCES

1. Cabeza R., Nyberg L. (1997) Imaging cognition: an empirical view of PET studies with normal subjects. *J. Cogn. Neurosci.*, **9**: 1–26.
2. Gillberg C. (1995) *Clinical Child Neuropsychiatry*, Cambridge University Press, Cambridge.
3. Clark P., Rutter M. (1979) Task difficulty and task performance in autistic children. *J. Child Psychol. Psychiatry*, **20**: 271–85.
4. Hermelin B., O'Connor N. (1970) *Psychological Experiments with Autistic Children*, Pergamon Press, New York.
5. Lord C., Rutter M. (1995) Autism and pervasive developmental disorders. In *Child and Adolescent Psychiatry*, 3rd ed. (Eds M. Rutter, E. Taylor, L. Hersov), pp. 569–593, Blackwell, Oxford.
6. Damasio A., Maurer R. (1978) A neurological model for childhood autism. *Arch. Neurol.*, **35**: 777–786.
7. Stone V. (2000) The role of the frontal lobe and the amygdala in the theory of mind. In *Understanding Other Minds: Perspectives from Autism*, 2nd ed. (Eds S. Baron-Cohen, H. Tager-Flushberg, D. Cohen), pp. 253–273, Oxford University Press, Oxford.
8. Ozonoff S., Pennington B., Rogers S. (1991) Executive function deficits in high-functioning autistic individuals: relationships to theory of mind. *J. Child Psychol. Psychiatry*, **32**: 1081–1105.
9. McEvoy R., Rogers S., Pennington B. (1993) Executive function and social communication deficits in young autistic children. *J. Child Psychol. Psychiatry*, **34**: 563–578.
10. Baron-Cohen S., Tager-Flushberg H., Cohen D. (2000) *Understanding Other Minds: Perspectives from Autism*, 2nd ed., Oxford University Press, Oxford.
11. Swanson J., Castellanos F., Murias M., LaHoste G., Kennedy J. (1998) Cognitive neuroscience of attention deficit hyperactivity disorder and hyperkinetic disorder. *Curr. Opin. Neurobiol.*, **8**: 263–271.
12. Taylor E. (1995) Syndromes of attention deficit and overactivity. In *Child and Adolescent Psychiatry*, 3rd ed. (Eds M. Rutter, E. Taylor, L. Hersov), pp. 285–307, Blackwell, Oxford.
13. Trommer B., Hoeppner J., Zecker S. (1991) The go-no go test in attention deficit disorder is sensitive to methylphenidate. *J. Child Neurol.*, **6**(Suppl.): S128–S131.
14. Carte E., Nigg J., Hinshaw S. (1996) Neuropsychological functioning, motor speed, and language processing in boys with ADHD. *J. Abnorm. Child Psychol.*, **24**: 481–98.
15. Casey B., Castellanos F., Giedd J., Marsh W., Hamburger S., Schubert A., Vauss Y., Vaituzis A., Dickstein D., Sarfatti S. *et al.* (1997) Implication of right frontostriatal circuitry in response inhibition and attention-deficit/hyperactivity disorder. *J. Am. Acad. Child Adolesc. Psychiatry*, **36**: 374–83.
16. Veiel H.R. (1997) A preliminary profile of neuropsychological deficits associated with major depression. *J. Clin. Exp. Neuropsychol.*, **19**: 587–603.

17. Miller E.N., Fujioka T.A., Chapman L.J., Chapman J.P. (1995) Hemispheric asymmetries of function in patients with major affective disorders. *J. Psychiatr. Res.*, **29**: 173–183.

18. Mialet J.P., Pope H.G., Yurgelun-Todd D. (1996) Impaired attention in depressive states: a non-specific deficit? *Psychol. Med.*, **26**: 1009–1020.

19. Bebio T., Herrmann M. (2000) Neuropsychological deficits in depressive disorders. *Fortschr. Neurol. Psychiatrie*, **68**: 1–11.

20. Kalski H., Punamaki R.L., Makinen-Pelli T., Saarinen M. (1999) Memory and metamemory functioning among depressed patients. *Appl. Neuropsychol.*, **6**: 96–107.

21. Emilien G., Penasse C., Waltregny A. (1998) Cognitive impairment in depressive disorders. Neuropsychological evaluation of memory and behavioural disturbances. *Encéphale*, **24**: 138–150.

22. Lemelin S., Baruch P., Vincent A., Everett J., Vincent P. (1997) Distractibility and processing resource deficit in major depression. Evidence for two deficient attentional processing models. *J. Nerv. Ment. Dis.*, **185**: 542–548.

23. Isley J.E., Moffoot A.P., O'Carroll R.E. (1995) An analysis of memory dysfunction in major depression. *J. Affect. Disord.*, **35**: 1–9.

24. Fossati P., Amar G., Raoux N., Ergis A.M., Allilaire J.F. (1999) Executive functioning and verbal memory in young patients with unipolar depression and schizophrenia. *Psychiatry Res.*, **89**: 171–187.

25. Schatzberg A.F., Posener J.A., DeBattista C., Kalehzan B.M., Rothschild A.J., Shear P.K. (2000) Neuropsychological deficits in psychotic versus nonpsychotic major depression and no mental illness. *Am. J. Psychiatry*, **157**: 1095–1100.

26. Merriam E.P., Thase M.E., Haas G.L., Keshavan M.S., Sweeney J.A. (1999) Prefrontal cortical dysfunction in depression determined by Wisconsin Card Sorting Test performance. *Am. J. Psychiatry*, **156**: 780–782.

27. Elliott R., Sahakian B.J., Herrod J.J., Robbins T.W., Paykel E.S. (1997) Abnormal response to negative feedback in unipolar depression: evidence for a diagnosis specific impairment. *J. Neurol. Neurosurg. Psychiatry*, **63**: 74–82.

28. McAllister-Williams R.H., Ferrier I.N., Young A.H. (1998) Mood and neuropsychological function in depression: the role of corticosteroids and serotonin. *Psychol. Med.*, **28**: 573–584.

29. Van Londen L., Goekoop J.G., Zwinderman A.H., Lanser J.B., Wiegant V.M., De Wied D. (1998) Neuropsychological performance and plasma cortisol, arginine vasopressin and oxytocin in patients with major depression. *Psychol. Med.*, **28**: 275–284.

30. Nelson E.B., Sax K.W., Strakowski S.M. (1998) Attentional performance in patients with psychotic and nonpsychotic major depression and schizophrenia. *Am. J. Psychiatry*, **155**: 137–139.

31. Jeste D.V., Heaton S.C., Paulsen J.S., Ercoli L., Harris J., Heaton R.K. (1996) Clinical and neuropsychological comparison of psychotic depression with nonpsychotic depression and schizophrenia. *Am. J. Psychiatry*, **153**: 490–496.

32. Kramer-Ginsberg E., Greenwald B.S., Krishnan K.R., Christiansen B., Hu J., Ashtari M., Patel M., Pollack S. (1999) Neuropsychological functioning and MRI signal hyperintensities in geriatric depression. *Am. J. Psychiatry*, **156**: 438–444.

33. Lawrie S.M., MacHale S.M., Cavanagh J.T., O'Carroll R.E., Goodwin G.M. (2000) The difference in patterns of motor and cognitive function in chronic fatigue syndrome and severe depressive illness. *Psychol. Med.*, **30**: 433–442.

34. Hasse-Sander I., Muller H., Schurig W., Kasper S., Möller H.J. (1998) Effects of electroconvulsive therapy on cognitive functions in therapy-refractory depression. *Nervenarzt*, **69**: 609–616.

35. Coleman E.A., Sackheim H.A., Prudie J., Devanand D.P., McElhiney M.C., Moody B.J. (1996) Subjective memory complaints prior to and following electroconvulsive therapy. *Biol. Psychiatry*, **39**: 346-356.

36. Little J.T., Kimbrell T.A., Wassermann E.M., Grafman J., Figueras S., Dunn R.T., Danielson A., Repella J., Huggins T., George M.S. *et al.* (2000) Cognitive effects of 1- and 20-hertz repetitive transcranial magnetic stimulation in depression: preliminary report. *Neuropsychiatry Neuropsychol. Behav. Neurol.*, **13**: 199–124.

37. Galderisi S., Mucci A., Catapano F., D'Amato A.C., Maj M. (1995) Neuropsychological slowness in obsessive-compulsive patients. Is it confined to tests involving the fronto-subcortical systems? *Br. J. Psychiatry*, **167**: 394–398.

38. Trichard C., Martinot J.L., Alagille M., Masure M.C., Hardy P., Ginestet D., Feline A. (1995) Time course of prefrontal lobe dysfunction in severely depressed in-patients: a longitudinal neuropsychological study. *Psychol. Med.*, **25**: 79–85.

39. Blumberg H.P., Stern E., Ricketts S., Martinez D., de Asis J., White T., Epstein J., Isenberg N., McBride P.A., Kemperman I. *et al.* (1999) Rostral and orbital prefrontal cortex dysfunction in the manic state of bipolar disorder. *Am. J. Psychiatry*, **156**: 1986–1988.

40. Ali S.O., Denicoff K.D., Altshuler L.L., Hauser P., Li X., Conrad A.J., Mirsky A.F., Smith-Jackson E.E., Post R.M. (2000) A preliminary study of the relation of neuropsychological performance to neuroanatomic structures in bipolar disorder. *Neuropsychiatry Neuropsychol. Behav. Neurol.*, **13**: 20–28.

41. Sax K.W., Strakowski S.M., Zimmerman M.E., DelBello M.P., Keck P.E. Jr., Hawkins J.M. (1999) Frontosubcortical neuroanatomy and the continuous performance test in mania. *Am. J. Psychiatry*, **156**: 139–141.

42. Mojtabai R., Bromet E.J., Harvey P.D., Carlson G.A., Graig T.J., Fennig S. (2000) Neuropsychological differences between first-admission schizophrenia and psychotic affective disorders. *Am. J. Psychiatry*, **157**: 1453–1460.

43. Green M.F., Nuechterlein K.H. (1999) Backward masking performance as an indicator of vulnerability to schizophrenia. *Acta Psychiatr. Scand.*, **99**(suppl. 395): 34–40.

44. Rund B.R., Borg N.E. (1999) Cognitive deficits and cognitive training in schizophrenic patients: a review. *Acta Psychiatr. Scand.*, **100**: 85–95.

45. Weickert T.W., Goldberg T.E., Gold J.M., Bigelow L.B., Egan M.D., Weinberger D.R. (2000) Cognitive impairments in patients with schizophrenia displaying preserved and compromised intellect. *Arch. Gen. Psychiatry*, **57**: 907–913.

46. Riley E.M., McGovern D., Mockler D., Doku V.C., Oceallaigh S., Fannon D.G., Tennakoon L., Santamaria M., Soni W., Morris R.G. *et al.* (2000) Neuropsychological functioning in first-episode psychosis—evidence of specific deficits. *Schizophr. Res.*, **43**: 47–55.

47. Erlenmeyer-Kimling L., Rock D., Roberts S.A., Janal M., Kestenbaum C., Cornblatt B., Adamo U.H., Gottesman I.I. (2000) Attention, memory, and motor skills as childhood predictors of schizophrenia-related psychoses: the New York High-Risk Project. *Am. J. Psychiatry*, **157**: 1416–1422.

48. Laurent A., Rochet T., D'Amato T., Anchisi A.M., Daumal M., Favre P., Bougerol T., Dalery J. (2000) Vulnerability to schizophrenia. III: Importance and limits of the Identical Pairs Continuous Performance Test. *Encéphale*, **26**: 48–55.

49. Hwang M.Y., Morgan J.E., Losconzcy M.F. (2000) Clinical and neuropsychological profiles of obsessive-compulsive schizophrenia: a pilot study. *J. Neuropsychiatry Clin. Neurosci.*, **12**: 91–94.

50. Berman I., Merson A., Viegner B., Losonczy M.F., Pappas D., Green A.I. (1998) Obsessions and compulsions as a distinct cluster of symptoms in schizophrenia: a neuropsychological study. *J. Nerv. Ment. Dis.*, **186**: 150–156.

51. Kohler C., Gur R.C., Swanson C.L., Petty R., Gur R.E. (1998) Depression in schizophrenia: I. Association with neuropsychological deficits. *Biol. Psychiatry*, **43**: 165–172.

52. Zalewski C., Johnson-Selfridge M.T., Ohriner S., Zarrella K., Seltzer J.C. (1998) A review of neuropsychological differences between paranoid and nonparanoid schizophrenia patients. *Schizophr. Bull.*, **24**: 127–145.

53. Aderibigbe Y.A., Gureje O. (1996) Symptom dimensions of schizophrenia: a selective integration of neurophysiological and neuropsychological correlates. *Neuropsychobiology*, **34**: 192–200.

54. O'Leary D.S., Flaum M., Kesler M.L., Flashman L.A., Arndt S., Andreasen N.C. (2000) Cognitive correlates of the negative, disorganized, and psychotic symptom dimensions of schizophrenia. *J. Neuropsychiatry Clin. Neurosci.*, **12**: 4–15.

55. Chen E.Y., Lam L.C., Chen R.Y., Nguyen D.G. (1996) Negative symptoms, neurological signs and neuropsychological impairments in 204 Hong Kong Chinese patients with schizophrenia. *Br. J. Psychiatry*, **168**: 227–233.

56. Suslow T., Junghanns K., Weitzsch C., Arolt V. (1998) Relations between neuropsychological vulnerability markers and negative symptoms in schizophrenia. *Psychopathology*, **31**: 178–187.

57. Abbruzzese M., Ferri S., Scarone S. (1997) The selective breakdown of frontal functions in patients with obsessive-compulsive disorder and in patients with schizophrenia: a double dissociation experimental finding. *Neuropsychologia*, **35**: 907–912.

58. Green M.F. (1996) What are the functional consequences of neurocognitive deficits in schizophrenia? *Am. J. Psychiatry*, **153**: 321–330.

59. Gallhofer B., Lis S., Meyer-Lindenberg A., Krieger S. (1999) Cognitive dysfunction in schizophrenia: a new set of tools for the assessment of cognition and drug effects. *Acta Psychiatr. Scand*, **99** (Suppl. 395): 118–128.

60. Bolton D., Raven P., Madronal-Luque R., Marks I.M. (2000) Neurological and neuropsychological signs in obsessive-compulsive disorder: interaction with behavioural treatment. *Behav. Res. Ther.*, **38**: 695–708.

61. Ko S.M. (1996) Obsessive-compulsive disorder—a neuropsychiatric illness. *Singapore Med. J.*, **37**: 186–188.

62. Beers S.R., Rosenberg D.R., Dick E.L., Williams T., O'Hearn K.M., Birmaher B., Ryan C.M. (1999) Neuropsychological study of frontal lobe function in psychotropic-naive children with obsessive-compulsive disorder. *Am. J. Psychiatry*, **156**: 777–779.

63. Abbruzzese M., Bellodi L., Ferri S., Scarone S. (1995) Frontal lobe dysfunction in schizophrenia and obsessive-compulsive disorder: a neuropsychological study. *Brain Cogn.*, **27**: 202–212.

64. Cavedini P., Ferri S., Scarone S., Bellodi L. (1998) Frontal lobe dysfunction in obsessive-compulsive disorder and major depression: a clinical-neuropsychological study. *Psychiatry Res.*, **78**: 21–28.

65. Tallis F. (1997) The neuropsychology of obsessive-compulsive disorder: a review and consideration of clinical implications. *Br. J. Clin. Psychol.*, **36**: 3–20.

66. Simpson S., Baldwin B. (1995) Neuropsychiatry and SPECT of an acute obsessive-compulsive syndrome patient. *Br. J. Psychiatry*, **166**: 390–392.
67. Purcell R., Maruff P., Kyrios M., Pantelis C. (1998) Neuropsychological deficits in obsessive-compulsive disorder: a comparison with unipolar depression, panic disorder, and normal controls. *Arch. Gen. Psychiatry*, **55**: 415–423.
68. Veale D.M., Sahakian B.J., Owen A.M., Marks I.M. (1996) Specific cognitive deficits in tests sensitive to frontal lobe dysfunction in obsessive-compulsive disorder. *Psychol. Med.*, **26**: 1261–1269.
69. Irle E., Exner C., Thielen K., Weniger G., Ruther E. (1998) Obsessive-compulsive disorder and ventromedial frontal lesions: clinical and neuropsychological findings. *Am. J. Psychiatry*, **155**: 255–263.
70. Tallis F., Pratt P., Jamani N. (1999) Obsessive-compulsive disorder, checking, and non-verbal memory: a neuropsychological investigation. *Behav. Res. Ther.*, **37**: 161–166.
71. Albert M., Feldman R., Willis A. (1974) The "subcortical dementia" of progressive supranuclear palsy. *J. Neurol. Neurosurg. Psychiatry*, **37**: 121–130.
72. Spinnler H., Della Sala S. (1999) Dementia: definition and diagnostic approach. In *Handbook of Experimental Neuropsychology* (Eds G. Denes, L. Pizzamiglio), pp. 689–697, Psychology Press, Hove.
73. Hofman A., Ott A., Breteler M., Bots M.L., Slooter A.J.C., van Harskamp F., van Dijn C.N., van Broeckhoven C., Grobbee E. (1997) Atherosclerosis, apolipoprotein E, and the prevalence of dementia and Alzheimer's disease in the Rotterdam Study. *Lancet*, **349**: 151–154.
74. Hachinski V. (1994) Vascular dementia—a radical redefinition. *Dementia*, **5**: 130–132.
75. Kertesz A., Polk M., Carr T. (1990) Cognition and white matter changes on magnetic resonance imaging in dementia. *Arch. Neurol.*, **47**: 387–391.
76. Ishii N., Nishihara Y., Imamura T. (1986) Why do frontal symptoms predominate in vascular dementia with lacunes? *Neurology*, **36**: 340–345.
77. Boller F., Muggia S. (1999) Non-Alzheimer dementias. In *Handbook of Experimental Neuropsychology* (Eds G. Denes, L. Pizzamiglio), pp. 747–774, Psychology Press, Hove.
78. Masur D., Sliwinski M., Lipton R., Blau A., Crystal H. (1994) Neuropsychological prediction of dementia and the absence of dementia in healthy elderly persons. *Neurology*, **44**: 1427–1432.
79. Jacobs D., Sano M., Dooneief G., Marder K., Bell K., Stern Y. (1995) Neuropsychological detection and characterization of preclinical Alzheimer's disease. *Neurology*, **45**: 957–962.
80. Ritchie K., Artero S., Touchon J. (2001) Classification criteria for mild cognitive impairment: a population-based validation study. *Neurology*, **56**: 37–42.
81. Crook T., Bartus R., Ferris S., Whitehouse P., Cohen GD., Gershon S. (1986) Age associated memory impairment: proposed diagnostic criteria and measures of clinical change—report of a National Institute of Mental Health work group. *Dev. Neuropsychol.*, **2**: 261–276.
82. Levy R., on behalf of the Aging-Associated Cognitive Decline Working Party (1994) Aging-associated cognitive decline. *Int. Psychogeriatrics*, **6**: 63–68.
83. Richards M., Touchon J., Ledésert B., Ritchie K. (1999) Cognitive decline in ageing: are AAMI and AACD distinct entities? *Int. J. Geriatr. Psychiatry*, **14**: 534–540.
84. Kaplan H.I., Sadock M.D. (1991) *Synopsis of Psychiatry*, 6th ed., Williams and Wilkins, Baltimore.

85. Bremner J.D., Randall P., Scott T.M., Bronen R.A., Seibyl J.P., Southwick S.M., Delaney R.C., McCarthy G., Charney D.S., Innis R.B. (1995) MRI-based measurement of hippocampal volume in patients with combat-related posttraumatic stress disorder. *Am. J. Psychiatry*, **152**: 973–981.

86. McEwen B.S., Sapolsky R.M. (1995) Stress and cognitive function. *Curr. Opin. Neurobiol.*, **5**: 205–216.

87. Hickling E.J., Gillen R., Blanchard E.B., Buckley T., Taylor A. (1998) Traumatic brain injury and posttraumatic stress disorder: a preliminary investigation of neuropsychological test results in PTSD secondary to motor vehicle accidents. *Brain Injury*, **12**: 265–274.

88. Beckham J.C., Crawford A.L., Feldman M.E. (1998) Trail making test performance in Vietnam combat veterans with and without posttraumatic stress disorder. *J. Traumatic Stress*, **11**: 811–819.

89. Barcelo F., Santome-Calleja A. (2000) A critical review of the specificity of the Wisconsin card sorting test for the assessment of prefrontal function. *Rev. Neurol.*, **30**: 855–864.

90. Schlösser R., Hutchinson M., Joseffer S., Rurinek H., Saarimaki A., Stevenson J., Dewey S.L., Brodic J.D. (1998) Functional magnetic resonance imaging of human brain activity in a verbal fluency test. *J. Neurol. Neurosurg. Psychiatry*, **64**: 492–498.

91. Kandel E.R. (1999) Biology and the future of psychoanalysis: a new intellectual framework for psychiatry revisited. *Am. J. Psychiatry*, **156**: 505–524.

92. Freud S. (1957) On narcissism: an introduction (1914). In *Complete Psychological Works*, standard ed., Vol. **14**, Hogarth Press, London.

93. Squire L.R., Shimamura A.P., Graf P. (1987) Strength and duration of priming effects in normal subjects and amnesic patients. *Neuropsychologie*, **25**: 195–210.

94. Buckner R.L. (1998) Functional anatomic correlates of object priming in humans revealed by rapid presentation event-related f-MRI. *Neuron*, **20**: 285–296.

95. Schachter D., Savage C., Alpert N., Rauch S., Albert M. (1996) Conscious recollection and the human hippocampal formation: evidence from position emission tomography. *Proc. Natl. Acad. Sci. USA*, **93**: 321–325.

96. Demb J.B., Desmond J.E., Wagner A.D. (1995) Semantic encoding and retrieval in the left inferior prefrontal cortex: a functional MRI study of task difficulty and process specificity. *J. Neurosci.*, **15**: 5870–5878.

97. Gabrieli J.D.E., Fleischman D.A., Keane M.M. (1995) Double dissociation between memory systems underlying explicit and implicit memory in the human brain. *Psychol. Sci.*, **6**: 76–82.

98. Lishman W.A. (1987) *Organic Psychiatry*, Blackwell, Oxford.

7

Neurobiology of Schizophrenia

Francine M. Benes[1] and Carol A. Tamminga[2]

[1]Laboratories for Structural Neuroscience, McLean Hospital, 115 Mill Street, Belmont,
MA 02478, USA
[2]Department of Psychiatry, University of Maryland, Maryland Psychiatric Research Center,
Box 21247, Baltimore, MD 21228, USA

INTRODUCTION

Signs and Symptoms of Schizophrenia

Schizophrenia is an episodic disorder of thought organization and content which manifests itself overtly in psychotic symptoms (hallucinations and delusions), in thought disorder, in cognitive disturbances and in reduced mental activity, including goal-directed thought and socialization [1–3]. These symptoms fluctuate across illness episodes and across the life history of persons with the illness [4, 5]. Symptoms characteristically begin in young adult years, although disease onset occasionally occurs in the very young and the very old. Florid illness continues through adult life. Often symptoms wane with ageing, making this appear to be a disease of child-bearing years [6–8]. The illness is said to present earlier and with greater severity in men than in women, although affecting equal numbers of each gender. Once the disease has begun, recovery rarely occurs; few persons with schizophrenia—perhaps less than 15%—are able to maintain a routine life including daily work, family life and social interactions.

Cognitive dysfunction accompanies overt symptoms, but it is not manifest in all performance domains [9, 10]. Particular mental functions, like attention, working memory, and executive function, are most affected [11]. Routine neuropsychological assessment of attention and working memory is characteristically abnormal in schizophrenia. Although the magnitude of cognitive dysfunction varies across affected individuals, the majority of persons with schizophrenia are affected to some degree [12–15]. Indeed, non-psychotic siblings of schizophrenic persons perform

Psychiatry as a Neuroscience. Edited by Juan José López-Ibor, Wolfgang Gaebel, Mario Maj and Norman Sartorius. © 2002 John Wiley & Sons Ltd.

abnormally on tasks of attention and short-term memory, especially if they have a diagnosis of a schizoid or schizotypal personality disorder [16, 17].

Signs of schizophrenia include neurophysiological alterations, which also affect not only the probands but also their unaffected relatives, to a milder degree. These signs include altered electroencephalographic (EEG) responses to a sensory cue, e.g. reduced P50, P300, and loss of prepulse inhibition (PPI) [18–21]. Smooth eye tracking, particularly the saccadic component, is abnormal [22, 23]. These signs of schizophrenia provide measures which can be objectively evaluated in the illness. Although these abnormalities are not diagnostically specific [24, 25], they can be used as putative markers for the heritable component of the illness nonetheless. Because the markers are manifest in family members, it is thought that they are linked to the genetic lineage of the diagnosis.

Data from several epidemiological studies suggest that the illness we know as schizophrenia may be only the "tip of the iceberg" of a larger group of disorders, variably called spectrum disorders [26–28] or schizotaxia [29]. This larger group of disorders appear to share the cognitive disturbances of schizophrenia, especially the attentional and short-term memory dysfunction, often negative symptoms and neurophysiological signs (e.g. altered eye tracking or PPI), even though not sharing the florid psychotic presentation. Perhaps 20% of persons with schizophrenia-like personality disorders have cognitive alterations that interfere with work and social life and may benefit from antipsychotic treatment [29], although these results are only preliminary. While the prevalence of schizophrenia in the worldwide population is 1%, spectrum disorders have a prevalence of 5%. The combined prevalence of the two is thus 6%, suggesting this is a highly significant illness with regard to overall morbidity and mortality.

Antipsychotic Drugs

In the late 1940s, two French psychiatrists serendipitously discovered that chlorpromazine (CPZ), which was then being used as a preanaesthetic medication, had selective antipsychotic actions [30]. Because the worldwide medical need was so great, the application of CPZ to treat schizophrenia spread quickly [31]. Many chemical congeners and pharmacologically related compounds were synthesized, tested worldwide and speedily introduced for the treatment of schizophrenia. These antipsychotic drugs, often called neuroleptics, modify the florid symptoms of hallucinations, delusions and disordered thought, but have a less complete impact on the cognitive dysfunctions of attention and working memory and on negative symptoms and come with significant motor and cardiovascular side effects. So, although these medicines were initially believed to be cures for the illness, longitudinal follow-up revealed that significant mental disabilities remained after treatment. These disabilities included untreated symptoms of the illness as well as drug-induced dysphoria, mental dulling and parkinsonism. This situation of limited treatment fuelled the search for and the discovery of new antipsychotic agents.

Shortly after the discovery of the antipsychotic action of CPZ, the laboratory of Arvid Carlsson in Sweden reported that the putative mechanism of antipsychotic action was dopamine receptor blockade [32, 33]. Subsequent research from this laboratory and from basic neuropharmacology laboratories around the world [34–36] strengthened this hypothesis. Supportive clinical data have appeared more recently [37]. Now dopamine receptor blockade is universally accepted as the primary mechanism of antipsychotic action. This development directly suggested a dopamine-related hypothesis of pathophysiology, proposed by Carlsson, which posits that dopaminergic transmission or an element of dopaminergic response may be elevated in the illness [32, 38]. This work was recognized in December 2000 by the Swedish Nobel Assembly in awarding its prize in Medicine to Arvid Carlsson.

In 1988, after many years of widespread use of antipsychotic drugs and at least 10 years without the introduction of any new pharmacological treatment for schizophrenia, careful study of clozapine, a mixed receptor antagonist of superior efficacy, revealed that it had a more comprehensive action and a "better" antipsychotic profile in schizophrenia than any other antipsychotic compound [39]. This observation was initially made in groups of schizophrenics who were not responding to treatment [39, 40] and was subsequently generalized to broader patient populations [41]. The revelation that there could be better medications for the treatment of schizophrenia spurred the pharmaceutical industry into developing a new line of compounds with mixed receptor profiles. These new antipsychotics have a distinct pharmacological profile which includes not only $5HT_{2A}$ and D_2 dopamine receptor affinity, but also, variably, blockade of several additional serotonin receptors, M_1 muscarinic and H_1 histaminic receptors, as well as partial agonist activity at $5HT_{1A}$ receptor, and reuptake blockade of the serotonin and norepinephrine reuptake pumps. At present, clinicians have a new generation of antipsychotic agents with equal antipsychotic potency, reduced side effects and, arguably, broader therapeutic profiles than traditional drugs [42]. Although clinicians always clamour for the "insulin" of psychosis, a drug which we do not currently have, these new drugs have contributed broadly to even greater recovery in schizophrenia.

Adoption Studies

An answer to the question of the aetiology of schizophrenia has been sought for decades. The non-biological formulations suggesting demon possession or schizophrenogenic mothers have gradually given way to fully scientific illness hypotheses. The question of the genetic basis of schizophrenia was addressed most compellingly by Seymour Kety and his colleagues in the twin registry studies carried out in Denmark [43, 44]. These scientists compared the incidence of the illness in monozygotic twins either raised together or separated at birth and raised in different environments. The discovery that incidence was similar in these groups demonstrated the power of inheritance in the aetiology of the illness. Subsequent family studies [45] and twin studies [46] confirmed and expanded these findings. Today a clear genetic risk for schizophrenia has been defined. The non-psychotic monozygotic twin of a schizophrenic person has a 35–45% chance of getting the illness him- or herself. While this implicates genetic transmission as a definite aetiological factor [47], it also suggests that other factors influence illness onset as well. Other environmental factors which increase the risk for schizophrenia include perinatal accidents, birth trauma, social stress and second-trimester viral illnesses in the mother [48].

Obstetrical Complications

The concept of a neurodevelopmental disturbance playing a role in schizo-phrenia is appealing, in part, because several clinical studies have demon-strated that patients with this disorder seem to have a higher than expected incidence of obstetrical complications in their birthing records [48–50]. More recently, a similar pattern has been demonstrated for patients with bipolar disorder [51]. Interestingly, it was recently concluded from a study of the $GABA_A$ receptor in the hippocampus of schizophrenics that there is a very broad window of opportunity for inducing such changes. This can be as early as the second trimester [49], during the perinatal period when the maturation of neuronal processes is actively occurring, or perhaps even much later during late adolescence and early adulthood when the prodrome of the illness is actually beginning [52].

Two-Factor Model

Recently, a "two-factor" model of schizophrenia [50] has postulated that both a genetic [43, 45, 53, 54] and an environmental risk factor explain the occurrence of this disorder. Family studies of psychotic disorders have demonstrated two basic patterns of inheritance. On the one hand, both affective disorders and schizophrenia are seen among the family members of schizoaffective patients [55, 56] while, on the other, schizotypal personality disorder tends to be seen in the first-degree relatives of those with schizophrenia [45]. Schizoaffective patients could be a genetically heterogeneous group of patients who carry the genes for both schizophrenia and affective disorder [56], while these latter two disorders may each reflect two distinct patterns of inheritance. An important question to ask is whether any of the post-mortem findings reported to date might reflect a susceptibility gene specific to one or the other disorder.

Among potential environment risk factors, obstetrical complications have been found to occur with considerable frequency in the birthing records not only of patients with schizophrenia [49, 50], but also of patients with manic depressive illness, particularly those with chronic psychotic features [51, 57]. As discussed above, however, non-specific stress during the prodrome of the illness, and perhaps even later, could play a role in the induction of histopathological changes in the brain. Based on these considerations, one could postulate that histopathological changes seen in *both* schizophrenia and affective disorder could potentially be related to a non-specific factor that is common to both disorders, while those that occur in only one disorder, but not the other, might reflect the presence of a specific susceptibility gene [58].

BRAIN IMAGING STUDIES

Modern imaging techniques enabling the visualization of in vivo brain structure, neurochemistry and function have literally opened up the living human brain for scientific study. While brain characteristics from postmortem tissue in schizophrenia have been described throughout the twentieth century, the translation of abnormal tissue characteristics into living dysfunction has been difficult. Neuropathology studies often focus on end-of-life neural changes in an illness, whereas in vivo brain imaging studies can be targeted to persons with early and still active illness. Nonetheless, resolution is at the cellular and molecular level with neuropathological techniques, whereas it is only at a 2- to 4-mm resolution with in vivo imaging techniques altogether, making these two techniques highly complementary. While in other body organs, like the heart, the mechanisms of function are reasonably clear from structure, the brain is more subtle in its translation of structure into function. Determining how brain regions, neuronal populations and transmitter systems form themselves into regional (micro and macro) networks to subserve motor and cognitive behaviours is a daunting task even with the techniques we have today.

Schizophrenia is an illness lacking a diagnostic neuropathology and where functional alteration in the behaviour of neural networks could be the basis for the clinical phenotype. Our knowledge of schizophrenia biology has been firmly advanced in recent years using brain imaging techniques to identify dysfunctional regions and their connectivity. Several regions of human brain have consistently been identified as abnormal across laboratories: (a) hippocampus, (b) anterior cingulate cortex (ACC), (c) dorsolateral prefrontal cortex and, occasionally, (d) the parietal and superior temporal cortices.

Hippocampus

Although there is an overall reduction in brain size in schizophrenia of approximately 3% and ventricular dilatation [59–63], hippocampal volume is differentially reduced in the illness. The magnitude is still not great, approximately 5%, but it is consistent across studies [64, 65] and remains when the volume is corrected for overall brain size [66]. Not only is the volume of the hippocampus reduced, but its shape is distorted as well, with the greatest distortion in the anterior/middle section [67]. The idea that abnormalities in the hippocampus can vary along its caudal–rostral extent, in addition to in its histological subfields, is apparent with these data. In imaging studies of monozygotic twins discordant for schizophrenia, the ill twin inevitably had the larger ventricles [65, 68] and the smaller hippocampal size, indicating an independence of this finding from genetic causes and its probable association with the expressed illness.

Functional characteristics of the hippocampus were reported in early functional imaging studies, even though resolution in these first studies was not optimal. Early it was reported that medication-free, floridly psychotic volunteers evidenced abnormal hippocampal metabolism [69], as did psychotic twin pairs [70]. As resolution has increased in functional magnetic resonance imaging (fMRI) studies, and positron emission tomography (PET) studies have incorporated MR-guided sampling, several interesting, possibly pivotal, observations have been made about hippocampal activity. First, Heckers et al. [71] noted impaired recruitment of hippocampal activation during task performance, along with an increase in baseline regional cerebral blood flow (rCBF). Thereafter, Medoff et al. [72] noted not only that basal activity was significantly increased, but that it was increased in medication-free schizophrenia volunteers, with "normalization" accompanying antipsychotic treatment. Moreover, the increase was present only in the anterior/middle region and not in the posterior compartment, compatible with the previous morphometric data [67]. Still further, in response to ketamine stimulation [providing N-methyl-D-aspartate (NMDA)-sensitive glutamate receptor inhibition], middle hippocampal rCBF was abnormally reduced in schizophrenia and remained unchanged in the control individuals. These imaging findings identify a functional abnormality in in vivo hippocampus in schizophrenia across laboratories, influenced by antipsychotic treatment and localized to the anterior half compared to the unaffected posterior portion. The abnormal sensitivity to NMDA receptor inhibition in schizophrenia is compatible with the idea that the schizophrenic hippocampus has a pre-existing reduction in glutamatergic activity at the NMDA receptor [73]. Because of the extensive interaction between the glutamate and GABAergic systems, interactive changes would be expected, making it difficult to determine whether the primary alteration is glutamatergic or GABAergic. Given that the structural and functional imaging data suggest regional differences across hippocampus, post-mortem tissue examination might well focus on anterior versus posterior differences in the hippocampus, in addition to subfield alterations.

Anterior Cingulate Cortex

Examination of the ACC in normal individuals performing tasks associated with attentional effort have always demonstrated the recruitment of this cortex on a regional basis, depending on task demands. Since attention is consistently noted to be abnormal in schizophrenia [16, 74, 75], the ACC has been carefully examined in the illness using functional imaging. Furthermore, ACC dysfunction with a variety of complex cognitive tasks has consistently been demonstrated in schizophrenia using a variety of functional imaging techniques.

Carter et al. [76] have demonstrated a failure in full activation of the ACC during tasks involving on-line attention and error detection in schizophrenia. Liddle et al. [77] have shown a consistent correlation of expression of positive thought disorder with both reduced inferior frontal cortical activity and increased anterior cingulate activity [77]. Using a novel hypothesis-led statistical technique, Fletcher [78] showed that schizophrenia is associated with failure of ACC modulation of fronto-temporal integration. In addition to the task-associated failure of ACC activation in schizophrenia, a positive correlation between ACC activity and magnitude of psychotic symptoms has been found [79, 80]. Holcomb et al. [81] have demonstrated reduced ACC activation during performance of an auditory recognition task, where performance was matched between the patient and the control groups and all were medication-free. Moreover, although a significant correlation between task difficulty and ACC rCBF occurs in the normal group, this expected correlation is entirely disrupted in the schizophrenia group [80]. In subjects where task performance was equivalent, the ACC was the only brain region where the schizophrenic and normal groups differed. When performance between groups was more disparate, the middle frontal cortex was also included in the area of dysfunction [81]. Overall, across laboratories, dysfunction in ACC activation is apparent in schizophrenia and has been associated with the expression of psychosis. As early as 1987 [82, 83], post-mortem studies had begun to show discrete changes in neural circuitry in ACC of schizophrenics, and subsequent studies extended these concepts to include the GABA [84], glutamate [85] and dopamine [86, 87] systems.

Dorsolateral Prefrontal Cortex

The middle frontal cortex has been studied using MR volumetrics, and results differ across laboratories [88–90]. Even in studies where frontal cortex grey and white matter volume is differentiated, results remain unclear, except for noting the variability and, if reported, the small change. The decrease in frontal cortex neuropil as assessed in post-mortem tissue [91], although possibly a chronic medication effect [92], appears to have insufficient penetration at this resolution to be apparent. However, the consistent reports of abnormal neurochemical changes in this region in post-mortem tissue is impressive [93–96].

A focus on function in the middle frontal cortex in schizophrenia developed early from one of the first observations using a functional imaging methodology. Ingvar and Franzen [97] measured neuronal activity in this region and found it to be reduced. Others followed up on this observation and reported reduced frontal activity, particularly during task performance [98–102]. The abnormality in working memory in schizophrenia and the elegant work of Goldman-Rakic in non-human primates, tying working memory performance to this region of frontal cortex, both gave these early findings considerable credibility [103].

However, several subsequent studies have challenged this presumption of a disease-linked abnormality in the dorsolateral prefrontal cortex. Middle frontal cortical activity is altered with antipsychotic drug treatment: antidopaminergic antipsychotics, such as haloperidol, reduce frontal cortex rCBF selectively in the middle frontal cortex and ACC [104]. Because few previous functional imaging studies used drug-free volunteers, aspects of the early results could be confounded by drug status. Moreover, several studies report that rCBF reduction in the middle frontal cortex occurs in schizophrenia with predominantly negative symptoms, but not in schizophrenia without negative symptoms [69, 105–107]. So, selecting a group of schizophrenia volunteers in whom negative-symptom individuals are over-represented could confound the outcome data. Furthermore, frontal cortical activation can be normal in schizophrenic persons whose task performance is matched to that of the control group [81, 108, 109]. This latter observation emphasizes the need to control for performance in functional imaging studies so as not to confound outcome with performance. At present, reduced activation patterns in the prefrontal cortex can be not only a correlate of schizophrenia, but also associated with antipsychotic treatment, negative symptoms or abnormal performance.

Other Regions

Several other regions of the brain have been selectively studied using various imaging methodologies. The superior temporal gyrus, including the plenum temporale, is reduced in size in schizophrenia [110–113]. In addition, data have identified a correlation between reduction in the size of this gyrus and the magnitude of positive symptoms in active illness episodes. It is not only the functional association between the superior temporal gyrus and the auditory cortex, but the proximity of the area to the medial temporal structures, which has sustained an interest in this area in the biology of schizophrenia.

The ascertainment of a reduction in size of the thalamus using imaging techniques [114] stimulated closer post-mortem histological studies, especially using stereology, in individual thalamus nuclei. Several groups have identified a reduction in neuronal number by using stereology in the dorsomedial nucleus of the thalamus [115, 116]; the anterior medial nucleus has been found by one group to be involved as well.

The inferior parietal cortex was found to have abnormal activation in a preliminary analysis of primary negative-symptom persons with schizophrenia [69], whereas in the overall group of active schizophrenics no signal was apparent from the inferior parietal cortex.

Findings from functional imaging studies will soon be supplemented by data from spectroscopy and ligand binding research. Multiple overlapping techniques carried out in the same set of patients and with concurrent behavioural assessment is the context in which future studies will be conducted. These data provide information on regional central nervous system involvement in schizophrenia, but also on the nature of the connections between different brain areas. Linked studies using imaging techniques and thereafter post-mortem histological studies provide answers to our questions of pathophysiology with their considerable synergy.

POST-MORTEM STUDIES

In the past 15 years, a wide variety of histopathological approaches have been applied to the study of schizophrenia, a disorder with no readily identifiable histopathological changes. The quest for a "neuropathology of schizophrenia" has been given new hope as increasingly sensitive and quantifiable approaches become available. Recent post-mortem studies are now routinely applying sophisticated approaches such as cell counting, immunocytochemistry (ICC), receptor binding autoradiography (RBA) and in situ hybridization (ISH), and are beginning to lay the groundwork for understanding how communication between neurons may be altered in schizophrenia. In the discussion that follows, recent histopathological studies in which various quantitative microscopic approaches have been employed are critically reviewed. As the reader will see, some exciting possibilities have begun to emerge regarding the underlying histopathology of schizophrenia; however, caution is needed because of the preliminary nature of all the recent post-mortem results.

The first section deals with stereomorphometric studies, which have the important strength of providing a broad vista of how the cortico-limbic system may be altered in schizophrenia. Such studies generally have the straightforward goal of determining whether neuronal cell loss is a feature of schizophrenia. However, the path created by the pursuit of an answer to this question has not been a smooth and untroubled one, even though important clues have begun to emerge. In the next three sections, cytochemical results from studies of the GABA, glutamate and dopamine systems, respectively, are used to address the fundamental question of whether there are changes in these neurotransmitter systems and, if so, whether these changes can suggest specific ways in which cortico-limbic circuitry may be altered in schizophrenia. In this regard, an important corollary issue is whether there is evidence of excitotoxicity in the schizophrenic brain. Hopefully, the reader will gain an appreciation of the complex nature of microscopic studies of schizophrenia and the fact that they are themselves in a developmental phase, one that offers great promise for eventually unravelling the riddle of how neural circuitry is altered in this disorder.

Stereomorphometric Studies

In the past 15 years, quantitative microscopic approaches have been used to assess the size of various regions of schizophrenic brain. Several groups have provided evidence for a reduction in the volume of the parahippocampal gyrus [117], entorhinal region [118], the prefrontal cortex [91], hippocampus [119], amygdala and globus pallidus [120]. It is important to emphasize, however, that volume changes may occur as a result of many different histopathological processes, some irreversible, but some reversible [52]. The presence of volume loss does not necessarily indicate that neuronal cell death has occurred. To rule in (or rule out) the presence of true neuronal degeneration, detailed cell counting is required; however, even with such information, the delineation of whether a subtle excitotoxic process may have occurred can be quite difficult. Unlike histopathological studies in the early part of the twentieth century, the "standard of practice" in this field today is to employ blind, quantitative techniques [52]. Almost all of the recent stereomorphometric studies of schizophrenic brain have presented a meticulous account as to how measurements were performed and how the resulting data were statistically analysed.

As predicted by the observation of volume loss (see below), cell counting studies have detected a reduction in neuronal numbers in the prefrontal cortex, anterior cingulate region [86, 121], primary motor cortices [121], the entorhinal region [118, 122] and hippocampus [123, 124]. Like the cortex, the medial dorsal thalamus [115, 125] and nucleus accumbens [114, 126] of schizophrenics have also been found to have a reduced number of neurons. Nevertheless, a reduction in either the density or the total numbers of neurons is also not sufficient to prove that a degenerative process has occurred. It is generally accepted that a "typical" degenerative process, like that seen in Alzheimer's disease, must be accompanied by a "gliotic reaction", i.e. an increase in the number of non-neuronal glial cells that are involved in the removal of cellular debris left by dying neurons. It is noteworthy that several cell counting studies have systematically evaluated whether the density of glial cells is increased in various regions and have found no evidence for a gliotic reaction [91, 118, 121, 127, 128]. While the absence of such a change in schizophrenia provides a compelling argument that a "typical" pattern of neuronal cell death does not ordinarily play a role in this disorder, there is still a possibility that an excitotoxic process may have occurred and may account for the lower density of neurons. One study has demonstrated a significant increase of astrocytes that are positive for glial fibrillary acidic protein (GFAP) in elderly schizophrenics with dementia, but not in those without significant cognitive decline [129]. These latter findings point to the importance of viewing histopathological changes in schizophrenic brain with respect to the entire life cycle of individuals with this disorder.

Our ability to understand the significance of neuronal loss without gliosis has been complicated by the fact that several recent cell counting studies have not demonstrated a reduction in the number of neurons in the hippocampal formation [130, 131] and the prefrontal area [91, 128]. One study surveyed the "entire cortical mantle" and failed to detect a reduction in the total numbers of neurons in schizophrenic subjects [116]. There are many different methodological factors that could potentially contribute to the differences in findings, including the nature of the patient and control samples, the manner in which the tissue has been prepared, the brain regions investigated and the type of cell counting methodology employed [132].

Neurotransmitter Systems

GABA System

The studies of the GABA system described in this section have been designed to provide the information regarding the disinhibitory interactions of this system with itself (GABA-to-GABA) and with the dopamine system. There are many different markers and methods that have been used to study the GABA system, including non-pyramidal cell counts [86, 133], assays of GABA concentrations [134], enzymatic [135] and ICC studies of glutamate decarboxylase (GAD) [136, 137], GABA receptor binding activity [84, 138–140], the GABA transporter [141–145], calcium binding [146–151] and other peptides, such as reelin [152, 153]. These studies have been providing overwhelming evidence that the GABA system is down-regulated in schizophrenia and, more recently, in bipolar disorder. Cell counting studies have indicated that an overt loss of GABAergic cells is a feature of bipolar disorder, but not schizophrenia. Nevertheless, patients with schizophrenia also show a defect of GABAergic neurotransmission, as suggested by the finding of an up-regulation of the $GABA_A$ receptor in ACC [84] and a decrease of GAD_{65}-immunoreactive terminals in the hippocampus of neuroleptic-free subjects [136]. In the latter study, a neuroleptic-dose-related increase of terminals suggested that antipsychotic medications may act, at least in part, by inducing sprouting of GABA terminals. This is consistent with a study showing a marked increase of GABA terminal staining in ACC of rats treated chronically with haloperidol [154].

Other cytochemical studies have employed ISH to examine the distribution of mRNA for GAD_{65} and GAD_{67} [155]. In the prefrontal cortex of patients with schizophrenia, a reduction in the number of cells expressing GAD_{67} mRNA has been reported by two different groups. More recently, a decrease in expression of GAD_{67} mRNA, but not that of GAD_{65}, has been noted [156]. A variety of studies have suggested that GAD_{67} is regulated through transcriptional mechanisms. For example, increased expression of mRNA for this protein has been found in relation to lesioning of the substantia nigra [156], or of climbing fibres of the cerebellum [157], and in response to systemic treatment with kainic acid [158]. In contrast, expression of GAD_{65} [159, 160] and immunoreactivity for GAD_{65} protein appear to be relatively stable [161] and to be controlled primarily through post-translational mechanisms [162]. In the hippocampus, ISH has shown decreased expression of GAD_{67} and GAD_{65} [163]; however, immunoreactivity for GAD_{65} protein in terminals was reduced only in neuroleptic-free patients [136]. Since mRNA for the two isoforms of GAD is expressed by 95% of the neurons in rat hippocampus [164], it seems likely that complex cellular mechanisms may be influencing the nature of the results observed in these post-mortem studies. The fact that changes in GAD_{67} mRNA in prefrontal cortex were observed not only in patients with schizophrenia, but also in those with bipolar disorder [153], suggests that these changes may be related to a non-specific factor associated with both disorders. Interestingly, differential expression of mRNAs associated with the two isoforms of GAD have been reported in relation to both acute and chronic stress [165], although in this case that for GAD_{67} is increased, rather than decreased as it is in schizophrenia and bipolar disorder. A recent study has attempted to model for the effects of pre- and/or postnatal stress by injecting rats with corticosterone [166]. Within 24 hours of the last injection, a decrease of mRNA for GAD_{67}, but not for GAD_{65}, was observed in the dentate gyrus, CA4, CA2 and CA1 of rats exposed both pre- and postnatally. Five days after the last injection, however, the levels of mRNA for GAD_{67} returned to normal, while those for GAD_{65} were markedly increased [166].

We have specifically investigated high affinity binding to the $GABA_A$ receptor complex. Using bicuculline as a selective antagonist, $[^3H]$muscimol binding was found to be increased in the hippocampus [139], ACC [84] and prefrontal cortex [138, 167] of patients with schizophrenia. It is noteworthy, however, that benzodiazepine receptor activity did not show differences, suggesting that there might be an uncoupling in the regulation of these two sites on the $GABA_A$ chloride ionophore complex [132]. One other study had reported a decrease of benzodiazepine receptor binding in the cortex [168], but it is not clear if the subjects in this study were treated with benzodiazepine agents prior to death. It is also important to note that this pattern does not preclude the presence of an allosteric uncoupling in the regulation of the receptor. In the prefrontal cortex [169] and ACC [84], increased $GABA_A$ receptor binding activity has been preferentially found on pyramidal but not on non-pyramidal cells, particularly in layers II and III. This pattern was thought to be consistent with the hypothesis that a compensatory up-regulation of this receptor was occurring in response to a decrease of GABAergic neurons and/or activity. When this form of analysis was applied to the hippocampus, a similar pattern was observed in sector CA1 [139]. In sector CA3, however, the increase of $GABA_A$ receptor binding activity was found on non-pyramidal but not on pyramidal cells, suggesting that a decrease of GABA-to-GABA interactions might be occurring in this sector in patients with schizophrenia.

Single photon emission computed tomography (SPECT) has also been employed in the attempt to study the $GABA_A$ receptor in schizophrenia using specific ligands, such $[^{123}I]$iomazenil for the benzodiazepine receptor. While two such studies have found no differences in patients with schizophrenia [170, 171], two others have found a reduction in this binding activity [172, 173]. Changes in the benzodiazepine receptor correlated with either cognitive impairment [173] or severity of illness [170].

Taken together, there are many different markers that have been used by our and other laboratories to examine the GABA system in post-mortem brains from patients with schizophrenia and, more recently, bipolar disorder. The results consistently indicate that a disruption of inhibitory GABAergic neurons occurs in selective regions of the cerebral cortex. In the hippocampus, however, there appear to be more complex alterations that involve both inhibitory and disinhibitory GABA cells [174, 175] and these changes would probably result in disruptions of the normal feedforward activity of this region.

Glutamate System

Studies using receptor binding autoradiography, ICC and ISH have suggested that there are changes in NMDA, α-amino-3-hydroxy-5-methyl-4-isoxazole propionic acid (AMPA) and kainic acid (KA) receptors in schizophrenia, but these are region-specific and complex. For example, a reduction of non-NMDA glutamate receptors, particularly the kainate subtype, has been observed in frontal cortex [176] and hippocampus, particularly in sectors CA4, CA3 and CA2 [177–180]. In addition to a decrease of binding activity [179], decreased expression of AMPA receptor subunit mRNAs [181], particularly the GluR1 and GluR2 [182], has also been reported in schizophrenia, although not all studies have detected this change [183].

For the NMDA receptor, non-competitive ligands, such as MK801 and TCP, that bind with high affinity to the phencyclidine (PCP) site in the calcium channel, have been employed and have tended to show increases in schizophrenia [184, 185], while other studies have found no differences [186, 187]. Using ISH, one study showed a reduction of mRNA for the NR2D subunit in schizophrenia [96], while another showed a reduction of NR1 mRNA [176, 188]. MK801 binding seems to require the NR1 and NR2A subunits, but not the NR2B or NR2D [189]. It is plausible that an increase of NR2D expression could give rise to an increase of binding to the PCP site, like that seen in schizophrenia. Some evidence suggests that mRNA levels correlated with cognitive impairment [188]. Based on a variety of observations, reduction of NMDA receptor-mediated function has been proposed to play a role in the pathophysiology of schizophrenia [190, 191]. Some investigators have specifically suggested that there may be a reduction of NMDA-sensitive receptors on GABAergic interneurons in the cingulate cortex of patients with schizophrenia [192]. These findings suggest an uncoupling in the regulation of the NMDA receptor, with the NMDA site being reduced and the PCP site being increased [193], like that seen for the $GABA_A$ receptor [140]. Overall, these studies of glutamate receptors in schizophrenia have suggested that there are decreases of the NMDA, AMPA and KA subtypes (for a review, see [194]). It is not clear, however, whether these decreases represent an up- or down-regulation of the glutamate system.

Synaptic Markers

Several studies have suggested that in schizophrenia there may be changes in the expression of various protein markers for synapses [195]. For example, synaptophysin immunoreactivity is decreased in the medial temporal lobe of schizophrenics [196]. This protein is a marker for presynaptic elements, and a decrease is consistent with the possibility that the volume loss seen in some brain imaging studies of the medial temporal lobe [65] might be associated with a reduced number of synapses. Contrary to this view, other protein markers for presynaptic terminals, such as synaptophysin, syntaxin and synaptosomal-associated protein 25kd (SNAP25), have been found to be increased in the cingulate cortex of schizophrenics, while no change was seen in the frontal, temporal or parietal cortices [197]. These latter data provide support for the viewpoint that there could be an increase of synaptic complexes in the neuropil of some cortical areas, such as the cingulate region, but decreases in others, such as the hippocampal formation and prefrontal cortex. Increased levels of growth-associated protein 43 (GAP43) have also been reported in associational cortices, such as the cingulate cortex, of schizophrenic brain [198]. This latter protein has been implicated in synaptic plasticity during early development and is particularly abundant in the cingulate region [199]. Accordingly, GAP43 could potentially contribute to an abnormal sprouting of axon terminals in this region of schizophrenics [200]. It is important to point out, however, that changes in the levels of any or all of these synaptic proteins can theoretically occur in the absence of overt change in the number of synapses. Accordingly, the above findings for synaptophysin, syntaxin, SNAP25 and GAP43 might represent changes that are restricted to the functional regulation of these proteins in axon terminals.

ANIMAL INVESTIGATIONS

Behavioural Paradigms

Prepulse Inhibition and Limbic Filtering

The startle reflex is a complex behavioural response to intensive stimuli that is defensive in nature [210]. An advantage of this paradigm is that it can be used to study a broad range of species, including humans. When the startling stimulus is preceded by a weak prestimulus, there is a suppression of the normal reflex [202]. This so-called prepulse inhibition (PPI) is not a form of conditioning, but rather seems to be a measure of sensorimotor gating that involves descending limbic cortico-striato-pallido-pontine circuitry. PPI has been found to be defective in schizophrenia [203]. Specifically, patients with this disorder show a failure to habituate the startle response and, although this is not specific to this disorder, it provides a useful window into how a complex circuit may be functionally regulated. Defects of PPI like that seen in schizophrenia could involve alterations in the integration of the dopamine, serotonin, glutamate and GABA neurotransmitter systems [201].

Electrophysiological studies in rodents have been directed at understanding how the gating of information is regulated at the synaptic and systems level [204]. Based on this approach, it seems likely that filtering mechanisms like those involved in PPI are quite complex and involve the interaction of multiple limbic regions, such as the hippocampus, amygdala and dorsomedial nucleus of the thalamus [205].

Fear Conditioning and the Amygdala

There are many different behavioural paradigms that could potentially be used in modelling for schizophrenia in rodent studies. Fear conditioning represents a particularly important one, as it measures potentiated startle responses under conditions of stress and provides a window into the activity of complex cortico-limbic circuits. The basolateral nuclear subdivision of the amygdala plays a complex role in associative learning and attention [206]. By regulating sensorimotor gating of the acoustic startle response [207], it probably contributes to fear conditioning, possibly through a mechanism involving its GABAergic interneurons [208]. Discrete subdivisions of this nucleus probably contribute different components to an integrated emotional response [209] and recall of emotional information [210]. Although the amygdala is probably not the actual site for long-term storage of memory, it appears to influence memory-storage mechanisms in other brain regions, such as the hippocampus and neocortex [210]. The amygdala is probably involved in aversive conditioning, while the hippocampus seems to play a role in contextual associative learning [211]. Like the hippocampus, the cingulate cortex also works cooperatively with the basolateral complex in mediating conditioned memory [212]. Overall, connections of the amygdala with the hippocampus and cingulate cortex appear to be necessary for the acquisition, but not the maintenance, of associative learning that occurs when fear is used as a conditioned stimulus.

Working Memory and Prefrontal Cortex

Cognitive psychologists and theorists recognize a type of memory that is active and relevant for very short periods of time [213]. Complex paradigms, such as the delayed response tasks (DRT), involve working memory, and their counterpart, the Wisconsin Card Sort Test (WCST), can be applied to human subjects. Subjects with prefrontal lesions and schizophrenia [99] show pronounced deficits in their ability to perform this task. Accordingly, schizophrenia has been postulated to involve a defect in the processing of information in the dorsolateral prefrontal cortex [213]. This model is consistent with various abnormalities, such as a decreased amount of neuropil [214] and GABAergic dysfunction [96, 138], that recent post-mortem studies have observed in schizophrenia.

Pharmacology

Dopamine

The dopaminergic system has been the most consistently targeted in schizophrenia. Blockade of dopamine receptors can reliably reduce psychosis in schizophrenia. On the basis of this observation, decades of research have been carried out focused on discovering abnormal dopaminergic function in schizophrenia. Other than a few "false starts" [215–217], the bulk of these studies have been either negative or non-contributory, i.e. demonstrating only a drug effect [34]. Still, because of the power and consistency of the drug treatment model, dopamine has continued to be taken as a pivotal player, although perhaps no longer considered singular in schizophrenia pathophysiology.

Carlsson's original construct gradually evolved to include the entire dopamine influenced cortico-striato-thalamo-cortical circuit potentially involved in schizophrenia. Moreover, as striatal pharmacology has become more fully described [218–220] at a systems and a cellular level, the need for a broader conceptualization of the neurotransmitter system involvement in schizophrenia has become apparent. Laruelle *et al.* [37] have used a clever in vivo ligand displacement technique to estimate synaptic dopamine release in striatum in schizophrenia. They have demonstrated increased dopamine release in response to amphetamine in schizophrenic subjects compared to control volunteers, but only in their florid state [221]. This has focused interest again on dopamine regulation in schizophrenia. Yet, most investigators now assume that regional changes in an entire system of neurotransmitters are likely to be involved in schizophrenia.

The recent characterization of a mouse knock-out, one which lacks the presynaptic dopamine transporter protein (DAT knock-out), has provided the field with a genetically altered mouse which is able to model the effects of increased dopaminergic activity and is available as an animal model for aspects of schizophrenia. Because the pharmacology of this model resembles the pharmacology of schizophrenia in several key respects, the link between increased dopamine neurotransmission and schizophrenia is strengthened. Considerable work is focused on additional characterization of this animal preparation.

Glutamate

Because PCP can cause schizophrenia-like symptoms in humans, and its weaker congener ketamine can exacerbate psychotic symptoms in schizophrenia, the idea that schizophrenic psychosis might be due to reduced NMDA-sensitive ionophore activity was proposed and began to be explored. Subsequent studies showing abnormalities in NMDA and non-NMDA glutamatergic measures in schizophrenia tissue (see section on Post-Mortem Studies) strengthen this idea. Some current data suggest that regional changes in glutamatergic transmission in hippocampus can alter function in that brain area [71, 72, 222] and by inference can affect the projection areas of hippocampus, implicating regional limbic areas of hippocampus, amygdala, anterior thalamus and ACC in schizophrenia pathophysiology. Several additional kinds of data from post-mortem, in vivo imaging and cognitive evaluation are consistent with the idea of glutamatergic involvement in schizophrenia.

Based on a hypothesis of reduced glutamatergic transmission at some population of NMDA-sensitive receptors being associated with schizophrenia, two animal preparations have been pursued as potential models for aspects of schizophrenia: (a) the PCP, MK801 or ketamine administration paradigm [223–227], and (b) the more elegant NK1 subunit knock-down genetically altered mouse model [228]. Both of these models (one pharmacological and the other genetically engineered) reduce NMDA-mediated glutamatergic transmission. PCP in its lower doses is a non-competitive antagonist of the NMDA receptor. Because of the behavioural actions of PCP and its agonists in humans, this action has been linked with psychosis generation. Moreover, competitive antagonists at the NMDA site are also psychotomimetic. Therefore, the behavioural and biochemical consequences of PCP administration are taken to be putative models of psychosis (reviewed in [42]). These include PPI disruption [229], disruption of memory and immediate early gene activation/suppression patterns [227]. The NK1 subunit knock-down genetically engineered mouse is viable (whereas the NK_1 knock-out is not). Because the NK1 subunit is necessary for the related ionophore to gate Ca^{++} as well as K^+, membership of at least one NK_1 subunit is essential in the multimeric NMDA receptor for its full function [230]. The knock-down mouse has NK1 expression reduced by over 90%, so it is likely to have NK_1-free NMDA receptors and reduced NMDA-mediated transmission. Since the pathology in this genetically engineered mouse parallels in one respect the pathology actually reported in schizophrenia hippocampus [73], this model has solid face validity. This mouse continues to be characterized and its role in testing theories and treatments continues to emerge.

Anatomic Networks

Amygdalo-Cingulo-Hippocampal Circuitry and Stress

In 1878, Broca [231] designated a rim-like confluence of cortex along the mid-sagittal surface of mammalian brain as the limbic lobe. Comprised primarily of the cingulate gyrus, hippocampal formation and amygdala, the limbic lobe has shown remarkable conservation during the phylogenesis of mammalian brain. Based on this observation, Broca postulated that these structures might be of central importance to the processing of the emotional components of cognitive behaviour. More recently, MacLean [232] extended this concept by suggesting that emotional disorders, such as schizophrenia, might involve abnormalities in the organization and functioning of the extended limbic system.

The amygdala is a particularly important cortico-limbic region that lies at the anterior tip of the temporal lobe. Considered by some to be an "arbitrarily defined set of cell groups", there are nevertheless subdivisions of this region that can be distinguished by their characteristic architecture, embryogenesis, neurotransmitter profiles, connectivity and functional roles. These include an olfactory part (central and main) that projects topographically to other regions involved in reproductive, defensive and ingestive behaviour systems in the hypothalamus, a central nucleus that projects to autonomic centres in the brainstem, and the fronto-temporal system that projects to the striatum, nucleus accumbens, hippocampus and cortex. The latter system is distinguished from the other more "primitive" components of the amygdala by its being a ventral extension of the claustrum; because of this, it is considered to be a derivative of frontal and temporal cortex. While the central subdivisions of the amygdala have projection neurons that employ GABA as a neurotransmitter, thus establishing their homology with the basal ganglia, the projection neurons of the basolateral complex, like those of the cortex, use glutamate as a transmitter.

The hippocampal formation plays a central role in the retrieval of information from memory storage [233–235]. Recent PET studies have examined the response of the hippocampus to episodic memory retrieval [71] in patients with schizophrenia and demonstrated that basal metabolic activity is increased in the hippocampus at rest. The patients in this study showed a significantly higher basal metabolic rate in the hippocampal formation. Under the conditions of low recall, however, there was no change in cerebral blood flow to the hippocampus, while under high recall conditions there was a slight decrease. The fact that the baseline was much higher than in normal subjects suggests the possibility that a "ceiling effect" might have occurred in the subjects included in this study. An alternative possibility, however, is that the hippocampus of schizophrenics may have a disturbance in the relay of information along the trisynaptic pathway, one that belies the overall increase of activity detected under baseline conditions.

Stress appears to play a central role in modulating the activity of both the amygdala [236] and the hippocampus [237]. The basolateral nucleus of the amygdala influences memory-modulating systems in relation to emotionally arousing events (for a review, see [210]). Both norepinephrine and dopamine show an increased release in the amygdala of stressed animals. For the dopamine system, acute stress is associated with a selective increase in the release of this transmitter from the ACC, also known as the medial prefrontal cortex in rodents [238, 239].

The connections between the amygdaloid complex and the ACC may be particularly important to understanding the pathophysiology of neuropsychiatric disorders. Layer II of the anterior cingulate region, where a variety of anomalies have been detected in schizophrenia (see above), receives a "massive" input from the basolateral complex of the amygdala [240]. In a series of post-mortem studies, an increase of vertical fibres was found in layer II of the ACC and the entorhinal region, but not the prefrontal cortex (for a review, see [241]). Since this latter region does not receive an appreciable input from the amygdala, it seemed possible that those fibres showing an increase in the anterior cingulate area might originate in a region, like the amygdala, that projects to the cingulate cortex, but not the prefrontal area [240]. Although post-mortem studies cannot establish a direct link between these two neuronal compartments, it seems likely that the basolateral nucleus and the anterior cingulate region may play an important role in the pathophysiology of schizophrenia and other neuropsychiatric disorders.

Cortico-Striato-Thalamo-Cortical Loops and Central Filtering

Neuroanatomists have known for some time that there is a continuous loop of connections between the cortex, striatum and thalamus. Since the dopamine projections to the striatum are arguably the most abundant ones in the brain, Carlsson *et al.* [242] have postulated that this neuromodulator contributes significantly to the pathophysiology of psychosis and its treatment with neuroleptic drugs via the cortico-striato-thalamo-cortical loop. Notable features of this model include descending glutamatergic projections from the cortex that exert an excitatory influence over GABAergic projection cells in the striatum [243]. This circuitry involves GABA-to-GABA projection pathways between the striatum and globus pallidus that inevitably result in disinhibitory effects converging on the thalamus. Such a mechanism would tend to reduce the filtering of sensory information passing through the thalamus to the cortex, although there are also parallel relays that would result in an overall increase of inhibitory inputs and therefore filtering activity in the thalamus. PPI is thought to involve the nucleus accumbens, a ventral subdivision of the corpus striatum [205], suggesting that more limbic components of the basal ganglia may be the more precise components of this circuitry involved in schizophrenia. In any case, the cortico-striato-thalamo-cortical loop is a very complex circuit that offers a multitude of mechanisms as possible drug targets in schizophrenia.

THE NEURODEVELOPMENTAL HYPOTHESIS

Disturbances of Cell Migration

The findings of a variety of changes in layer II of the anterior cingulate and prefrontal cortices suggested the possibility that there might be a disturbance in the migration of neurons in the developing cortex of subjects with schizophrenia [244]. To investigate this possibility further, the distribution of nicotinamide adenine dinucleotide phosphate (NADPH) diaphorase was examined in the prefrontal cortex of normal controls and schizophrenics [93]. The results demonstrated a significantly higher density of cells showing this marker in the subcortical white matter than in the cortical mantle [245]. Of significance to the current discussion is the fact that NADPH diaphorase has been co-localized to subpopulations of interneurons that are GABAergic in nature [246–254].

Reelin and Cortical Lamination

Another line of investigation that has pointed to a possible neurodevelopmental mechanism playing a role in the pathophysiology of schizophrenia has come from studies of reelin, a protein extracted from the Reeler mouse mutant. Reelin is believed to be secreted by a subclass of interneurons called

Cajal-Retzius cells that may be GABAergic in nature [255, 256]. These neurons are the first to appear and are localized in layer I [257]. During early development of the cortex, they interact with Martinotti cells in deeper laminae and may play a role in the formation of laminar patterns [257]. In both schizophrenia and bipolar disorder, reelin and GAD_{67} mRNA have been found to be decreased in layer I and, to a lesser extent, layer II [152]. These latter findings are consistent with both a cell counting study [86] and high-resolution analyses of $GABA_A$ receptor binding activity [169] showing preferential changes in layer II of the prefrontal cortex. The authors of these studies propose that a down-regulation of reelin expression in this region of schizophrenic and bipolar brain may be due to either a genetic or an epigenetic factor. Since this protein is reduced in both schizophrenia and bipolar disorder, it seems more likely that the changes noted might be related to an environmental factor common to both. In this regard, it is noteworthy that obstetrical complications have been found to occur in both schizophrenia [49] and bipolar disorder [51, 57], making it plausible that an insult early in life could influence the expression of this protein during adulthood.

Postnatal Ingrowth of Extrinsic Afferents

Important questions regarding the role of a neurodevelopmental disturbance in the induction of altered phenotypes of GABA cells are when and how such changes become manifest during the life cycle in individuals who carry the susceptibility genes for schizophrenia and bipolar disorder. One possibility is that the GABA cells are abnormal from birth; however, the clinical observation that most subjects with schizophrenia are relatively normal during childhood and early adolescence argues against this possibility. It is important to emphasize, however, that studies in rat suggest that the cortical GABA system continues to develop until the equivalent of early adolescence [258–262]. Taking these observations together, a second possibility is that the GABA cells are relatively normal during childhood when they are also relatively immature, but become abnormal as their maturation process is completed. A vulnerability gene or genes associated with schizophrenia or bipolar disorder could initiate such a change. In this latter case, it would be assumed that both disorders would share common genes and these would be capable of altering the normal functioning of GABA cells. A third possibility is that the GABA cells are either relatively normal or abnormal during childhood, but their activity is quiescent as they await the ingrowth of an extrinsic fibre system, such as the dopaminergic afferents to the medial prefrontal cortex [263, 264]. These latter fibres continue forming increased numbers of appositions with GABAergic interneurons until the early adult period [265].

Influence of Pre- and Postnatal Stress

The role of stress in the induction of changes in the cortical GABA system in schizophrenia and bipolar disorder is an interesting issue to explore. For example, glucocorticoid hormones have the ability to bind to the $GABA_A$ receptor [266] and have been found to directly increase its activity [267, 268]. In this regard, it is noteworthy that the binding of [^{3}H]corticosterone is greatest in sector CA2 [269, 270], where schizophrenics and bipolars both show a marked decrease of non-pyramidal neurons and the largest increase of $GABA_A$ receptor binding (see above). It is important to point out, however, that stress is believed to *increase* rather than decrease the activity of the GABA system [272–274], although it is possible that chronic stress, particularly when preceded by stress in utero, might result in an eventual decrease in the activity of this transmitter system. This possibility is particularly intriguing when the marked sensitivity of GABAergic neurons to excitotoxic injury [275] is taken into account. It is believed that cell death in this setting probably requires both an increase of excitatory activity and an increased release of glucocorticoid hormone [276].

Another important component to the stress response is the increased release of dopamine that occurs in the medial prefrontal cortex [238, 239]. Relevant to this discussion is the fact that an increase of dopamine varicosities forming appositions with GABAergic interneurons has been induced by exposing rats both pre- and postnatally to stress-related doses of corticosterone [87]. Thus, it is possible that the postnatal maturation of GABA cells in the cortex may be normally influenced by the ingrowth of dopamine fibres, but abnormally affected when this occurs in individuals for whom pre- and postnatal stress are comorbid factors. In this latter case, it would have to be assumed that any gene or genes involving the dopamine system and perhaps also cortical GABA cells would be affected by prenatal exposure to stress and would be permanently sensitized in such individuals.

CONCLUSIONS

It should be evident from the above discussion that the past 20 years have produced an exponential growth in our understanding of the pathophysiology of schizophrenia. The availability of increasingly sophisticated brain imaging and molecular approaches have made it possible to investigate the structure and function of the human brain under both normal and abnormal conditions. So, what have we learned about schizophrenia? Although the genetic component of this disorder has remained elusive, brain imaging studies have demonstrated that schizophrenia probably involves multiple brain regions, including the prefrontal region, anterior cingulate cortex, hippocampus and amygdala. Post-mortem studies are suggesting that superficial layers of these cortical areas and sectors CA4, CA3 and CA2, but not CA1, show more prominent, though not exclusive, changes in schizophrenia. There is not as yet a consensus as to whether the metabolism in these various regions is over- or underactive, and there continues to be conflicting evidence as to whether the glutamate system is up- or down-regulated. There is, however, a growing consensus that GABAergic inter-neurons within the cortico-limbic system are probably unable to provide sufficient amounts of inhibitory modulation to excitatory projection neurons and possibly also to other GABA cells in the hippocampal formation.

REFERENCES

1. Sartorius N., Shapiro R., Jablensky A. (1974) The international pilot study of schizophrenia. *Schizophr. Bull.*, **11**: 21–34.
2. Andreasen N.C., Grove W.M. (1986) Thought, language, and communication in schizophrenia: diagnosis and prognosis. *Schizophr. Bull.*, **12**: 348–359.
3. Carpenter W.T. Jr., Buchanan R.W. (1994) Schizophrenia. *N. Engl. J. Med.*, **330**: 681–690.
4. Ciompi L., Muller C. (1976) *Lebenslauf und Alter der Schizophrenen. Eine katamnestische Langzeitstudie bis ins Senium.* Springer, Berlin.
5. Bleuler M. (1978) *The Schizophrenic Disorders: Long-Term Patient and Family Studies*, Yale University Press, New Haven.
6. Tsuang M.T., Woolson R.F., Fleming J.A. (1979) Long-term outcome of major psychoses. I. Schizophrenia and affective disorders compared with psychiatrically symptom-free surgical conditions. *Arch. Gen. Psychiatry*, **36**: 1295–1301.
7. Harding C.M., Brooks G.W., Ashikaga T., Strauss J.S., Breier A. (1987) The Vermont longitudinal study of persons with severe mental illness. II: Long-term outcome of subjects who retrospectively met DSM-III criteria for schizophrenia. *Am. J. Psychiatry*, **144**: 727–735.
8. Harding C.M., Brooks G.W., Ashikaga T., Strauss J.S., Breier A. (1987) The Vermont longitudinal study of persons with severe mental illness, I: Methodology, study sample, and overall status 32 years later. *Am. J. Psychiatry*, **144**: 718–726.
9. Goldberg T.E., Gold J.M., Greenberg R., Griffin S., Schulz S.C., Pickar D., Kleinman J.E., Weinberger D.R. (1993) Contrasts between patients with affective disorders and patients with schizophrenia on a neuropsychological test battery. *Am. J. Psychiatry*, **150**: 1355–1362.
10. Chapman L.J., Chapman J.P., Kwapil T.R., Eckblad M., Zinser M.C. (1994) Putatively psychosis-prone subjects 10 years later. *J. Abnorm. Psychol.*, **103**: 171–183.
11. Green M.F. (1996) What are the functional consequences of neurocognitive deficits in schizophrenia? *Am. J. Psychiatry*, **153**: 321–330.
12. Cornblatt B.A., Erlenmeyer-Kimling L. (1985) Global attentional deviance as a marker of risk for schizophrenia: specificity and predictive validity. *J. Abnorm. Psychol.*, **94**: 470–486.
13. Cornblatt B.A., Lenzenweger M.F., Erlenmeyer-Kimling L. (1989) The continuous performance test, identical pairs version: II. Contrasting attentional profiles in schizophrenic and depressed patients. *Psychiatry Res.*, **29**: 65–85.

14. Braff D.L., Heaton R., Kuck J., Cullum M., Moranville J., Grant I., Zisook S. (1991) The generalized pattern of neuropsychological deficits in outpatients with chronic schizophrenia with heterogeneous Wisconsin Card Sorting Test results. *Arch. Gen. Psychiatry*, **48**: 891–898.
15. Braff D.L. (1993) Information processing and attention dysfunctions in schizophrenia. *Schizophr. Bull.*, **19**: 233–259.
16. Goldberg T.E., Ragland J.D., Torrey E.F., Gold J.M., Bigelow L.B., Weinberger D.R. (1990) Neuropsychological assessment of monozygotic twins discordant for schizophrenia. *Arch. Gen. Psychiatry*, **47**: 1066–1072.
17. Cannon T., Zorrila L., Shtasel D., Gur R.E., Gur R.C., Marco E., Moberg P., Price A. (1994) Neuropsychological functioning in siblings discordant for schizophrenia and healthy volunteers. *Arch. Gen. Psychiatry*, **51**: 651–661.
18. Pfefferbaum A., Wenegrat B.G., Ford J.M., Roth W.T., Kopell B.S. (1984) Clinical application of the P3 component of event-related potentials. II. Dementia, depression and schizophrenia. *Electroencephalogr. Clin. Neurophysiol.*, **59**: 104–124.
19. Blackwood D.H., St. Clair D.M., Muir W.J., Duffy J.C. (1991) Auditory P300 and eye tracking dysfunction in schizophrenic pedigrees. *Arch. Gen. Psychiatry*, **48**: 899–909.
20. Javitt D.C., Steinschneider M., Schroeder C.E., Arezzo J.C. (1996) Role of cortical N-methyl-D-aspartate receptors in auditory sensory memory and mismatch negativity generation: implications for schizophrenia. *Proc. Natl. Acad. Sci. USA*, **93**: 11 962–11 967.
21. Braff D.L., Swerdlow N.R., Geyer M.A. (1999) Symptom correlates of prepulse inhibition deficits in male schizophrenic patients. *Am. J. Psychiatry*, **156**: 596–602.
22. Holzman P.S., Solomon C.M., Levin S., Waternaux C.S. (1984) Pursuit eye movement dysfunctions in schizophrenia. Family evidence for specificity. *Arch. Gen. Psychiatry*, **41**: 136–139.
23. Clementz B.A., Sweeney J.A., Hirt M., Haas G. (1990) Pursuit gain and saccadic intrusions in first-degree relatives of probands with schizophrenia. *J. Abnorm. Psychol.*, **99**: 327–335.
24. Thaker G.K., Ross D.E., Buchanan R.W., Moran M.J., Lahti A., Kim C.E., Medoff D. (1996) Does pursuit abnormality in schizophrenia represent a deficit in the predictive mechanism? *Psychiatry Res.*, **59**: 221–237.
25. Thaker G.K., Ross D.E., Cassady S.L., Adami H.M., LaPorte D., Medoff D.R., Lahti A. (1998) Smooth pursuit eye movements to extraretinal motion signals: deficits in relatives of patients with schizophrenia. *Arch. Gen. Psychiatry*, **55**: 830–836.
26. Siever L.J., Gunderson J.G. (1983) The search for a schizotypal personality: historical origins and current status. *Compr. Psychiatry*, **24**: 199–212.
27. Thaker G.K., Adami H., Moran M., Lahti A.C., Cassady S.L. (1993) Psychiatric illnesses in families of subjects with schizophrenia-spectrum personality disorders: high morbidity risks for unspecified functional psychoses and schizophrenia. *Am. J. Psychiatry*, **150**: 66–71.
28. Kendler K.S., Neale M.C., Walsh D. (1995) Evaluating the spectrum concept of schizophrenia in the Roscommon Family Study. *Am. J. Psychiatry*, **152**: 749–754.
29. Tsuang M.T., Stone W.S., Seidman L.J., Faraone S.V., Zimmet S., Wojcik J., Kelleher J.P., Green A.I. (1999) Treatment of nonpsychotic relatives of patients with schizophrenia: four case studies. *Biol. Psychiatry*, **45**: 1412–1418.
30. Delay J., Deniker P. (1952) 38 cas de psychoses traités par la cure prolongée et continue de 4500 RP. In *Comptes-Rendus du Ième Congrès des Aliénistes et Neurologistes de Langue Française*, Luxembourg, July 21–27, pp. 503–513, Masson, Paris.

31. Davis J.M. (1969) Review of antipsychotic drug literature. In *Diagnosis and Drug Treatment of Psychiatric Disorders* (Eds D.F. Klein, J.M. Davis), pp. 52–138, Williams and Wilkins, Baltimore.

32. Carlsson A., Lindquist L. (1963) Effect of chlorpromazine or haloperidol on formation of 3-methoxytyramine and normetanephrine in mouse brain. *Acta Pharmacol. Toxicol.*, **20**: 140–145.

33. Anden N.E., Butcher S.G., Corrodi H., Fuxe K., Ungerstedt U. (1970) Receptor activity and turnover of dopamine and noradrenaline after neuroleptics. *Eur. J. Pharmacol.*, **11**: 303–314.

34. Snyder S.H. (1972) Catecholamines in the brain as mediators of amphetamine psychosis. *Arch. Gen. Psychiatry*, **27**: 169–179.

35. Creese I. (1976) Dopamine receptor binding predicts clinical and pharmacological potencies of antischizophrenic drugs. *Science*, **192**: 481–483.

36. Sweeney J., Haas G., Shuhua L. (1992) Neuropsychological and eye movement abnormalities in first-episode and chronic schizophrenia. *Schizophr. Bull.*, **18**: 283–293.

37. Laruelle M., Abi-Dargham A., van Dyck C.H., Gil R., D'Souza C.D., Erdos J., McCance E., Rosenblatt W., Zoghbi S.S., Baldwin R.M. *et al.* (1996) Single photon emission computerized tomography imaging of amphetamine-induced dopamine release in drug-free schizophrenic subjects. *Proc. Natl. Acad. Sci. USA*, **93**: 235–240.

38. Carlsson A. (1975) Receptor mediated control of dopamine metabolism. In *Pre- and Postsynaptic Receptors* (Eds E. Usdin, W.E. Bunney), pp. 49–65, Dekker, New York.

39. Kane J., Honigfeld G., Singer J., Meltzer H. (1988) Clozapine for the treatment-resistant schizophrenic. A double-blind comparison with chlorpromazine. *Arch. Gen. Psychiatry*, **45**: 789–796.

40. Conley R.R., Tamminga C.A., Beasley C. (1997) Olanzapine versus chlorpromazine in therapy-refractory schizophrenia. *Schizophr. Res.*, **24**: 190.

41. Kane J.M. (1999) Management strategies for the treatment of schizophrenia. *J. Clin. Psychiatry*, **60**(Suppl. 12): 13–17.

42. Tamminga C.A. (1998) Principles of the pharmacology of schizophrenia. In *Neurobiology of Psychiatric Disorders* (Ed. B.S. Bunney), pp. 272–285, Oxford Univeristy Press, New York.

43. Kety S., Rosenthal D., Wender P., Schulsinger F. (1968) The type and prevalence of mental illness in the biological and adoptive families, of adopted schizophrenics. In *The Transmission of Schizophrenia* (Eds D. Rosenthal, S. Kety), pp. 25–37, Pergamon Press, Oxford.

44. Kety S.S., Rosenthal D., Wender P.H., Schulsinger F., Jacobsen B. (1976) Mental illness in the biological and adoptive families of adopted individuals who have become schizophrenic. *Behav. Genet.*, **6**: 219–225.

45. Kendler K.S., Gruenberg A., Tsuang M.T. (1985) Psychiatric illness in first-degree relatives of schizophrenic and surgical control patients. *Arch. Gen. Psychiatry*, **42**: 770–779.

46. Kendler K.S. (1985) A twin study of individuals with both schizophrenia and alcoholism. *Br. J. Psychiatry*, **147**: 48–53.

47. Kendler K.S., Diehl S.R. (1993) The genetics of schizophrenia: a current, genetic-epidemiologic perspective. *Schizophr. Bull.*, **19**: 261–285.

48. Lewis S.W., Murray R.M. (1987) Obstetric complications, neurodevelopmental deviance, and risk of schizophrenia. *J. Psychiatr. Res.*, **21**: 413–421.

49. Jacobsen B., Kinney D.K. (1980) Perinatal complications in adopted and non-adopted schizophrenics and their controls: preliminary results. *Acta Psychiatr. Scand.*, **238**: 103–123.
50. Parnas J., Schulsinger F., Teasdale W., Schulsinger H., Feldman P.M., Mednick S.A. (1982) Perinatal complications and clinical outcome. *Br. J. Psychiatry*, **140**: 416–420.
51. Kinney D.K., Yurgelun-Todd D.A., Tohen M., Tramer S. (1998) Pre- and peri-natal complications and risk for bipolar disorder: a retrospective study. *J. Affect. Disord.* **50**: 117–124.
52. Benes F.M. (1988) Post-mortem structural analyses of schizophrenic brain: study designs and the interpretation of data. *Psychiatr. Dev.*, **6**: 213–226.
53. Gottesman I.I., Shields J. (1972) *Schizophrenia and Genetics: A Twin Study Vantage Point*, Academic Press, New York.
54. Kety S. (1983) Mental illness in the biological and adoptive relatives of schizophrenic adoptees: findings relevant to genetic and environmental factors in etiology. *Am. J. Psychiatry*, **140**: 720–727.
55. Fowler R.C. (1978) Remitting schizophrenia as a variant of affective disorder. *Schizophr. Bull.*, **4**: 68–77.
56. Levitt J.J., Tsuang M.T. (1988) The heterogeneity of schizoaffective disorder: implications for treatment. *Am. J. Psychiatry*, **145**: 926–936.
57. Kinney D.K., Yurgelun-Todd D.A., Levy D.L., Medoff D., Lajonchere C.M., Radford-Paregol M. (1993) Obstetrical complications in patients with bipolar disorder and their siblings. *Psychiatry Res.*, **48**: 47–56.
58. Benes F.M. (1995) A neurodevelopmental approach to the understanding of schizophrenia and other mental disorders. In *Developmental Psychopathology*, Vol. 1 (Eds D. Cicchetti, D.J. Cohen), pp. 227–253, Wiley, New York.
59. Johnstone E.C., Crow T.J., Frith C.D., Husband J., Kreel L. (1976) Cerebral ventricular size and cognitive impairment in chronic schizophrenia. *Lancet*, **2**: 924–926.
60. Shelton R.C., Weinberger D.R. (1987) Brain morphology in schizophrenia. In *Psychopharmacology: The Third Generation of Progress* (Eds H.Y. Meltzer), pp. 773–781, Raven Press, New York.
61. Daniel D.G., Goldberg T.E., Gibbons R.D., Weinberger D.R. (1991) Lack of a bimodal distribution of ventricular size in schizophrenia: a Gaussian mixture analysis of 1056 cases and controls. *Biol. Psychiatry*, **30**: 887–903.
62. Van Horn J.D., McManus I.C. (1992) Ventricular enlargement in schizophrenia. A meta-analysis of studies of the ventricle:brain ratio (VBR). *Br. J. Psychiatry*, **160**: 687–697.
63. Lawrie S.M., Abukmeil S.S. (1998) Brain abnormality in schizophrenia. A systematic and quantitative review of volumetric magnetic resonance imaging studies. *Br. J. Psychiatry*, **172**: 110–120.
64. Bogerts B., Ashtari M., Degreef G., Alvir J.M., Bilder R.M., Lieberman J.A. (1990) Reduced temporal limbic structure volumes on magnetic resonance images in first episode schizophrenia. *Psychiatry Res.*, **35**: 1–13.
65. Suddath R.L., Christison G.W., Torrey E.F., Casanova M.F., Weinberger D.R. (1990a) Anatomical abnormalities in the brains of monozygotic twins discordant for schizophrenia. *N. Engl. J. Med.*, **322**: 789–794.
66. Nelson M.D., Saykin A.J., Flashman L.A., Riordan H.J. (1998) Hippocampal volume reduction in schizophrenia as assessed by magnetic resonance imaging: a meta-analytic study. *Arch. Gen. Psychiatry*, **55**: 433–440.

67. Csernansky J.G., Joshi S., Wang L., Haller J.W., Gado M., Miller J.P., Grenander U., Miller M.I. (1998) Hippocampal morphometry in schizophrenia by high dimensional brain mapping. *Proc. Natl. Acad. Sci. USA*, **95**: 11 406–11 411.
68. Reveley A.M., Reveley M.A., Clifford C.A., Murray R.M. (1982) Cerebral ventricular vize in twins discordant for schizophrenia. *Lancet*, **i**: 540–541.
69. Tamminga C.A., Thaker G.K., Buchanan R., Kirkpatrick B., Alphs L.D., Chase T.N., Carpenter W.T. (1992) Limbic system abnormalities identified in schizophrenia using positron emission tomography with fluorodeoxyglucose and neocortical alterations with deficit syndrome. *Arch. Gen. Psychiatry*, **49**: 522–530.
70. Berman K.F., Torrey E.F., Daniel D.G., Weinberger D.R. (1992) Regional cerebral blood flow in monozygotic twins discordant and concordant for schizophrenia. *Arch. Gen. Psychiatry*, **49**: 927–934.
71. Heckers S., Rauch S.L., Goff D., Savage C.R., Schacter D.L., Fischman A.J., Alpert N.M. (1998) Impaired recruitment of the hippocampus during conscious recollection in schizophrenia. *Nature*, **1**: 318–323.
72. Medoff D.R., Holcomb H.H., Lahti A.C., Tamminga C.A. (2001) Probing the human hippocampus using rCBF: contrasts in schizophrenia. *Hippocampus* (in press).
73. Gao X.M., Sakai K., Roberts R.C., Conley R.R., Dean B., Tamminga C.A. (2000) Ionotropic glutamate receptors and expression of N-methyl-D-aspartate receptor subunits in subregions of human hippocampus: effects of schizophrenia. *Am. J. Psychiatry*, **157**: 1141–1149.
74. Gruzelier J., Seymour K., Wilson L., Jolley A., Hirsch S. (1988) Impairments on neuropsychologic tests of temporohippocampal and frontohippocampal functions and word fluency in remitting schizophrenia and affective disorders. *Arch. Gen. Psychiatry*, **45**: 623–629.
75. Green M.F., Nuechterlein K.H., Gaier D.J. (1992) Sustained and selective attention in schizophrenia. *Prog. Exp. Personality Psychopathol. Res.*, **15**: 290–313.
76. Carter C.S., Braver T.S., Barch D.M., Botvinick M.M., Noll D., Cohen J.D. (1998) Anterior cingulate cortex, error detection, and the on-line monitoring of performance. *Science*, **280**: 747–749.
77. Liddle P.F., Friston K.J., Frith C.D., Hirsch S.R., Jones T., Frackowiak R.S. (1992) Patterns of cerebral blood flow in schizophrenia. *Br. J. Psychiatry*, **160**: 179–186.
78. Fletcher P. (1998) The missing link: a failure of fronto-hippocampal integration in schizophrenia. *News and Views*, **1**: 266–267.
79. Liddle P.F. (1996) Functional imaging—schizophrenia. *Br. Med. Bull.*, **52**: 486–494.
80. Tamminga C.A., Lahti A.C., Medoff D.R., Holcomb H.H. (2000) The functional involvement of the anterior cingulate cortex in schizophrenic psychosis. In *Contemporary Psychiatry* (Eds F. Henn, N. Sartorius, H. Helmchen, H. Lauter), pp. 101–110, Springer, Berlin.
81. Holcomb H.H., Lahti A.C., Medoff D.R., Weiler M., Dannals R.F., Tamminga C.A. (2000) Brain activation patterns in schizophrenic and comparison volunteers during a matched-performance auditory recognition task. *Am. J. Psychiatry*, **157**: 1634–1645.
82. Benes F.M., Bird E.D. (1987) An analysis of the arrangement of neurons in the cingulate cortex of schizophrenic patients. *Arch. Gen. Psychiatry*, **44**: 608–616.
83. Benes F.M., Majocha R., Bird E.D., Marotta C.A. (1987) Increased vertical axon numbers in cingulate cortex of schizophrenics. *Arch. Gen. Psychiatry*, **44**: 1017–1021.

84. Benes F.M., Vincent S.L., Alsterberg G., Bird E.D., SanGiovanni J.P. (1992) Increased GABAA receptor binding in superficial layers of cingulate cortex in schizophrenics. *J. Neurosci.*, **12**: 924–929.

85. Benes F.M., Sorensen I., Vincent S.L., Bird E.D., Sathi M. (1992b) Increased density of glutamate-immunoreactive vertical processes in superficial laminae in cingulate cortex of schizophrenic brain. *Cereb. Cortex*, **2**: 503–512.

86. Benes F.M., McSparren J., Bird E.D., Vincent S.L., SanGiovanni J.P. (1991) Deficits in small interneurons in prefrontal and anterior cingulate cortex of schizophrenic and schizoaffective patients. *Arch. Gen. Psychiatry*, **48**: 996–1001.

87. Benes F.M., Todtenkopf M.S., Taylor J.B. (1997) Differential distribution of tyrosine hydroxylase fibers on small and large neurons in layer II of anterior cingulate cortex of schizophrenic brain. *Synapse*, **25**: 80–92.

88. Schlaepfer T.E., Harris G.J., Tien A.Y., Peng L.W., Lee S., Federman E.B., Chase G.A., Barta P.E., Pearlson G.D. (1994) Decreased regional cortical gray matter volume in schizophrenia. *Am. J. Psychiatry*, **151**: 842–848.

89. Buchanan R.W., Vladar K., Barta P.E., Pearlson G.D. (1998) Structural evaluation of the prefrontal cortex in schizophrenia. *Am. J. Psychiatry*, **155**: 1049–1055.

90. Sullivan E.V, Mathalon D.H., Lim K.O., Marsh L., Pfefferbaum A. (1998) Patterns of regional cortical dysmorphology distinguishing schizophrenia and chronic alcoholism. *Biol. Psychiatry*, **43**: 118–131.

91. Selemon L.D., Rajkowska G., Goldman-Rakic P.S. (1995) Abnormally high neuronal density in the schizophrenic cortex. A morphometric analysis of prefrontal area 9 and occipital area 17. *Arch. Gen. Psychiatry*, **52**: 805–818.

92. Lidow M.S., Song Z.M., Castner S.A., Allen P.B., Greengard P., Goldman-Rakic P.S. (2001) Antipsychotic treatment induces alterations in dendrite- and spine-associated proteins in dopamine-rich areas of the primate cerebral cortex. *Biol. Psychiatry*, **49**: 1–12.

93. Akbarian S., Bunney W.E., Potkin S.G., Wigal S.B., Hagman J.D., Sandman C.A., Jones E.G. (1993) Altered distribution of nicotinamide-adenine dinucleotide phosphate-diaphorase cells in frontal lobe of schizophrenics implies disturbances of cortical development. *Arch. Gen. Psychiatry*, **50**: 227–230.

94. Akbarian S., Kim J.J., Potkin S.G., Hagman J.O., Tafazzoli A., Bunney W.E., Jones E.G. (1995) Gene expression for glutamic acid decarboxylase is reduced without loss of neurons in prefrontal cortex of schizophrenics. *Arch. Gen. Psychiatry*, **52**: 258–278.

95. Akbarian S., Sucher N.J., Bradley D., Tafazzoli A., Trinh D., Hetrick W.P., Potkin S.G., Sandman C.A., Bunney W.E. Jr., Jones E.G. (1996) Selective alterations in gene expression for NMDA receptor subunits in prefrontal cortex of schizophrenics. *J. Neurosci.*, **16**: 19–30.

96. Lewis D.A. (2000) GABAergic local circuit neurons and prefrontal cortical dysfunction in schizophrenia. *Brain Res. Brain Res. Rev.*, **31**: 270–276.

97. Ingvar D.H., Franzen G. (1974) Abnormalities of cerebral blood flow distribution in patients with chronic schizophrenia. *Acta Psychiatr. Scand.*, **50**: 425–462.

98. Buchsbaum M.S., Ingvar D.H., Kessler R., Waters R.N., Cappelletti J., van Kammen D.P., King A.C., Johnson J.L., Manning R.G., Flynn R.W. *et al.* (1982) Cerebral glucography with positron tomography. *Arch. Gen. Psychiatry*, **39**: 251–259.

99. Berman K.F., Zec R.F., Weinberger D.R. (1986) Physiologic dysfunction of dorsolateral prefrontal cortex in schizophrenia: II. Role of neuroleptic treatment, attention, and mental effort. *Arch. Gen. Psychiatry*, **43**: 126–135.

100. Andreasen N.C., Rezai K., Alliger R.J., Swayze V.W., Flaum M., Kirchner P., Cohen G., O'Leary D.S. (1992) Hypofrontality in neuroleptic-naive patients and in patients with chronic schizophrenia. *Arch. Gen. Psychiatry*, **49**: 943–958.

101. Andreasen N.C., Rezai K., Alliger R.J., Swayze V.W., Flaum M., Kirchner P., Cohen G., O'Leary D.S. (1992) Hypofrontality in neuroleptic-naive patients and in patients with chronic schizophrenia. Assessment with xenon 133 single-photon emission computed tomography and the Tower of London. *Arch. Gen. Psychiatry*, **49**: 943–958.

102. Buchsbaum M.S., Haier R.J., Potkin S.G., Nuechterlein K.H., Bracha H.S., Katz M., Lohr J., Wu J., Lottenberg S., Jerabek P.A. *et al.* (1992) Frontostriatal disorder of cerebral metabolism in never-medicated schizophrenics. *Arch. Gen. Psychiatry*, **49**: 935–942.

103. Goldman-Rakic P.S. (1994) Working memory dysfunction in schizophrenia. *J. Neuropsychiatry Clin. Neurosci.*, **6**: 348–357.

104. Holcomb H.H., Cascella N.G., Thaker G.K., Medoff D.R., Dannals R.F., Tamminga C.A. (1996) Functional sites of neuroleptic drug action in the human brain: PET/FDG studies with and without haloperidol. *Am. J. Psychiatry*, **153**: 41–49.

105. Liddle P.F. (1987) The symptoms of chronic schizophrenia: a re-examination of the positive-negative dichotomy. *Br. J. Psychiatry*, **151**: 145–151.

106. Heckers S., Goff D., Schacter D.L., Savage C.R., Fischman A.J., Alpert N.M., Rauch S.L. (1999) Functional imaging of memory retrieval in deficit vs. non-deficit schizophrenia. *Arch. Gen. Psychiatry*, **56**: 1117–1123.

107. Menon V, Anagnoson R.T., Glover G.H., Pfefferbaum A. (2001) Functional magnetic resonance imaging evidence for disrupted basal ganglia function in schizophrenia. *Am. J. Psychiatry*, **158**: 646–649.

108. Kaplan R.D., Szechtman H., Franco S., Szechtman B., Nahmias C., Garnett E.S., List S., Cleghorn J.M. (1993) Three clinical syndromes of schizophrenia in untreated subjects: relation to brain glucose activity measured by positron emission tomography (PET). *Schizophr. Res.*, **11**: 47–54.

109. Nordahl T.E., Kusubov N., Carter C., Salamat S., Cummings A.M., O'Shora-Celaya L., Eberling J., Robertson L., Huesman R.H., Jagust W. *et al.* (1996) Temporal lobe metabolic differences in medication-free outpatients with schizophrenia via the PET-600. *Neuropsychopharmacology*, **15**: 541–554.

110. Shenton M.E., Kikinis R., Jolesz F.A., Pollak S.D., LeMay M., Wible C.G., Hokama H., Martin J., Metcalf D., Coleman M. *et al.* (1992) Abnormalities of the left temporal lobe and thought disorder in schizophrenia. A quantitative magnetic resonance imaging study. *N. Engl. J. Med.*, **327**: 604–612.

111. Menon R.R., Barta P.E., Aylward E.H., Richards S.S., Vaughn D.D., Tien A.Y., Harris G.J., Pearlson G.D. (1995) Posterior superior temporal gyrus in schizophrenia: grey matter changes and clinical correlates. *Schizophr. Res.*, **16**: 127–135.

112. Shenton M.E., McCarley R.W., Tamminga C.A. (1995) Cortex, IX. Heschl's gyrus and the planum temporale. *Am. J. Psychiatry*, **152**: 966.

113. Pearlson G.D. (1997) Superior temporal gyrus and planum temporale in schizophrenia: a selective review. *Prog. Neuropsychopharmacol. Biol. Psychiatry*, **21**: 1203–1229.

114. Buchsbaum M.S., Someya T., Teng C.Y., Abel L., Chin S., Najafi A., Haier R.J., Wu J., Bunney W.E. Jr. (1996) PET and MRI of the thalamus in never-medicated patients with schizophrenia. *Am. J. Psychiatry*, **153**: 191–199.

115. Pakkenberg B. (1990) Pronounced reduction of total neuron number in mediodorsal thalamic nucleus and nucleus accumbens in schizophrenic brain. *Arch. Gen. Psychiatry*, **47**: 1023–1028.
116. Pakkenberg B. (1992) The volume of the mediodorsal thalamic nucleus in treated and untreated schizophrenics. *Schizophr. Res.*, **7**: 95–100.
117. Brown R., Colter N., Corsellis J.A.N., Crow T.J., Frith C.D., Jagoe R., Johnstone E.C., Marsh L. (1986) Post-mortem evidence for structural brain changes in schizophrenia. Differences in brain weight, temporal horn area and parahippocampal gyrus width as compared with affective disorder. *Arch. Gen. Psychiatry*, **43**: 36–42.
118. Falkai P., Bogerts B., Rozumek M. (1988) Limbic pathology in schizophrenia: the entorhinal region—a morphometric study. *Biol. Psychiatry*, **24**: 515–521.
119. Bogerts B., Falkai P., Tutsch J. (1986) Cell numbers in the pallidum and hippocampus of schizophrenics. In *Biological Psychiatry* (Ed. C. Shagass), pp. 1178–1180, Elsevier, Amsterdam.
120. Bogerts B., Meertz E., Schonfeldt-Bausch R. (1985) Basal ganglia and limbic system pathology in schizophrenia. A morphometric study of brain volume and shrinkage. *Arch. Gen. Psychiatry*, **42**: 784–791.
121. Benes F.M., Davidson J., Bird E.D. (1986) Quantitative cytoarchitectural studies of cerebral cortex of schizophrenics. *Arch. Gen. Psychiatry*, **43**: 31–35.
122. Jakob H., Beckmann H. (1986) Prenatal developmental disturbances in the limbic allocortex in schizophrenics. *J. Neural Transm.*, **65**: 303–326.
123. Falkai P., Bogerts B. (1986) Cell loss in the hippocampus of schizophrenics. *Eur. Arch. Psychiatry Neurol. Sci.*, **236**: 154–161.
124. Jeste D., Lohr J.B. (1989) Hippocampal pathologic findings in schizophrenia. *Arch. Gen. Psychiatry*, **46**: 1019–1024.
125. Dom R. (1976) Neostriatal and thalamic interneurons. Their role in the pathophysiology of Huntington's chorea, Parkinson's disease and catatonic schizophrenia. Doctoral dissertation. Katholieke Universiteit, Leuven.
126. Pakkenberg B. (1989) What happens in the leucotomised brain? A postmortem morphological study of brains from schizophrenic patients. *J. Neurol. Neurosurg. Psychiatry*, **52**: 156–161.
127. Falkai P., Honer W.G., David S., Bogerts B., Majtenyi C., Bayer T.A. (1999) No evidence for astrogliosis in brains of schizophrenic patients. A post-mortem study. *Neuropathol. Appl. Neurobiol.*, **25**: 48–53.
128. Selemon L.D., Rajkowska G., Goldman-Rakic P.S. (1998) Elevated neuronal density in prefrontal area 46 in brains from schizophrenic patients: application of a three-dimensional, stereologic counting method. *J. Comp. Neurol.*, **392**: 402–412.
129. Arnold S.E., Trojanowski J.Q. (1996) Cognitive impairment in elderly schizophrenia: a dementia (still) lacking distinctive histopathology. *Schizophr. Bull.*, **22**: 5–9.
130. Benes F.M., Sorensen I., Bird E.D. (1991) Reduced neuronal size in posterior hippocampus of schizophrenic patients. *Schizophr. Bull.*, **17**: 597–608.
131. Heckers S., Heinsen H., Geiger B., Beckmann H. (1991) Hippocampal neuron number in schizophrenia. A stereological study. *Arch. Gen. Psychiatry*, **48**: 1002–1008.
132. Benes F.M. (1997) Is there evidence for neuronal loss in schizophrenia? *Int. Rev. Psychiatry*, **9**: 429–436.
133. Benes F.M., Kwok E.W., Vincent S.L., Todtenkopf M.S. (1998) A reduction of nonpyramidal cells in sector CA2 of schizophrenics and manic depressives. *Biol. Psychiatry*, **44**: 88–97.

134. Bird E.D., Barnes J., Iversen L., Spokes E.G., Mackay A.V.P., Shepherd M. (1977) Increased brain dopamine and reduced glutamic acid decarboxylase and choline acetyl transferase activity in schizophrenia and related psychoses. *Lancet*, **ii**: 1157–1159.

135. Hanada S., Mita T., Nishinok N., Tankaka C. (1987) ^{3}H-muscimol binding sites increased in autopsied brains of chronic schizophrenics. *Life Sci.*, **40**: 259–266.

136. Todtenkopf M.S., Benes F.M. (1998) Distribution of glutamate decarboxylase65 immunoreactive puncta on pyramidal and nonpyramidal neurons in hippocampus of schizophrenic brain. *Synapse*, **29**: 323–332.

137. Benes F.M., Todtenkopf M.S., Logiotatos P., Williams M. (2001) Glutamate decarboxylase65-immunoreactive terminals in cingulate and prefrontal cortices of schizophrenic and bipolar brain. *J. Chem. Neuroanatomy* (in press).

138. Benes F.M., Vincent S.L., Marie A., Khan Y. (1996) Up-regulation of GABAA receptor binding on neurons of the prefrontal cortex in schizophrenic subjects. *Neuroscience*, **75**: 1021–1031.

139. Benes F.M., Khan Y., Vincent S.L., Wickramasinghe R. (1996) Differences in the subregional and cellular distribution of GABAA receptor binding in the hippocampal formation of schizophrenic brain. *Synapse*, **22**: 338–349.

140. Benes F.M., Wickramasinghe R., Vincent S.L., Khan Y., Todtenkopf M. (1997) Uncoupling of GABA(A) and benzodiazepine receptor binding activity in the hippocampal formation of schizophrenic brain. *Brain Res.*, **755**: 121–129.

141. Simpson M.D., Slater P., Deakin J.F., Royston M.C., Skan W.J. (1989) Reduced GABA uptake sites in the temporal lobe in schizophrenia. *Neurosci. Lett.*, **107**: 211–215.

142. Reynolds G.P., Czudek C., Andrews H. (1990) Deficit and hemispheric asymmetry of GABA uptake sites in the hippocampus in schizophrenia. *Biol. Psychiatry*, **27**: 1038–1044.

143. Simpson M.D., Slater P., Deakin J.F. (1998) Comparison of glutamate and gamma-aminobutyric acid uptake binding sites in frontal and temporal lobes in schizophrenia. *Biol. Psychiatry*, **44**: 423–427.

144. Pierri J.N., Chaudry A.S., Woo T.U., Lewis D.A. (1999) Alterations in chandelier neuron axon terminals in the prefrontal cortex of schizophrenic subjects. *Am. J. Psychiatry*, **156**: 1709–1719.

145. Woo T.U., Whitehead R.E., Melchitzky D.S., Lewis D.A. (1998) A subclass of prefrontal gamma-aminobutyric acid axon terminals are selectively altered in schizophrenia. *Proc. Natl. Acad. Sci. USA*, **95**: 5341–5346.

146. Conde F., Lund J.S., Jacobowitz D.M., Baimbridge K.G., Lewis D.A. (1994) Local circuit neurons immunoreactive for calretinin, calbindin D-28k or parvalbumin in monkey prefrontal cortex: distribution and morphology. *J. Comp. Neurol.*, **341**: 95–116.

147. Beasley C.L., Reynolds G.P. (1997) Parvalbumin-immunoreactive neurons are reduced in the prefrontal cortex of schizophrenics. *Schizophr. Res.*, **24**: 349–355.

148. Woo T.U., Miller J.L., Lewis D.A. (1997) Schizophrenia and the parvalbumin-containing class of cortical local circuit neurons. *Am. J. Psychiatry*, **154**: 1013–1015.

149. Kalus P., Senitz D., Beckmann H. (1997) Altered distribution of parvalbumin-immunoreactive local circuit neurons in the anterior cingulate cortex of schizophrenic patients. *Psychiatry Res.*, **75**: 49–59.

150. Daviss S.R., Lewis D.A. (1995) Local circuit neurons of the prefrontal cortex in schizophrenia: selective increase in the density of calbindin-immunoreactive neurons. *Psychiatry Res.*, **59**: 81–96.

151. Iritani S., Kuroki N., Ikeda K., Kazamatsuri H. (1999) Calbindin immunoreactivity in the hippocampal formation and neocortex of schizophrenics. *Prog. Neuropsychopharmacol. Biol. Psychiatry*, **23**: 409–421.

152. Impagnatiello F., Guidotti A.R., Pesold C., Dwivedi Y., Caruncho H., Pisu M.G., Uzunov D.P., Smalheiser N.R., Davis J.M., Pandey G.N. *et al.* (1998) A decrease of reelin expression as a putative vulnerability factor in schizophrenia. *Proc. Natl. Acad. Sci. USA*, **95**: 15718–15723.

153. Guidotti A., Auta J., Davis J.M., Gerevini V.D., Dwivedi Y., Grayson D.R., Impagnatiello F., Pandey G., Pesold C., Sharma R. *et al.* (2000) Decrease in reelin and glutamic acid decarboxylase67 (GAD67) expression in schizophrenia and bipolar disorder: a postmortem brain study *Arch. Gen. Psychiatry*, **57**: 1061–1069.

154. Vincent S.L., Adamec E., Sorensen I., Benes F.M. (1994) The effects of chronic haloperidol administration on GABA-immunoreactive axon terminals in rat medial prefrontal cortex. *Synapse*, **17**: 26–35.

155. Kaufman D.L., Houser C.R., Tobin A.J. (1991) Two forms of the γ-aminobutyric acid synthetic enzyme glutamate decarboxylase have distinct intraneuronal distributions and cofactor interactions. *J. Neurochem.*, **56**: 720–723.

156. O'Connor L.N., Brene S., Herrera-Marschitz M., Persson H., Ungerstedt U. (1991) Short-term dopaminergic regulation of GABA release in dopamine deafferentated caudate-putamen is not directly associated with glutamic acid decarboxylase gene expression. *Neurosci. Lett.*, **128**: 66–70.

157. Litwak J., Mercugliano M., Chesselet M.F., Oltmans G.A. (1990) Increased glutamic acid decarboxylase (GAD) mRNA and GAD activity in cerebellar Purkinje cells following lesion-induced increases in cell firing. *Neurosci. Lett.*, **116**: 179–183.

158. Feldblum S., Ackerman R.F., Tobin A.J. (1990) Long-term increase of glutamate decarboxylase mRNA in a rat model of temporal lobe epilepsy. *Neuron*, **5**: 361–371.

159. Ding R., Asada H., Obata K. (1998) Changes in extracellular glutamate and GABA levels in the hippocampal CA3 and CA1 areas and the induction of glutamic acid decarboxylase-67 in dentate granule cells of rats treated with kainic acid. *Brain Res.*, **800**: 105–113.

160. Feldblum S., Anoal M., Lapsher S., Cumoulin A., Privat A. (1998) Partial deafferentation of the developing rat spinal cord delays the spontaneous repression of GAD67 mRNAs in spinal cells. *Perspect. Dev. Neurobiol.*, **5**: 131–143.

161. Martin D.L., Martin S.B., Wu S.J., Expina N. (1993) Regulatory properties of brain glutamate decarboxylase (GAD): the apoenzyme of GAD is present principally as the smaller of the two molecular forms of GAD in the brain. *J. Neurosci.*, **11**: 2725–2731.

162. Miller L.P., Walters J.R., Martin D.L. (1991) Post-mortem changes implicate adenine nucleotides and puridoxal-5'-phosphate in regulation of brain glutamate decarboxylase. *Nature*, **266**: 847–848.

163. Heckers S., Stone D., Walsh J., Schick J., Koul P., Benes F.M. (2001) Decreased hippocampal expression of glutamic acid decarboxylase (GAD) 65 and 67 mRNA in bipolar disorder, but not schizophrenia. Submitted for publication.

164. Stone D.J., Walsh J., Benes F.M. (1999) Localization of cells preferentially expressing GAD(67) with negligible GAD(65) transcripts in the rat hippocampus. A double in situ hybridization study. *Brain Res. Mol. Brain Res.*, **71**: 201–209.

165. Bowers G., Cullinan W.E., Herman J.P. (1998) Region-specific regulation of glutamic acid decarboxylase (GAD) mRNA expression in central stress circuits. *J. Neurosci.*, **18**: 5938–5947.

166. Stone D.J., Walsh J.P., Benes F.M. (2000) Effects of pre- and postnatal stress on the rat GABA system. *Hippocampus* (in press).

167. Dean B., Hussain T., Hayes W., Scarr E., Kitsoulis S., Hill C., Opeskin K., Copolov D.L. (1999) Changes in serotonin2A and GABA(A) receptors in schizophrenia: studies on the human dorsolateral prefrontal cortex. *J. Neurochem.*, **72**: 1593–1599.

168. Squires R.F., Lajtha A., Saederup E., Palkovits M. (1993) Reduced [3-H]-flunitrazepam bindings in cingulate cortex and hippocampus of postmortem schizophrenic brains. *Neurochem. Res.*, **18**: 219–223.

169. Benes F.M., Vincent S., Marie A., Khan Y. (1996) Upregulation of GABA-A receptor binding on pyramidal neurons of prefrontal cortex in schizophrenic subjects. *Neuroscience*, **75**: 1021–1031.

170. Busatto G.F., Pilowsky L.S., Costa D.C., Ell P.J., David A.S., Lucey J.V., Kerwin R.W. (1997) Correlation between reduced in vivo benzodiazepine receptor binding and severity of psychotic symptoms in schizophrenia. *Am. J. Psychiatry*, **154**: 56–63.

171. Abi-Dargham A., Laruelle M., Krystal J., D'Souza C., Zoghbi S., Baldwin R.M., Seibyl J., Mawlawi O., de Erasquin G., Charney D. *et al.* (1999) No evidence of altered in vivo benzodiazepine receptor binding in schizophrenia. *Neuropsychopharmacology*, **20**: 650–661.

172. Verhoeff N.P., Soares J.C., D'Souza C.D., Gil R., Degen K., Abi-Dargham A., Zoghbi S.S., Fujita M., Rajeevan N., Seibyl J.P. *et al.* (1999) [^{123}I]iomazenil SPECT benzodiazepine receptor imaging in schizophrenia. *Psychiatry Res.*, **91**: 163–173.

173. Ball S., Busatto G.F., David A.S., Jones S.H., Hemsley D.R., Pilowsky L.S., Costa D.C., Ell P.J., Kerwin R.W. (1998) Cognitive functioning and GABAA/benzodiazepine receptor binding in schizophrenia: a ^{123}I-iomazenil SPET study. *Biol. Psychiatry*, **43**: 107–117.

174. Benes F.M. (1999) Evidence for altered trisynaptic circuitry in schizophrenic hippocampus. *Biol. Psychiatry*, **46**: 589–599.

175. Berretta S., Munno D.W., Benes F.M. (2000) Amygdalar activation alters the hippocampal GABA system: "partial" modelling for postmortem changes in schizophrenia. *J. Comp. Neurol.* (in press).

176. Sokolov B.P. (1998) Expression of NMDAR1, GluR1, GluR7, and KA1 glutamate receptor mRNAs is decreased in frontal cortex of "neuroleptic-free" schizophrenics: evidence on reversible up-regulation by typical neuroleptics. *J. Neurochem.*, **71**: 2454–2464.

177. Harrison P.J., McLaughlin D., Kerwin R.W. (1991) Decreased hippocampal expression of a glutamate receptor gene in schizophrenia. *Lancet*, **337**: 450–452.

178. Kerwin R.W., Patel S., Meldrum B.S., Czudek C., Reynolds G.P. (1988) Asymmetrical loss of glutamate receptor subtype in left hippocampus in schizophrenia. *Lancet*, **i**: 583–584.

179. Kerwin R., Patel S., Meldrum B. (1990) Quantitative autoradiographic analysis of glutamate binding sites in the hippocampal formation in normal and schizophrenic brain post mortem. *Neuroscience*, **39**: 25–32.

180. Porter R.H., Eastwood S.L., Harrison P.J. (1997) Distribution of kainate receptor subunit mRNAs in human hippocampus, neocortex and cerebellum, and

bilateral reduction of hippocampal GluR6 and KA2 transcripts in schizophrenia. *Brain Res.*, **751**: 217–231.

181. Eastwood S.L., Kerwin R.W., Harrison P.J. (1997) Immunoautoradiographic evidence for a loss of alpha-amino-3-hydroxy-5-methyl-4-isoxazole propionate-preferring non-N-methyl-D-aspartate glutamate receptors within the medial temporal lobe in schizophrenia. *Biol. Psychiatry*, **41**: 636–643.

182. Eastwood S.L., McDonald B., Burnet P.W., Beckwith J.P., Kerwin R.W., Harrison P.J. (1995) Decreased expression of mRNAs encoding non-NMDA glutamate receptors GluR1 and GluR2 in medial temporal lobe neurons in schizophrenia. *Brain Res. Mol. Brain Res.*, **29**: 211–223.

183. Breese C.R., Freedman R., Leonard S.S. (1995) Glutamate receptor subtype expression in human postmortem brain tissue from schizophrenics and alcohol abusers. *Brain Res.*, **674**: 82–90.

184. Kornhuber J., Mack-Burkhardt F., Riederer P., Hebenstreit G.F., Reynolds G.P., Andrews H.B., Beckmann H. (1989) [^{3}H]MK-801 binding sites in postmortem brain regions of schizophrenic patients. *J. Neural Transm.*, **77**: 231–236.

185. Simpson M.D., Slater P., Royston M.C., Deakin J.F.W. (1992) Alterations in phencyclidine and sigma binding sites in schizophrenic brains. *Schizophr. Res.*, **6**: 41–48.

186. Shibuya H., Mori H., Toru M. (1992) Sigma receptors in schizophrenic cerebral cortices. *Neurochem. Res.*, **17**: 983–990.

187. Weissman A.D., Casanova M.F., Kleinman J.E., London E.D., De Souza E.B. (1991) Selective loss of cerebral cortical sigma, but not PCP binding sites in schizophrenia. *Biol. Psychiatry*, **29**: 41–54.

188. Humphries C., Mortimer A., Hirsch S., de Belleroche J. (1996) NMDA receptor mRNA correlation with antemortem cognitive impairment in schizophrenia. *Neuroreport*, **7**: 2051–2055.

189. Lynch D.R., Anegawa N.J., Verdoorn T., Pritchett D.B. (1994) N-methyl-D-aspartate receptors: different subunit requirements for binding of glutamate antagonists, glycine antagonists and channel-blocking agents. *Mol. Pharmacol.*, **45**: 540–545.

190. Moghaddam B. (1994) Recent basic findings in support of excitatory amino acid hypotheses of schizophrenia. *Prog. Neuropsychopharmacol. Biol. Psychiatry*, **18**: 859–870.

191. Tamminga C.A. (1998) Schizophrenia and glutamatergic transmission. *Crit. Rev. Neurobiol.*, **12**: 21–36.

192. Olney J.W., Farber N.B. (1995) Glutamate receptor dysfunction and schizophrenia. *Arch. Gen. Psychiatry*, **52**: 998–1007.

193. Benes F.M. (1996) The role of glutamate in the pathophysiology of schizophrenia. In *Excitatory Amino Acids and the Cerebral Cortex* (Eds F. Conti, T.P. Hicks), pp. 361–374, MIT Press, Cambridge.

194. Meador-Woodruff J.H., Healy D.J. (2000) Glutamate receptor expression in schizophrenic brain. *Brain Res. Brain Res. Rev.*, **31**: 288–294.

195. Honer W.G. (1999) Assessing the machinery of mind: synapses in neuropsychiatric disorders. *J. Psychiatry Neurosci.*, **24**: 116–121.

196. Eastwood S.L., Harrison P.J. (1999) Detection and quantification of hippocampal synaptophysin messenger RNA in schizophrenia using autoclaved, formalin-fixed, paraffin wax-embedded sections. *Neuroscience*, **93**: 99–106.

197. Gabriel S.M., Haroutunian V., Powchik P., Honer W.G., Davidson M., Davies P., Davis K.L. (1997) Increased concentrations of presynaptic proteins in the

cingulate cortex of subjects with schizophrenia. *Arch. Gen. Psychiatry*, **54**: 559–566.

198. Sower A.C., Bird E.D., Perrone-Bizzozero N.I. (1995) Increased levels of GAP-43 protein in schizophrenic brain tissues demonstrated by a novel immuno-detection method. *Mol. Chem. Neuropathol.*, **24**: 1–11.

199. Benowitz L., Routtenberg A. (1987) A membrane phosphoprotein associated with neural development, axonal regeneration, phospholipid metabolism and synaptic plasticity. *Trends Neurosci.*, **10**: 527–532.

200. Stevens J.R. (1992) Abnormal reinnervation as a basis for schizophrenia: an hypothesis. *Arch. Gen. Psychiatry*, **49**: 238–243.

201. Swerdlow N.R., Geyer M.A. (1998) Using an animal model of deficient sensor-imotor gating to study the pathophysiology of new treatments and schizo-phrenia. *Schizophr. Bull.*, **24**: 285–301.

202. Graham F. (1975) The more or less startling effects of weak prestimuli. *Psycho-physiology*, **12**: 238–248.

203. Braff D.L., Grillon C., Geyer M. (1978) Gating and habituation of the startle reflex in schizophrenic patients. *Psychophysiology*, **15**: 339–343.

204. Grace A.A. (2000) Gating of information flow within the limbic system and the pathophysiology of schizophrenia. *Brain Res. Rev.*, **31**: 330–341.

205. Bakshi V.P., Geyer M.A. (1998) Multiple limbic regions mediate the disruption of prepulse inhibition produced in rats by the noncompetitive NMDA antag-onist dizocilpine. *J. Neurosci.*, **18**: 8394–8401.

206. Gallagher M., Graham P.W., Holland P.C. (1990) The amygdala central nu-cleus and appetitive Pavlovian conditioning: lesions impair one class of con-ditioned behavior. *J. Neurosci.*, **10**: 1906–1911.

207. Wan F.J., Swerdlow N.R. (1997) The basolateral amygdala regulates sensor-imotor gating of acoustic startle in the rat. *Neuroscience*, **76**: 715–724.

208. Stutzmann G.E., LeDoux J.E. (1999) GABAergic antagonists block the inhibitory effects of serotonin in the lateral amygdala: a mechanism for modulation of sensory inputs related to fear conditioning. *J. Neurosci.*, **19**: RC8.

209. Killcross S., Robbins T.W., Everitt B.J. (1997) Different types of fear-condi-tioned behaviour mediated by separate nuclei within amygdala. *Nature*, **388**: 377–380.

210. Cahill L., Haier R.J., Fallon J., Alkire M.T., Tang C., Keator D., Wu J., McGaugh J.L. (1996) Amygdala activity at encoding correlated with long-term, free recall of emotional information. *Proc. Natl. Acad. Sci. USA*, **93**: 8016–8021.

211. Selden N.R., Everitt B.J., Jarrard L.E., Robbins T.W., (1991) Complementary roles for the amygdala and hippocampus in aversive conditioning to explicit and contextual cues. *Neuroscience*, **42**: 335–350.

212. Poremba A., Gabriel M. (1997) Amygdalar lesions block discriminative avoid-ance learning and cingulothalamic training-induced neuronal plasticity in rabbits. *J. Neurosci.*, **17**: 5237–5244.

213. Goldman-Rakic P. (1991) Prefrontal cortical dysfunction in schizophrenia: the relevance of working memory. In *Psychopathology and the Brain* (Eds B.J. Car-roll, J.E. Barrett), pp. 1–23, Raven Press, New York.

214. Selemon L.D., Goldman-Rakic P.S. (1999) The reduced neuropil hypothesis: a circuit based model of schizophrenia. *Biol. Psychiatry*, **45**: 17–25.

215. Seeman P., Ulpian C., Bergeron C., Riederer P., Jellinger K., Gabriel E., Rey-nolds G.P., Tourtellotte W.W. (1984) Bimodal distribution of dopamine recep-tor densities in brains of schizophrenics. *Science*, **225**: 728–731.

216. Wong D.F., Wagner H.N. Jr., Tune L.E., Dannals R.F., Pearlson G.D., Links J.M., Tamminga C.A., Broussolle E.P., Ravert H.T., Wilson A.A. (1986) Positron emission tomography reveals elevated D2 dopamine receptors in drug-naive schizophrenics. *Science*, **234**: 1558–1563.
217. Seeman P., Guan H.-C., Van Tol H.H.M. (1993) Dopamine D4 receptors elevated in schizophrenia. *Nature*, **365**: 441–445.
218. Carlsson M., Carlsson A. (1990) Interactions between glutamatergic and monoaminergic systems within the basal ganglia—implications for schizophrenia and Parkinson's disease. *Trends Neurosci.*, **13**: 272–276.
219. Graybiel A.M. (1990) Neurotransmitters and neuromodulators in the basal ganglia. *Trends Neurosci.*, **13**: 244–254.
220. Greengard P., Allen P.B., Nairn A.C. (1999) Beyond the dopamine receptor: the DARPP-32/protein phosphatase-1 cascade. *Neuron*, **23**: 435–447.
221. Laruelle M., Abi-Dargham A., Gil R., Kegeles L., Innis R. (1999) Increased dopamine transmission in schizophrenia: relationship to illness phases. *Biol. Psychiatry*, **46**: 56–72.
222. Tamminga C.A., Cascella N., Fakouhi T.D., Hertig R.L. (1992) Enhancement of NMDA-mediated transmission in schizophrenia: effects of milacemide. In *Novel Antipsychotic Drugs* (Ed. H.Y. Meltzer), pp. 171–177, Raven Press, New York.
223. Domino E.F. (1980) History and pharmacology of PCP and PCP-related analogs. *J. Psychedel. Drugs*, **12**: 223–227.
224. Tamminga C.A., Tanimoto K., Kuo S., Chase T.N., Contreras P.C., Rice K.C., Jackson A.E., O'Donohue T.L. (1987) PCP-induced alterations in cerebral glucose utilization in rat brain: blockade by metaphit, a PCP-receptor-acylating agent. *Synapse*, **1**: 497–504.
225. Javitt D.C., Zukin S.R. (1991) Recent advances in the phencyclidine model of schizophrenia. *Am. J. Psychiatry*, **148**: 1301–1308.
226. Gao X.M., Tamminga C.A. (1996) Phencyclidine produces changes in NMDA and kainate receptor binding in rat hippocampus over a 48-hour time course. *Synapse*, **23**: 274–279.
227. Gao X.M., Hashimoto T., Tamminga C.A. (1998) Phencyclidine (PCP) and dizocilpine (MK801) exert time-dependent effects on the expression of immediate early genes in rat brain. *Synapse*, **29**: 14–28.
228. Mohr A.R., Gainetdinov R.R., Caron M.G., Koller B.H. (1999) Mice with reduced NMDA receptor expression display behaviors related to schizophrenia. *Cell*, **98**: 427–436.
229. Geyer M.A. (1998) Behavioral studies of hallucinogenic drugs in animals: implications for schizophrenia research. *Pharmacopsychiatry*, **31**(Suppl. 2): 73–79.
230. Monyer H., Burnashev N., Laurie D.J., Sakmann B., Seeburg P.H. (1994) Developmental and regional expression in the rat brain and functional properties of four NMDA receptors. *Neuron*, **12**: 529–540.
231. Broca P. (1878) Anatomie comparée des circonvolutions cérébrales: le grand lobe limbique et la scissure limbique dans la série des manmifères. *Rev. Anthropol.*, **1**: 385–498.
232. MacLean P.D. (1954) Studies on limbic system (visceral brain) and their bearing on psychosomatic problems. In *Recent Developments in Psychosomatic Medicine* (Ed. E.R.C. Wittkower), pp. 101–125, Sir Isaac Pribram and Sons, London.
233. Squire L.R., Knowlton B., Musen G. (1993) The structure and organization of memory. *Annu. Rev. Psychol.*, **44**: 453–495.

234. Eichenbaum H. (1997) Declarative memory: insights from cognitive neurobiology. *Annu. Rev. Psychol.*, **48**: 547–572.
235. Eichenbaum H. (1999) Conscious awareness, memory and the hippocampus. *Nature Neurosci.*, **2**: 775–776.
236. Stutzmann G.E., McEwen B.S., LeDoux J.E. (1998) Serotonin modulation of sensory inputs to the lateral amygdala: dependency on corticosterone. *J. Neurosci.*, **18**: 9529–9538.
237. Sapolsky R.M. (1986) Glucocorticoid toxicity in the hippocampus: temporal aspects of synergy with kainic acid. *Neuroendocrinology*, **43**: 386.
238. Thierry A.M., Tassin J.P., Blanc G., Glowinski J. (1976) Selective activation of the mesocortical DA system by stress. *Nature*, **263**: 242–244.
239. Roth R.H., Tam S.Y., Ida Y., Yang J.X., Deutch A.Y. (1988) Stress and the mesocorticolimbic dopamine systems. *Ann. N.Y. Acad. Sci.*, **537**: 138–147.
240. Van Hoesen G.W., Morecraft R.J., Vogt B.A. (1993) Connections of the monkey cingulate cortex. In *Neurobiology of Cingulate Cortex and Limbic Thalamus* (Eds B.A. Vogt, M. Gabriel), pp. 249-284, Birkhäuser, Boston.
241. Benes F.M., Berretta S. (2000) Amygdalo-entorhinal inputs to the hippocampal formation in relation to schizophrenia. *Ann. N.Y. Acad. Sci. USA*, **911**: 293–304.
242. Carlsson A., Waters N., Waters S., Carlsson M. (2000) Network interactions in schizophrenia – therapeutic implications. *Brain Res. Rev.*, **31**: 342–349.
243. Carlsson A. (1988) The current status of the dopamine hypothesis of schizophrenia. *Neuropsychopharmacology*, **1**: 179–186.
244. Benes F.M. (1993) Neurobiological investigations in cingulate cortex of schizophrenic brain. *Schizophr. Bull.*, **19**: 537–549.
245. Andersen S.A., Volk D.W., Lewis D.A. (1996) Increased density of microtubule associated protein 2-immunoreactive neurons in the prefrontal white matter of schizophrenic subjects. *Schizophr. Res.*, **19**: 111–119.
246. Chesselet M.F., Robbins E. (1989) Characterization of striatal neurons expressing high levels of glutamic acid decarboxylase messenger RNA. *Brain Res.*, **492**: 237–244.
247. Spike R.C., Todd A.J., Johnston H.M. (1993) Coexistence of NADPH diaphorase with GABA, glycine, and acetylcholine in rat spinal cord. *J. Comp. Neurol.*, **335**: 320–333.
248. Valtschanoff J.G., Weinberg R.J., Kharazia V.N., Nakane M., Schmidt H.H. (1993) Neurons in rat hippocampus that synthesize nitric oxide. *J. Comp. Neurol.*, **331**: 111–121.
249. Valtschanoff J.G., Weinberg R.J., Kharazia V.N., Schmidt H.H., Nakane M., Rustioni A. (1993) Neurons in rat cerebral cortex that synthesize nitric oxide: NADPH diaphorase histochemistry, NOS immunocytochemistry, and colocalization with GABA. *Neurosci. Lett.*, **157**: 157–161.
250. Davila J.C., Megias M., Andreu M.J., Real M.A., Guirado S. (1995) NADPH diaphorase-positive neurons in the lizard hippocampus: a distinct subpopulation of GABAergic interneurons. *Hippocampus*, **5**: 60–70.
251. Gabbott P.L., Bacon S.J. (1995) Co-localisation of NADPH diaphorase activity and GABA immunoreactivity in local circuit neurones in the medial prefrontal cortex (mPFC) of the rat. *Brain Res.*, **699**: 321–328.
252. Gabbott P.L., Bacon S.J. (1996) Local circuit neurons in the medial prefrontal cortex (areas 24a,b,c, 25 and 32) in the monkey: I. Cell morphology and morphometrics. *J. Comp. Neurol.*, **364**: 567–608.

253. Gabbott P.L., Bacon S.J. (1996) Local circuit neurons in the medial prefrontal cortex (areas 24a,b,c, 25 and 32) in the monkey: II. Quantitative areal and laminar distributions. *J. Comp. Neurol.*, **364**: 609–636.

254. Gabbott P.L., Dickie B.G., Vaid R.R., Headlam A.J., Bacon S.J. (1997) Local-circuit neurones in the medial prefrontal cortex (areas 25, 32 and 24b) in the rat: morphology and quantitative distribution. *J. Comp. Neurol.*, **377**: 465–499.

255. Pesold C., Impagnatiello F., Pisu M.G., Uzunov D.P., Costa E., Guidotti. A. (1998) Reelin is preferentially expressed in neurons synthesizing γ-aminobutyric acid in cortex and hippocampus in adult rats. *Proc. Natl. Acad. Sci. USA*, **95**: 3221–3226.

256. Pesold C., Liu W.S., Guidotti A., Costa E., Caruncho H.J. (1999) Cortical bitufted, horizontal and Martinotti cells preferentially express and secrete reelin into perineuronal nets, nonsynaptically modulating gene expression. *Proc. Natl. Acad. Sci. USA*, **96**: 3217–3222.

257. Marin-Padilla M. (1984) Neurons of layer I. A developmental analysis. In *Cerebral Cortex* (Eds. A. Peter, E.G. Jones), pp. 447–478, Plenum Press, New York.

258. Coyle J.T., Yamamura H.I. (1976) Neurochemical aspects of the ontogenesis of GABAergic neurons in the rat brain. *Brain Res.*, **118**: 429–440.

259. Candy J.M., Martin I.L. (1979) The postnatal development of the benzodiazepine receptor in the cerebral cortex and cerebellum of the rat. *J. Neurochem.*, **32**: 655–658.

260. Johnston M.V., Coyle J.T. (1980) Ontogeny of neurochemical markers for noradrenergic, GABAergic and cholinergic neurons in neocortex lesioned with methylazoxymethanol acetate. *J. Neurochem.*, **34**: 1429–1441.

261. Johnston M.V. (1988) Biochemistry of neurotransmitters in cortical development. In *Cerebral Cortex* (Eds A. Peter, E.G. Jones), pp. 211–236, Plenum Press, New York.

262. Vincent S.L., Pabreza L., Benes F.M. (1994) Postnatal maturation of GABA-immunoreactive neurons of rat medial prefrontal cortex. *Soc. Neurosci. Abstract*, 20.

263. Verney C., Berger B., Adrien J., Vigny A., Gay M. (1982) Development of the dopaminergic innervation of the rat cerebral cortex. A light microscopic immunocytochemical study using anti-tyrosine hydroxylase antibodies. *Brain Res.*, **281**: 41–52.

264. Kalsbeek A., Voorn P., Buijs R.M., Pool C.W., Uylings H.B. (1988) Development of the dopaminergic innervation in the prefrontal cortex of the rat. *J. Comp. Neurol.*, **269**: 58–72.

265. Benes F.M., Vincent S.L., Molloy R., Khan Y. (1996) Increased interaction of dopamine-immunoreactive varicosities with GABA neurons of rat medial prefrontal cortex occurs during the postweanling period. *Synapse*, **23**: 237–245.

266. Sutanto W., Handelmann G., de Bree F., de Kloet E.R. (1989) Multifaceted interaction of corticosteroids with the intracellular receptors and with membrane GABAA receptor complex in the rat brain. *J. Neuroendocrinol.*, **1**: 243–247.

267. Majewska M.D., Bisserbe J.C., Eskay L.R. (1985) Glucocorticoids are modulators of GABAA receptors in brain. *Brain Res.*, **339**: 178–182.

268. Lambert J.J., Peters J.A., Cottrell G.A. (1987) Actions of synthetic and endogenous steroids on the GABAA receptor. *Trends Pharmacol. Sci.*, **8**: 224–227.

269. McEwen B.S., Bregon A., Davis P.G., Krey L.C., Luine V.N., BcGinnis M.Y., Paden C.M., Parsons B., Rainbow T.C. (1982) Steroid hormones: humoral

signals which alter brain cell properties and functions. *Rec. Prog. Horm. Res.*, **38**: 41–92.

270. Stumpf W.E., Heiss C., Sar M., Duncan G.E., Draver C. (1989) Dexamethasone and corticosterone receptor sites. *Histochemistry*, **92**: 201–210.

271. Woodbury D.M. (1952) Effects of adrenal steroids: separability of anticonvulsant from hormonal effects. *J. Pharmacol. Exp. Ther.*, **153**: 337–343.

272. Feldman W., Robinson S. (1968) Electrical activity of the brain in adrenalectomized rats with implanted electrodes. *J. Neurol. Sci.*, **6**: 1–8.

273. Pfaff D.W., Silva M.T.A., Weiss J.M. (1971) Telemetered recording of hormone effects on hippocampal neurons. *Science*, **172**: 394–395.

274. Miller A.L., Chaptal C., McEwen B.S., Beck J.R.E. (1978) Modulation of high affinity GABA uptake into hippocampal synaptosomes by glucocorticoids. *Psychoneuroendocrinology*, **3**: 155–164.

275. Schwarcz R., Coyle J.T. (1977) Neurochemical sequelae of kainate injections in corpus striatum and substantia nigra of the rat. *Life Sci.*, **20**: 431–436.

276. Sapolsky R.M. (1992) *Stress, the Aging Brain, and the Mechanisms of Neuron Death*, MIT Press, Cambridge.

8

Biological Research in Anxiety Disorders

Thomas W. Uhde and Ravi Singareddy

*Department of Psychiatry and Behavioral Neurosciences, School of Medicine,
Wayne State University, Detroit, MI 48231, USA*

INTRODUCTION

The study of stress, fear and anxiety was the major focus of research among the early neuroscientists interested in behaviour. This is not surprising, because fear, anxiety and alarm play a fundamental role in survival. Thus, research investigating the phenomenology and neurobiology of anxiety, fear, startle, arousal, alarm, vigilance and alerting functions has been conducted for decades.

In the late nineteenth century, James [1, 2] investigated the neurobiology of fear and rage. He proposed a direct connection between peripheral bodily changes and emotion and launched the concept that some individuals might be unusually responsive to interoceptive cues. A modern analogue of this concept (i.e. anxiety sensitivity) has received renewed interest in the literature. According to this modernized theory, selected somatic sensations serve as powerful stimuli for fear or alarm in some patients with anxiety disorders [3–5]. Certain subtypes of symptoms may be particularly linked to anxiety vulnerability [6], although "anxiety sensitivity" per se is an unreliable predictor of anxiety responses to chemical substances known to induce panic attacks [7]. There is also evidence that anxiety sensitivity may be a heritable trait, particularly in women [8]. Thus, while James's hypothesis stimulated interest in the neurobiology of emotion, particularly the autonomic nervous system, more recent research teams have rekindled and expanded these notions to include genetic and gene–environmental interactions.

In the early twentieth century, Cannon [9, 10] demonstrated that emotional stimuli might induce adrenal gland secretion. In a series of

Psychiatry as a Neuroscience. Edited by Juan José López-Ibor, Wolfgang Gaebel, Mario Maj and Norman Sartorius. © 2002 John Wiley & Sons Ltd.

experiments, Cannon showed that cats exposed to barking dogs release epinephrine. Cannon's experiments inspired research investigating the neuroendocrinological basis of stress, much of which prevailed in the 1950s and 1960s (for reviews, see [11–13]).

Interest in biological factors underlying anxiety was again stimulated by the work of Cohen and White [14], who noted exercise intolerance and increased production of lactate levels in the blood of individuals with neurocirculatory asthenia, the diagnostic forerunner of panic disorder (PD). The work of Mandel Cohen can be linked to today's ongoing research related to chemical models of anxiety, particularly in relation to lactate-induced and CO_2-inhalation-induced panic attacks.

The observations of Klein [15, 16], who proposed two distinct types of anxiety (generalized and panic anxiety) with differential drug responsivity, became the impetus for much of today's investigations into the biological basis of anxiety disorders. Complementing Klein's work was that of Pitts and McClure [17], who developed a method for inducing anxiety by administering intravenous lactate. These separate lines of investigation converged to influence the modern era of anxiety disorder research. In fact, pharmacological and related challenge paradigms remain a valuable strategy for the study of anxiety, fear, alarm, startle and arousal functions in humans.

Among the DSM-IV anxiety disorders, PD, obsessive-compulsive disorder (OCD) and post-traumatic stress disorder (PTSD) have been most intensively investigated, although several research teams have conducted elegant studies investigating the neurobiology of social anxiety disorder and generalized anxiety disorder. Despite these efforts, no definitive pathophysiological or genetic abnormality has been found for any anxiety disorder. Recent advances in the development of research tools, such as real-time functional magnetic resonance imaging (fMRI) [18, 19] and microarrays [20–22], hold great promise for our ability to define more precisely the neurocircuitry and genetic–environmental causations of selective anxiety disorders.

This chapter provides an overview of PD, OCD and PTSD. These anxiety disorders were selected because for each of them an extensive base of knowledge exists in two or more of the following areas: neurochemistry, neuroendocrinology or neuroimmunology, and neurophysiology. For each disorder, however, we selected subtopics that represent unique or particularly salient features of that disorder. For example, under neuroendocrinology–neuroimmunology, we discuss the hypothalamic–pituitary–adrenal (HPA) axis system in PD and PTSD, hypothalamic–growth hormone (GH)–somatomedin (HGS) function in PD, and post-streptococcal auto-immunity in OCD. Thus, we provide an update of information that is particularly relevant or novel for each anxiety disorder, rather than offering a catalogue of common information. Because of the emergent critical value of neuroimaging and genomic strategies to investigate anxiety–fear–alarm–arousal mechanisms, we also provide a brief synopsis of what is known about the genetics and neuroanatomy–neurocircuitry of PD, OCD and PTSD.

PANIC DISORDER

Until the 1960s, PD was subsumed under various names, such as anxiety neurosis, neurocirculatory asthenia, soldier's heart, and Da Costa's syndrome (for review, see [13]). Originally thought to be a rare condition, PD is now known to be a prevalent mental disorder—12-month prevalence is approximately 1% [23]—with devastating socioeconomic consequences, such as job loss, financial dependence, excessive health care utilization [24–27], and a markedly adverse effect on quality of life [28, 29]. Of particular concern is that PD is associated with a high prevalence of suicidal behaviours [30].

A range of biological and psychosocial theories have been proposed to explain the onset and course of panic attacks and the secondary complications of anticipatory anxiety and agoraphobia. Among the anxiety disorders, PD was the first to be extensively studied from a biological perspective. Three decades of research have led to several conclusions: (a) PD is a familial condition, with considerable evidence of a genetic transmission; (b) neuroanatomical substrates that mediate panic attacks, conditioned fear responses and avoidance behaviours are complex, overlapping and highly redundant; (c) abnormalities in respiratory system function are common in PD; (d) panic attacks, the core pathological feature of PD, occur during both awake and sleep states; (e) differential behavioural and biochemical responses to selective agents implicate noradrenergic, serotonergic, benzodiazepine-γ-aminobutyric acid (GABA) and adenosinergic systems in the neurobiology of PD; and (f) blunted GH responses to clonidine are the most consistently observed neuroendocrine abnormality in PD.

Neurogenetics

First-degree relatives of patients with PD have up to a 21-fold greater lifetime risk of PD than relatives of unaffected probands [31–37]. The concordance rate in monozygotic twins has been uniformly reported to be higher than that in dizygotic twins [38], suggesting a genetic contribution. However, the concordance rate for panic in monozygotic twins is less than 50%, indicating that genes are not the only cause of the disorder. On the basis of twin studies and other lines of evidence, it appears that a *susceptibility to*, rather *inheritance of*, panic is transmitted from affected parents to offspring.

Several candidate genes have been proposed and have either been excluded by candidate gene probe and linkage studies [39, 40] or have yet to be confirmed [41–44]. Increasingly, it appears that PD, as well as other constructs related to behavioural inhibition, develops as a by-product of multiple genes and gene–environmental interactions [20, 31, 45, 46].

Neuroanatomy

Most of the neuroimaging studies in PD patients have reported regional reductions in cerebral blood flow (CBF) or metabolism. Reiman *et al.* [47] found a decreased left/right parahippocampal blood flow ratio with positron emission tomography (PET) using [^{15}O]H$_2$O in lactate-vulnerable PD patients. Subsequently, Nordahl *et al.* [48], using PET with ^{18}F-labelled deoxyglucose (FDG), found a decreased left/right hippocampal ratio of metabolism in PD patients compared to normal controls. In contrast, an increase in glucose metabolism was found in the left hippocampal and parahippocampal area in a study comparing cerebral metabolic activity using PET-FDG in six female lactate-sensitive PD patients compared to healthy female volunteers [49]. Other studies have shown reduction in global CBF [50, 51] as well as involvement of right superior temporal, right inferior parietal [49], frontal [52] and occipital cortex [53] in chemically sensitive PD patients.

Overall, the majority of research indicates an alteration in the hippocampus and the adjacent cortex (parahippocampus) in PD patients. These changes in CBF and metabolism could be due to vasoconstricting effects of hyperventilation-induced hypocapnia, which is common in PD patients, especially during lactate-induced panic [54]. However, there is also evidence that PD patients are more sensitive to the vasoconstrictive effects of hyperventilation-induced hypocapnia than are non-panic subjects [51, 55, 56]. Gorman *et al.* [51] speculate, however, that additional factors other than hyperventilation-induced hypocapnia are involved in the mediation of cerebral vasoconstriction.

An extensive literature indicates that the amygdala plays a crucial role in signs and symptoms of anxiety and fear (reviewed in [57]). The amygdala receives sensory information through its lateral and basolateral nuclei. In turn, these nuclei project to the central nucleus of the amygdala, which then projects to hypothalamic and brainstem target areas implicated in anxiety and fear [58, 59]. Thus, the central nucleus of amygdala has extensive efferents to many brain regions that influence key signs and/or symptoms associated with panic or panic-like syndromes. For example, the central nucleus of the amygdala has projections to brain regions that directly or indirectly regulate behavioural "vigilance", "alarm" and "arousal" (e.g. noradrenergic nucleus locus coeruleus) and defensive behaviours (e.g. central grey region [51, 57]), respiratory rate (e.g. parabrachial nucleus), pupillary, heart rate and HPA axis functions (e.g. lateral nucleus and para-ventricular nucleus of the hypothalamus, respectively).

Based on these and other preclinical observations, several investigators have suggested that PD patients suffer from a dysregulation in anxiety–fear–alarm–arousal–startle systems, which conceivably could have different points of initial "activation" or origin of pathology, in brain areas such as, but not limited to, the central nucleus of the amygdala, bed nucleus of the stria terminalis, hippocampus, thalamus, hypothalamus, anterior cingulate, periaquiductal grey or other brain regions [51, 58–67].

It should be underscored that the biological functions of anxiety and fear (as well as arousal, startle and alarm) serve complementary functions in terms of promoting survival in humans and animals. However, several lines of evidence indicate that the neural or endocrine substrates subserving anxiety–fear–alarm–startle–arousal functions can be differentially "activated" by independent temporal, developmental and environmental factors (see also [57, 68–73]).

Neurophysiology

Respiratory System

Respiratory system dysfunction in PD is suggested by the observation that, compared to normal controls, PD patients have an increased sensitivity to exogenous lactate and CO_2 inhalation.

In the original study by Pitts and McClure [17], intravenous administration of sodium lactate produced panic in susceptible individuals, but not in normal subjects. Several subsequent studies have shown that 50–70% of PD patients, compared to approximately 10% of normal volunteers, have panic attacks after intravenous sodium lactate infusion [74, 75].

Numerous studies have attempted to identify the panicogenic mechanism of exogenous lactate. These include changes in acid–base status [76], serum ionized calcium or phosphate [77, 78], intravascular volume and CBF [79, 80]. Hyperventilation, however, is probably the most consistent behavioural and physiological correlate of lactate-induced panic [54, 78, 81]. These findings suggest that lactate-induced panic is associated with changes in respiratory *drive* functions.

It is now well established that CO_2 inhalation induces panic attacks and that these events resemble naturally occurring panic [82]. CO_2 inhalation induces a significantly greater number of panic attacks and more severe ratings of anxiety in patients with PD than in normal control subjects [83–91]. Among the various strategies to investigate CO_2 reactivity, re-breathing air and inhalation of 5%, 7% and 35% CO_2 have been employed in the study of PD. Although the relative rates of CO_2-induced panic differ depending on the methodology, independent studies have consistently demonstrated a greater sensitivity to CO_2 in PD patients compared with normal control subjects [82–84, 86–92].

There is some evidence to suggest that single-breath 35% CO_2 inhalation, in contrast to other CO_2 concentrations or to re-breathing techniques, may be the most effective method for identifying differences in CO_2 reactivity across different diagnostic groups [92, 93]. Single-breath 35% CO_2 inhalation distinguishes patients with PD from patients with major depression [94], OCD [92, 95] and generalized anxiety disorder [96], with the greatest rates reported in the PD patients. Interestingly, a recent study found that 5-7% CO_2 inhalation triggered panic attacks at similar rates in both patients with PD and those with premenstrual dysphoric disorder, and that both groups had increased sensitivity compared with normal control subjects and de-pressed patients [86]. The existence of either comorbid depressive disorder or generalized anxiety disorder renders PD patients more vulnerable to the effects of 35% CO_2 inhalation [96, 97].

Medications effective in PD block the panicogenic effects of 35% CO_2 [89, 98–100] and decrease sensitivity to CO_2 [101].

In summary, there is firm evidence that patients with PD have an in-creased sensitivity to exogenous lactate and CO_2 inhalation. The mechan-isms underlying these increased sensitivities remain unclear. Klein [102] and several other authors [20, 66, 84, 103] have proposed abnormalities in CO_2 concentrations or CO_2 receptor sensitivity, primarily hypersensitivity. Even if chemoreceptor up-regulation proves to be a core abnormality in PD, it is reasonable to assume that a combination of factors and different patho-logical processes may cause CO_2 receptor abnormalities. In addition, systems that mediate CO_2-induced anxiety interface with other systems known to be involved in anxiety and startle, such as the locus coeruleus and HPA axis. What particular sequence or requisite neurochemical or biological events must be present to cause panic attacks remain unknown, although alterations in respiratory drive and CO_2 receptor function would seem, on the basis of current information, to play a key role. In fact, CO_2-induced panic attacks, once triggered, appear to be inevitably associated with increases in minute ventilation and respiratory rate [86]. Nonetheless, it should be underscored that not all PD patients experience panic attacks or demonstrate other evidence of CO_2 over-reactivity [82, 90]. Taken together, these observations suggest that those genetic, biological and environmental factors that confer increased sensitivity to CO_2 inhalation (or lactate) are not *identical* to those factors that cause PD. Some investigators have found an increased respiratory sensitivity to CO_2 inhalation in subjects at high risk for PD (defined as the presence of PD in first-degree relatives) compared with people at low risk (absence of PD in first-degree relatives) [104–108]. Future research will determine whether increased CO_2 inhalation sensitivity can be used as a biological marker for susceptibility for panic attacks in non-anxious individuals, with or without an increased familial risk for PD. High throughput gene screening will also permit the identification of possible genes associated with the lactate-sensitive and CO_2-sensitive endophenotypes, which may represent a more productive research approach to identifying candidate genes than simply studying patients with "categorical" diagnoses such as PD.

Sleep

Common sleep complaints in PD patients are insomnia, restless or broken sleep and sleep panic attacks [109–116]. Sleep panic attacks are the most disturbing and disabling sleep problem in PD. Not surprisingly, PD patients with sleep panic attacks report higher rates of insomnia, especially non-restorative sleep and frequent awakenings, than do PD patients who do not suffer such attacks [115, 117–119].

In terms of sleep architecture, most polysomnographic studies have not found major abnormalities in PD [114, 116, 120]. For example, the widely reported shortened rapid eye movement (REM) latency observed in depression is not characteristic of PD. Particularly noteworthy, however, is the co-existence of sleep panic attacks in a majority of patients with otherwise classic daytime, "wake" panic attacks. Sleep electroencephalography (EEG) studies indicate that sleep panic attacks, often reported by PD patients as their most distressing symptom, emerge during the transition from late stage 2 to early stage 3 sleep [121], when dreaming is absent and cognitions are minimal.

Interestingly, unlike patients with major depression, PD patients experience a worsening of anxiety, including the precipitation of panic attacks, after 24 hours of sleep deprivation [121–123]. Furthermore, Uhde and coworkers reported that PD patients with recurrent sleep panic attacks tend to develop a conditioned fear of sleep, and, as a result, develop sleep deprivation [121, 124, 125]. The subgroup of PD patients with comorbid sleep panic attacks (30–65%, depending on the diagnostic criteria), therefore, are particularly at risk for developing a positive feedback loop of worsening psychopathology. That is, sleep panic attacks promote a conditioned fear of sleep, and of the sleep environment [121], which leads to avoidance of sleep and sleep deprivation, followed by an increase in the frequency and intensity of both daytime "wake" and nocturnal sleep panic attacks.

Based on these observations, our laboratory speculates that patients with sleep panic attacks share a common biological diathesis, and possibly a common genetic heritability, with PD patients who report CO_2-induced and relaxation-induced panic attacks. Future research will also focus on the relationship between possible subsets of symptoms, within the spectrum of "wake" and "sleep" panic attacks, that predict liability to the development of conditioned fear and avoidance behaviours.

Neurochemistry

Noradrenergic System

In the late 1970s, Redmond and Huang [61] found an association between the activation of the locus coeruleus, the major noradrenergic nucleus in the brain, and fear behaviours in stump-tail monkeys. Subsequently, several groups of investigators [126–131] proposed noradrenergic dysfunction, primarily overactivity, in PD. A number of probes were used to assess the noradrenergic system in PD.

Yohimbine, an α_2 adrenoceptor antagonist, has consistently been shown to induce behavioural and cardiovascular hyperactivity in PD patients [128, 132, 133], suggesting α_2 adrenoceptor supersensitivity. The anxiogenic response to yohimbine is particularly linked to panic attacks. Moreover, the increased behavioural sensitivity to yohimbine in PD is distinctly different from the anxiogenic responses observed in other anxiety and neuropsychiatric disorders [134–136].

A blunted cardiovascular response to clonidine, an α_2 adrenoceptor agonist, has been reported in PD patients, but this has not been consistently replicated [129, 131, 137]. In contrast, blunted GH responses to clonidine have been reported and independently confirmed by several research teams (for original data and review, see [64]). This finding, however, is not limited to PD and has been observed in patients with depression [138], generalized anxiety disorder and OCD (reviewed in [64, 139]).

The regulation of GH release is complex and is influenced by noradrenergic, cholinergic, dopaminergic, GABAergic and serotonergic systems, as well as by GH releasing factor (GRF), somatostatin release-inhibiting factor (SRIF) and GH itself via feedback loops. However, not all agents that stimulate GH release are blunted in PD patients, indicating that there is no intrinsic, primary abnormality in the HGS axis in PD [64]. Interestingly, patients with PD continue to demonstrate blunted GH responses to clonidine even after effective treatment with fluoxetine [140]. It is possible, therefore, that the blunted GH response to clonidine is a "trait" marker for disturbances in anxiety–fear–alarm–arousal systems, although a linkage to genes known to regulate GH or GH receptors has not been reported in PD.

Taken together, these data are consistent with the theory that PD (and probably several other anxiety disorders) is characterized by noradrenergic overactivity, resulting in down-regulation of α_2 adrenoceptors at the level of the hypothalamus. These data also suggest that alterations in noradrenergic activity (and its behavioural analogues of increased arousal and alarm) may be linked to many anxiety and mood disorders, and are probably not specific to PD.

There is inconsistent evidence in favour of β receptor involvement in PD. Beta-blockers are generally ineffective in the treatment of PD, although the β adrenergic receptor agonist isoproterenol has been shown to induce panic attacks in susceptible individuals at the same rate as sodium lactate [75].

Adenosinergic System

As reviewed elsewhere [141–146], "chemical models" (i.e. the induction of anxiety via the administration of drugs or peptides) have been employed as a research tool to investigate neurotransmitter systems in PD. Our research team has been particularly active in developing and studying the caffeine challenge test as a tool for the study of anxiety disorders, particularly PD. We also have proposed that acute caffeine intoxication and chronic caffeinism, respectively, are nearly perfect mimickers of PD and generalized anxiety disorder [146, 147]. Finally, several lines of evidence indicate that PD patients have an increased sensitivity to caffeine. Because of its relevance to both clinical practice and the study of adenosinergic function in PD, a summary of the behavioural and biochemical effects of caffeine is provided below.

Without making any reference to "panic attacks", Greden [148] reported three cases in which the clinical profile of caffeinism was essentially identical to that of anxiety neurosis, the diagnostic forerunner of PD [13]. Interestingly, in one case, Greden [148] reported that an individual who had recently consumed large amounts of caffeine developed dyspnoea, lightheadedness and changes in cardiac rhythm, suggestive of a panic-like event. In four cases, Uhde [147, 149] found that the effect of high levels of caffeine consumed over short or long periods of time, respectively, was indistinguishable from DSM-III/IV panic attacks or generalized anxiety symptomatology. Interestingly, in one case excessive caffeine induced a sleep panic attack. That caffeine can induce symptoms of anxiety is hardly a new observation [150, 151], although it probably remains one of the most unrecognized of common problems in general medical practice. Other than minor age-appropriate life stressors, none of our four subjects had suffered from anxiety disorders earlier and all four improved with the gradual decrease in their daily caffeine intake. These observations are noteworthy for two reasons: they suggest (a) that caffeine can induce symptoms of anxiety in *medically and psychiatrically healthy* people, and (b) that caffeine-induced anxiety, depending on prior levels and patterns of consumption, can trigger *panic attacks or generalized anxiety* that are identical to symptoms observed in patients with panic and generalized anxiety disorders.

While excessive caffeine can trigger pathological anxiety in healthy individuals, including panic attacks, there remains considerable evidence to suggest that PD patients are unusually sensitive, compared to patients with other anxiety disorders and normal controls, to the anxiogenic effects of caffeine. What is the evidence for this view?

Our laboratory found that PD patients consume less caffeine than normal control subjects; moreover, a significantly greater percentage of PD patients (67%) reported giving up coffee compared with either normal controls (13–20%, matched for age, gender and socioeconomic status) or depressed patients (22%) [149, 152]. Panic patients reported that they gave up caffeinated beverages and foods because of their anxiogenic and related stimulant effects. Finally, there were several significantly positive correlations between daily caffeine consumption and measures of "anxiety", "insomnia", "alertness" and "distress" (but not "well-being") in PD patients, which were not found in depressed patients or normal controls (for review, see [149]). More recent unpublished findings in our laboratory have replicated these earlier observations in PD patients; furthermore, we have found that patients with another anxiety disorder (i.e. social anxiety disorder) do not consume less caffeine or discontinue its use because of its psychostimulant effects.

To confirm the apparent increased sensitivity to caffeine (based on self-report measures) in PD, we conducted a number of double-blind, placebo-controlled experiments in humans. In normal controls, we found a dose-related increase in ratings of anxiety, as well as plasma cortisol and lactate, following 0 mg (placebo), 240 mg, 480 mg and 720 mg *orally administered* caffeine. Interestingly, two normal controls experienced panic attacks for the first time in their life at the 720-mg dose. These findings, taken together with earlier case reports [147, 149], suggest that oral caffeine at a dose of 720 mg or more can trigger panic attacks in healthy people who typically consume low-to-average (≤250 mg daily) amounts of caffeine. In contrast, with one exception (see below), no normal control subject [153] has experienced a panic attack (or anything resembling "severe" anxiety) at doses below 480 mg per os or 5 mg/kg intravenously. The exception involved a normal subject who was awakened with a *sleep panic attack* 1 minute after receiving 5 mg/kg caffeine intravenously during stage 2 sleep [154].

Collectively, we find panic-induced rates of 0%, 0%, 3.1% and 16.7%, respectively, in *healthy normal control subjects* following administration of 0 mg (placebo) and 240, 480, and 720 *oral milligram equivalent doses* of caffeine [i.e. assuming that oral (mg)/intravenous (mg/kg) doses of 240/3, 480/5 and 720/7, respectively, are roughly equivalent]. Based on the apparent panicogenic "threshold" of 480 mg caffeine in normal controls, we separately compared the behavioural and biochemical effects of caffeine (480 mg per os) in 57 patients with PD compared with 27 normal control subjects. While not all subjects received placebo, no subject, whether patient or normal control, had (in this or any other study) a panic attack after placebo administration. Caffeine also failed to induce panic attacks in any normal control. After caffeine, however, 36.9% of the patient group reported panic attacks. Moreover, as reviewed elsewhere [146], PD patients had significantly greater increases in plasma cortisol and lactate compared with normal control subjects. The Yale group [155] also found differential behavioural sensitivity, as reflected by caffeine-induced panic attack rates of 71% and 0%, respectively, in PD patients and normal controls.

Interestingly, two research teams [156, 157], using taste threshold as the dependent variable, found that caffeine lowers the level for quinine detection to a greater degree in PD patients than in normal controls. Using this paradigm, PTSD patients were not found to have different caffeine-mediated changes in quinine threshold compared with normal controls.

A range of studies employing different methods (dietary assessment, self-report ratings, pharmacological challenge and taste threshold testing) strongly support the view that PD patients have a genuine increased sensitivity to caffeine compared with normal controls (well-documented) and patients with other anxiety disorders, such as social anxiety disorder [158] and PTSD [157].

In animal and tissue preparations, caffeine has direct or indirect effects on multiple neurotransmitter systems implicated in the neurobiology of fear–anxiety–arousal–startle functions (e.g. benzodiazepine-GABAergic, noradrenergic, dopaminergic). In addition, caffeine inhibits phosphodiesterase, resulting in increases in cyclic adenosine monophosphate (AMP) and alterations in intracellular calcium stores. Most of the neurotransmitter, phosphodiesterase, cyclic AMP and calcium effects, however, occur in animals at tissue concentrations that far exceed those seen in humans consuming less than toxic levels of caffeine. In contrast, caffeine, at doses commonly consumed in humans, produces tissue concentrations associated with robust adenosine receptor antagonist action [152, 159]. Moreover, adenosine and caffeine, as expected, have opposite effects, respectively, in terms of decreasing/increasing arousal, blood pressure, seizure threshold, heart rate, and the biological effects of the stress response (for reviews, see [146, 149]).

In summary, it is highly likely that caffeine produces anxiogenic and panicogenic effects in humans, possibly particularly in PD patients, via blockade of one of several adenosinergic receptors. It is also possible that different adenosinergic receptors—A1, A2a, A2b, A3 [160]—mediate different components of caffeine's anxiogenic-panicogenic spectrum [161, 162]. Although adenosine reuptake blockers that have low penetration into brain may prove ineffective in the treatment of PD [163], drug discovery efforts will continue to focus on the development of agonists that have preferential action at different adenosine receptor subtypes.

Serotonergic System

Several lines of evidence in both animals and humans suggest an important role for the serotonergic system, encompassing probably more than 14 receptor subtypes, in anxiety–fear–alarm–arousal functions. The challenge for clinical investigators is how to investigate pre- versus postsynaptic receptor subtype function in brain specific areas.

Pharmacological challenge with the serotonin (5-HT) releasing agent fenfluramine has been reported to be anxiogenic and to produce greater increase in plasma prolactin and cortisol in PD patients [164]. Similarly, several studies (but not all) using m-chloromethylpiperazine (m-CPP), a postsynaptic 5-HT_2 receptor agonist, have reported increased anxiety in PD (reviewed in [165]). However, challenge with the 5-HT precursor L-tryptophan [166] and 5-hydroxytryptophan (5-HTP) [167, 168] as well as tryptophan depletion [169] studies have been unable to establish a definitive role for 5-HT dysfunction in PD.

Because the 5-HT transporter system in platelets is similar to that in the brain, several investigators have studied [^{3}H]imipramine or [^{3}H]paroxetine binding in platelets of PD patients compared to normal controls or patients with other neuropsychiatric syndromes. Lewis et al. [170] found decreased imipramine binding in PD, an observation that could not be replicated by Uhde's group [171]. More recently, using paroxetine binding (the preferred ligand for the investigation of 5-HT transporter status), Maguire et al. [172] and Stein et al. [173] failed to find abnormal paroxetine binding in PD. However, Marazziti et al. [174] reported decreased paroxetine binding, which normalized within 1 year in conjunction with clinical improvement.

Despite these mixed results, the selective 5-HT reuptake inhibitors (SSRIs) are clearly effective in PD. It is likely, therefore, that the use of specific 5-HT receptor probes [175] in the study of PD will lead to a more precise understanding of the role of different receptor subtypes in the pathogenesis and therapy of the disorder. While there is no validated animal model of PD per se [64], there are compelling animal data implicating 5-HT_{1A} receptors in the neurobiology of fear (for reviews, see [176–178]). Briefly, knock-outs of 5-HT$_{1A}$ receptors produce behavioural inhibition and fearful behaviours in a number of animal models (for review of conflict tests, see [179]), such as open field [180], novel environments [181], elevated maze [181], foot shock [181] and forced swim test [182], as well as increased heart rate responses to foot shock and novelty suppressed feeding [178]. Interestingly, buspirone, a partial 5-HT$_{1A}$ agonist, has limited anti-anxiety efficacy (and in our clinic is used only as an adjunctive treatment for patients with *any* anxiety disorder). Nonetheless, these collective findings suggest a role for 5-HT function, and selective 5-HT receptor subtypes (e.g. 5-HT$_{1A}$), in the neurobiology of anxiety–fear–arousal–startle systems, if not specifically in PD.

In the future, as susceptibility genes, neurotransmitter-receptor subtypes, and neuroendocrine systems are more causally linked to different types of behaviour (e.g. avoidance) or symptomatology (e.g. panic attacks, impulsivity), it is likely that DSM-IV and ICD-10 nomenclature [183] will be replaced with more meaningful diagnostic anxiety "endophenotypes" [46, 184, 185]. This will move psychiatric nomenclature away from the current "descriptive" model to one aligned with an increasingly more sophisticated understanding of how gene, gene–environment and biological systems interact separately and together to trigger, maintain and turn off specific anxiety and anxiety-related behaviours in humans.

Benzodiazepine-GABAergic System

That the benzodiazepine-GABAergic system plays a role in the biological functions of fear in animals is well established in the literature (for reviews, see [186, 187]). The hypothesis that alteration in benzodiazepine-GABAergic receptor function is relevant to arousal (and, conversely, sedation) in humans is also well established, although it has not been confirmed that *any specific* abnormality in the benzodiazepine-GABAergic system is inevitably involved in the pathophysiology of PD or any other anxiety disorder.

Administration of both oral and intravenous flumazenil, a benzodiazepine receptor antagonist, to PD patients produces clinically unimpressive behavioural effects. Nutt *et al.* [188] reported increased ratings of anxiety in PD patients, and Woods *et al.* [189] failed to demonstrate anxiolytic effects. Strohle *et al.* [190] investigated the effects of flumazenil compared with placebo and lactate. This team found that 8 of 10 patients had lactate-induced panic attacks, whereas no patients experienced panic attacks after saline or flumazenil. Coupland *et al.* [191] examined whether the behavioural response to flumazenil might identify patients vulnerable to situational panic attacks. In this study, the rate and severity of anxiety following flumazenil was not significantly different between patients with social phobia and normal controls. Given that flumazenil, a pure or neutral benzodiazepine antagonist, impressively reduces the sedative and anxiolytic actions of exogenously administered benzodiazepine, triggers withdrawal symptoms in long-term benzodiazepine users [192] and blocks the proconvulsant and anxiogenic actions of inverse agonists, the findings with flumazenil in panic patients suggest that PD is unlikely to be caused by a simple "deficiency" or an "excess", respectively, of endogenous benzodiazepine-like agonist(s) or inverse-agonist(s).

It should be emphasized that these inconsistent behavioural effects of flumazenil do not preclude a role for endogenous or even dietary sources [193, 194] of benzodiazepines in the pathophysiology of PD. Changes in benzodiazepine receptor sensitivity or distribution, as a primary disturbance or secondary to tonic GABAergic or neurosteroid influence, remain viable possibilities [195–197]. In fact, several research teams have independently found, using radiolabelled iomazenil (single photon emission tomography, SPECT) or flumazenil (PET), significant abnormalities in benzodiazepine receptor binding [198–201]. Moreover, benzodiazepine compounds are the only agents to block all chemical models of PD (for review, see [145]). PD patients also have altered benzodiazepine sensitivity to benzodiazepine-induced disruption of saccadic eye movements [188, 202, 203], although this abnormality is not specific to PD and may be seen across a spectrum of anxiety syndromes [203].

Thus, while the appealing notion of under- or overproduction of an unknown endogenous benzodiazepine compound is an unlikely *direct* cause of PD, there is overwhelming evidence to support a key role for benzodiazepine-GABAergic systems in PD.

Cholecystokinin

Cholecystokinin (CCK) concentrations are lower in the cerebrospinal fluid (CSF) [204] and lymphocytes [205] of patients with PD. These findings could possibly result from an up-regulation of CCK receptors in PD patients compared with healthy normal controls.

Consistent with this notion, infusions of CCK tetrapeptide, CCK-4, and pentagastrin, a synthetic analogue of CCK-4, produce greater rates of panic and more severe ratings of anxiety in PD patients compared with normal control subjects [206–210]. These anxiogenic effects are blocked by CCK_B antagonists such as L-365260 and CI-988 [211, 212], tricyclic antipanic agents such as imipramine [213], β adrenergic blockers such as propranolol [214], but not $5\text{-}HT_3$ antagonists such as ondansetron [208]. Studies investigating CCK_B antagonists for the treatment of *natural panic attacks* in PD have been disappointing [215–217]. Moreover, even though PD patients are clearly more sensitive to the behavioural effects of CCK_B agonists compared with normal controls, the panicogenic effects of CCK_B agonists are not specific to PD. Pentagastrin produces panic attacks in normal controls [206, 209, 210, 218–221] and in patients with social anxiety disorder [208, 209] and OCD [220]. Interestingly, the panicogenic effects of pentagastrin in patients with OCD are unassociated with a worsening of obsessions or compulsions.

Taken together, these observations implicate CCK neuropeptides in the chemical induction of anxiety and panic attacks. However, the robust panicogenic properties of CCK_B receptor agonists are not specific for PD. Moreover, the neurobiological relationship between CCK-4-induced and pentagastrin-induced panic to *natural or spontaneous panic* attacks, if any, remains to be elucidated.

Given the failure to date to develop a new class of CCK_B antagonist anxiolytic compounds, it is reasonable to question the value of chemical models as a drug discovery strategy. For drug discovery, it is critical that all research teams employ rigorous, consistent and reliable criteria whenever using chemical models in the investigation of anxiety disorders. It remains quite possible that entirely new CCK_B antagonist compounds, with appropriate absorption and pharmacokinetic properties, will be developed in the future.

Neuroendocrinology

Studies evaluating the HPA axis system in PD have examined plasma and urinary cortisol levels at baseline and under different challenge conditions. Overall, the degree of HPA axis dysfunction in PD, if any, is relatively unimpressive, particularly in relation to the abnormalities reported in patients with major depression.

Evidence for increased plasma and/or urinary free cortisol levels has been inconsistent [143, 222–224]. In a recent study of 24-hour blood sampling of adrenocorticotropic hormone (ACTH) and cortisol in PD, some patients had elevated overnight cortisol secretion and increased activity in ultradian secretory episodes, but these findings were subtle [225].

Several studies have reported significant rates of dexamethasone nonsuppression in patients with PD, but many of these studies were conducted in PD complicated by depression or severe agoraphobia (reviewed in [226]). Finally, blunted ACTH responses to corticotropin releasing hormone (CRH) have been reported in some older studies [223, 227], but a more recent study found normal or slightly enhanced responses in non-depressed patients with PD [228].

Despite these unimpressive findings with traditional indices, research teams have reported significantly greater plasma cortisol increases in PD patients, compared to normal controls, after the administration of some (*m*-CPP [228], caffeine [146], yohimbine [230]) but not all (lactate [231], CO_2 [232]) chemical models of anxiety. Interestingly, the presence of high cortisol levels with low pCO_2 has been reported in PD as a baseline predictor of panicking versus non-panicking after lactate. Moreover, in the caffeine challenge test, PD patients have significantly greater increases in cortisol compared to normal control subjects, although cortisol rises do not distinguish between the panickers and the non-panickers.

Most evidence, therefore, indicates that HPA axis dysfunction, even when present in panic patients, is modest in degree. When there is evidence of dysfunction, it is generally in the direction of "increased" activity. However, while increases in plasma cortisol may be associated with some panic attacks, HPA activation is not a seminal neuroendocrine correlate of panic attacks. That similar panicogenic, but quite divergent cortisol responses, are associated with different chemical models suggests that (a) two or more fundamentally different pathways can mediate panic attacks or (b) HPA activation (i.e. increased cortisol levels), when associated with panic attacks, involves higher-level (i.e. upstream) sites within a single panicogenic pathway, compared with site(s) in the neuronal circuit that are unassociated with increases in cortisol.

Research supporting increased HPA activation in PD is primarily derived from the measurement of plasma cortisol levels prior to and after the administration of chemical agents known, at sufficient doses, to trigger panic attacks in humans. Almost all of the data accumulated in PD patients are, in fact, gathered under conditions where the *internal experience and behavioural responses* are different (i.e. *greater or more severe*) than what is experienced in the normal control subject. As a case in point, our laboratory has consistently reported that caffeine (480 mg per os) induces panic attacks in PD patients but *not* in normal control subjects. Moreover, PD patients have significantly greater increases in plasma cortisol after caffeine (480 mg per os) compared to normal controls, although *within* the patient group there is no difference in the cortisol increment in panicking versus non-panicking patients. Most investigators would view these data as evidence for increased HPA activation in the patients. But what would happen if a healthy normal control experienced a panic attack for the first time in his life?

Using a higher caffeine dose (720 mg per os) (not given to PD patients), two of six normal controls experienced panic attacks [153]. These panicking normal controls had a greater than five-fold peak change (peak concentration minus baseline mean) in cortisol ($\Delta 15.8 \pm 1.9\,\mu g/dl$ SE) compared with the non-panicking healthy volunteers ($\Delta 2.8 \pm 2.2\,\mu g/dl$). Obviously, differences in doses (i.e. 480 mg in panicking patients versus 720 mg in panicking normal controls), subjective state (i.e. experiencing versus non-experiencing panic attacks) and prior history (e.g. number and distribution of lifetime panic attacks) make it impossible to ascertain the individual and interactive contributions of dose, life stressors and other relevant factors to the changes in cortisol. It is of interest, however, that the average caffeine-induced mean peak change in plasma cortisol in our *panicking* PD patients across all studies is 6.0 μg/dl, considerably less than the approximately 16.0 μg/dl peak change found in our two *panicking* normal control subjects.

It is theoretically possible, therefore, that some PD patients are unable to mount a *normal* HPA axis response *during* panic attacks. If so, this raises the possibility that what appears to be a *relative* increase in HPA activation after the chemical induction of panic attacks is not evidence for increased HPA axis function but, rather, *either* an *abnormal decreased* ability to mount an adequate HPA response during panic attacks or a *normal down-regulation* of the axis as a result of repeated prior episodes of panic. Future research needs to investigate the clinical phenomenology and molecular mechanisms that mediate both sensitization and tolerance in stress-induced and *panic-induced* activations of HPA axis function.

It is beyond the scope of this review, but we have speculated that psychological factors (e.g. chronic worry) and external stressors, if sufficiently severe, may result in alterations in growth and stature [125]. Several lines of evidence in humans and animals support this notion [233, 234]. If it is confirmed by independent laboratories, the locus coeruleus and HGS systems become an ideal analogue for investigating "mind–body–brain" dynamics.

OBSESSIVE-COMPULSIVE DISORDER

OCD was thought to be rare, but recent epidemiological data indicate a 1.9–3.3% prevalence in the general population [235]. OCD is often quite disabling and associated with significant work and social impairment and a negative impact on family life [236]. The discovery in 1967 of the effectiveness of clomipramine (a 5-HT reuptake inhibitor) in the treatment of OCD was a major advance, which heralded a new era in the study of serotonergic mechanisms in this and related anxiety disorders.

Neurogenetics

Black *et al.* [237] reported increased anxiety disorders in first-degree relatives of probands with OCD compared with the relatives of normal controls. These findings suggested that OCD confers an increased familial risk for anxiety disorders, although, in this study, not specifically for OCD.

However, Pauls *et al.* [238] later found significantly increased rates of OCD and subsyndromal OCD (10.3% and 7.9%, respectively) in relatives of probands with OCD compared with relatives of normal controls (1.9% and 2%, respectively). Moreover, a recent twin study in women [239] found that self-reported measures of obsessions and compulsions were heritable (26% and 33%, respectively) and related in part to common genetic factors.

Rates of tics are significantly greater among the relatives of OCD patients compared to the first-degree relatives of "psychiatrically unaffected" individuals [238]. Other lines of evidence [240] also suggest a comorbid, often familial relationship between OCD and tic disorders. In addition to tic disorders, another research team [241] found that body dysmorphic disorder and pathological grooming habits (nail biting, trichotillomania, or skin picking) are also transmitted in the families of patients with OCD, which is unrelated to the presence or absence of the somatoform or grooming condition in the probands.

As has been done for PD, several candidate genes have been proposed for OCD [242–246]. Initial investigations suggested a role for the catechol-*O*-methyltransferase (COMT) and 5-HT transporter promoter genes [243, 247], although a subsequent study provided only partial support for an association with the COMT gene locus [248]. For genetic approaches to the investigation of OCD, the reader is referred to Wolff *et al.* [184].

Neuroanatomy

Several imaging studies have found that basal ganglia volume is decreased in patients with OCD compared with healthy controls [249, 250]. However, these findings have not been consistently replicated [251, 252].

PET and SPECT investigations have demonstrated abnormalities in the orbitofrontal cortex (OFC), anterior cingulate gyrus, and basal ganglia (especially caudate nuclei and thalamus) in patients with OCD (for reviews, see [253, 254]). Moreover, PET studies demonstrate a decline in OFC and caudate activity toward normal control values when OCD patients are effectively treated with either SSRIs or behavioural therapy [253, 255–259]. Similarly, SPECT studies have shown normalization of OFC activity [260, 261] with SSRI treatment, whereas, by contrast, abnormalities in the OFC, caudate and thalamus are further magnified with symptom provocation [262–267].

Converging data, therefore, suggest that orbitofrontal–basal ganglia–thalamus–orbitofrontal circuits are important in the mediation of OCD symptoms [256, 268–271]. Interestingly, early evidence implicating these structures came from autopsy findings. Victims of the influenza pandemic who developed obsessive-compulsive traits had prominent lesions in their basal ganglia [272]. Several neurological disorders of basal ganglia, such as

Sydenham's chorea and Huntington's disease, are also associated with obsessive-compulsive symptoms.

Neurophysiology

Many patients with OCD report poor quality sleep, although the range and quality of subjective sleep disturbance is quite broad (e.g. many patients report no problems whatsoever, whereas other patients have major problems initiating and maintaining sleep). From a clinical perspective, most subjective complaints can be linked to clinical aspects of the illness. For example, adolescents and adults whose night-time activities are preoccupied with thoughts about germs or performing cleaning rituals may demonstrate significant increases in sleep latency, decreases in total sleep time or abnormalities in sleep continuity [121].

Early studies [273] suggested that OCD might be associated with a shortened REM latency, similar in degree to patients with major depression. However, two subsequent studies failed to replicate this early observation [274, 275]. Despite these later negative findings, Huwig-Poppe et al. [276] recently reported that the tryptophan depletion test, a strategy that decreases 5-HT levels, produces a more marked disturbance in sleep continuity in patients with OCD compared with normal control subjects. These findings, in addition to supporting a role for 5-HT in OCD, suggest that the tryptophan depletion test [277] may be a valuable strategy for investigating serotonergic functions in sleep (or sleep deprivation) of patients with other anxiety disorders.

Interestingly, patients with OCD do not appear to have a consistent change (either improvement or worsening) of obsessions or compulsions after sleep deprivation [278], which stands in contrast to the worsening and improvement seen in anxiety and depression, respectively, in patients with PD and major depression [121]. Thus, both the tryptophan depletion test and sleep deprivation offer interesting research tools for investigating the neurobiology of anxiety disorders, particularly when combined with neuroimaging and genetic information [279].

Clinical experience suggests that sleep problems, when evident in OCD, improve in parallel with the successful treatment of core symptoms (i.e. obsessions and compulsions), although no research team, to our knowledge, has confirmed this impression with polysomnography.

Neurochemistry

The efficacy of SSRIs in OCD stimulated interest in the serotonergic system.

CSF levels of 5-hydroxyindole acetic acid (5-HIAA), a 5-HT metabolite, are elevated in some [280] but not all studies [281, 282]. Administration of *m*-CPP, a 5-HT agonist, has been found to exacerbate OCD symptoms in some studies [283, 284], but other research teams [285–287] have not replicated these findings. However, effective treatment with SSRIs is associated with decreases in CSF 5-HIAA [281] and normalization of the neuroendocrine and behavioural responses to *m*-CPP [288, 289], supporting a role for 5-HT systems in the pathophysiology of OCD.

There is evidence of possible involvement of opioids [290], oxytocin [291], vasopressin [292], and gonadal steroids [293] in OCD. Although it is likely that other neurotransmitters (e.g. dopamine, norepinephrine), in addition to 5-HT, are involved in the pathophysiology of OCD, the convergence of data from a range of different studies and methodologies consistently supports a key role for serotonergic systems in OCD.

Neuroimmunology

Early observations of obsessive-compulsive-like symptoms in patients with Sydenham's chorea (a manifestation of rheumatic fever with neurological symptoms) suggested an autoimmune basis for childhood-onset OCD [294–296]. More recently, Swedo *et al.* [297] coined the term *paediatric autoimmune neuropsychiatric disorder associated with streptococcal infections* (PANDAS) to characterize patients whose OCD symptoms appear to have been triggered by group A β-haemolytic streptococcal (GABHS) infections.

Patients with PANDAS may present not only with OCD, but also with tics, as well as attention deficit hyperactivity disorder (ADHD)-like symptoms [297]. That PANDAS can present with attention problems and hyperactivity led the Yale group [298] to investigate antistreptococcal titres in patients with chronic tic disorder, OCD or ADHD and controls. Interestingly, they found that ADHD predicted antistreptolysin O and antideoxyribonuclease B titres, after covarying for the presence of comorbid OCD or chronic tic disorder. Peterson *et al.* [298] also found that higher antistreptococcal titres were associated with increased brain volumes in the globus pallidus and putamen of OCD and ADHD patients, but not in patients with chronic tic disorder or control subjects. The cause–effect relationship between streptococcal infections and the onset and course of symptoms such as obsessions, compulsions, attention problems and hyperactivity remains unclear.

Of particular interest are findings with the expression of D8/17, an antigen of B lymphocytes, in OCD. D8/17 is associated with greater susceptibility to rheumatic fever, as a complication of GABHS infection. D8/17 expression is significantly higher in children with PANDAS and in children with Sydenham's chorea compared with a healthy comparison group [296]. Investigators have also found that patients with childhood-onset OCD or

Tourette's syndrome have significantly greater D8/17 expression than healthy controls [299]. Taken together, these combined observations provide formidable evidence for an autoimmune (specifically, post-streptococcal) aetiology in childhood-onset OCD.

Ongoing research is evaluating the effects of plasma exchange (plasma-pheresis) and intravenous immunoglobulin (IVIG) treatment in patients with PANDAS. Although requiring confirmation, preliminary results are quite promising [300].

Because antibiotic therapy is used to block recurrences of rheumatic fever, penicillin prophylaxis might theoretically also be effective in the treatment and/or prevention of infection-induced exacerbations of PANDAS. In contrast to the preliminary positive reports with plasma exchange and IVIG, initial findings with penicillin prophylaxis have not been promising [301]. It is unknown, therefore, whether penicillin prophylaxis will ultimately have a role in the treatment of specific subtypes of OCD (PANDAS) or tic disorders.

POST-TRAUMATIC STRESS DISORDER

PTSD is a chronic anxiety disorder whose symptoms have been described since the inception of war. Kessler *et al.* [302] found a 7.8% lifetime prevalence of the disorder (men 5%, women 10.4%) in the general population.

Neurogenetics

Both heritable and non-genomic factors influence susceptibility to PTSD [303]. Using the Vietnam Era Twin Registry, True *et al.* [304] found that genetic factors contributed 13–34% of re-experiencing symptoms and 28–34% of symptoms related to avoidance and/or arousal clusters. In a related study, the Washington University team [305] found that 15.3% of the risk for PTSD was shared in common with alcohol and drug dependence. Many of the comorbid problems associated with PTSD (e.g. alcohol abuse), therefore, might be related to both distinct and shared genetic and non-genomic factors.

Perhaps particularly relevant is the study of genetic factors which increase the likelihood that a person will be exposed to a traumatic event. Several lines of evidence in humans and animals indicate that certain heritable personality or behavioural traits may increase or decrease one's likelihood to participate in behaviours which themselves may confer relatively increased or decreased liability to be exposed to major life or traumatic events [306–309].

As for PD and OCD, several candidate genes have been proposed for PTSD, particularly those related to dopamine regulation [310], but have not been confirmed by independent research teams [311]. In the future, it may be more productive to investigate genetic factors associated with certain symptoms (e.g. recurrent nightmares) or biological markers (e.g. cortisol) associated with, but not diagnostic of, PTSD (for review, see [312]), rather than to study the genetic risk for categorical syndromes per se (i.e. PTSD).

Neuroanatomy

Neuroanatomical loci in both subcortical (e.g. hypothalamus and amygdala) and cortical (e.g. prefrontal, anterior cingulate, and orbitofrontal cortex) regions are implicated in the pathophysiology of PTSD. MRI investigations have found right-hippocampal volume reductions in combat-related PTSD [313], left-hippocampal volume decreases in childhood sexual abuse-related PTSD [314, 315], and bilateral hippocampal volume reductions in veterans with PTSD [316]. Interestingly, hippocampal volume changes correlate with short-term verbal memory deficits in combat-related PTSD [313].

PET studies reveal decreased metabolic rates in the temporal and prefrontal cortex of patients with combat-related PTSD and in the parietal cortex of patients with comorbid PTSD and substance abuse [318, 319]. Increased blood flow in the amygdala, insula, orbitofrontal cortex and anterior cingulate and decreased flow in mid-temporal, left inferior frontal and medial prefrontal cortex have been reported in combat veterans with versus without PTSD [319, 320]. Interestingly, a decrease in blood flow in the medial prefrontal cortex is observed in PTSD patients when exposed to reminders of their original trauma [319, 320].

These imaging studies implicate a number of brain regions including, but not limited to, the hippocampus, medial prefrontal cortex, parietal cortex and anterior cingulate. That abnormalities in these anatomical regions have been reported in PTSD is relevant to the spectrum of problems associated with PTSD (for reviews, see [70, 320–325]. The hippocampus plays a role in learning and memory (perhaps related to amnesia and flashbacks, for example) and contextual conditioning (possibly related to the generalization of fear cues to associated environmental context) and the medial prefrontal cortex mediates extinction (e.g. inability to eradicate fearful responses to cues no longer associated with trauma). Whether the apparent decreased hippocampal size in PTSD is a consequence of trauma or a risk factor for the development of PTSD will be an important subject for future research.

Neurophysiology

Sensory input and memory processing appear to be disturbed in PTSD. Disturbances in sensory processing, which are believed to play an important role in hyperarousal symptoms (e.g. exaggerated startle response), have been studied using evoked potentials. Abnormal P300 (300 milliseconds after the stimuli [326]) as well as P50 components of evoked potentials have been reported in patients with PTSD [327]. These findings suggest that sensory processing disturbances are independent of attentional deficits, because sound does not achieve conscious awareness in 50 milliseconds [328]. The first positive deflection of auditory evoked potentials exhibits reduced sensory gating in both women with rape-related PTSD and men with combat-related PTSD, suggesting that patients with PTSD have difficulty filtering auditory stimuli [329].

In terms of memory and learning (relevant to the decreased size of the hippocampus in PTSD, see preceding section), many studies have found evidence of short-term explicit or declarative memory disturbances, independent of attentional problems, in patients with PTSD [330–332]. Disturbances in memory and learning may be under-appreciated in individuals with major life stressors that do not meet the full criteria for PTSD.

Traditional physiological indices such as blood pressure, heart rate, skin conductance and electromyographic activity of facial muscles at baseline and in response to various trauma-related stimuli have been extensively investigated in PTSD. Almost two-thirds of patients with PTSD have demonstrated exaggerated psychophysiological reactivity to internal or external trauma-related cues in comparison to non-traumatized control subjects, traumatized combat veterans without either PTSD or other anxiety disorders, and traumatized individuals with other anxiety disorders [333-335]. However, baseline measures have been similar in both PTSD subjects and normal controls [335].

Ross *et al.* [336] have referred to sleep disturbance as the "hallmark" of PTSD and suggest that REM dysfunction may be a critical factor in both daytime flashbacks and night-time anxiety dreams. However, polysomnographic findings of sleep among PTSD subjects have been inconsistent [337, 338]. Higher-percentage [339] and abnormal REM sleep [340], as well as increase in movement during REM sleep [340], have been reported in PTSD, although these findings have not been consistently replicated [341].

Even though a seminal role of sleep dysregulation in the pathophysiology of PTSD cannot be established, it is clear that patients with PTSD have disturbed sleep and frequent sleep complaints [338].

Neurochemistry

Adrenergic System

Some studies have reported increased 24-hour urinary concentrations of both norepinephrine (noradrenaline) and epinephrine (adrenaline) in patients with combat- and sexual abuse-related PTSD [342–344]. Moreover, fewer total α_2 adrenergic receptor sites per platelet have been reported in adults and children with PTSD compared with controls [345, 346], suggesting that chronic elevation of circulating catecholamines causes a down-regulation of available receptor sites [346]. In contrast to this, other studies have found no significant difference in baseline catecholamine levels between subjects with and those without PTSD [347–349].

However, exposure to trauma-related stimuli increases plasma concentration of norepinephrine, epinephrine and their metabolites in PTSD [350, 351]. Similarly, administration of yohimbine (an α_2 adrenergic antagonist) triggers flashbacks and other PTSD symptoms in most PTSD subjects (for review, see [328, 335, 352]). Additionally, in vitro studies have found a greater and more rapid loss of platelet α_2 adrenergic receptors in combat veterans with PTSD after incubating intact platelets with high levels of epinephrine [345], suggesting that α_2 adrenergic receptors in these individuals are unusually sensitive to agonist stimulation. Studies focused on both baseline and in vitro challenges of β adrenergic receptor measures in patients with PTSD have been inconsistent [328, 353].

Serotonergic System

The evidence indicating serotonergic system dysfunction in PTSD comes from investigations reporting decreased serum 5-HT concentration [354], decreased density of platelet 5-HT uptake sites [355] and a blunted prolactin response to D-fenfluramine (central 5-HT hypoactivity) [356] in PTSD patients. m-chlorophenylpiperazine, a 5-HT agonist, which primarily affects 5-HT$_2$ and 5-HT$_{1C}$ receptors, produces panic attacks and flashbacks in some but not all PTSD subjects [357]. Probably the most consistent evidence to suggest a role of serotonergic systems in the pathophysiology of PTSD is the favourable treatment response to SSRIs.

Neuroendocrinology

The most widely investigated stress-responsive neuroendocrine system is the HPA axis, although other hypothalamic–pituitary hormonal systems are probably equally sensitive to external cues of distress and fear [64]. Nonetheless, the HPA axis system is preferentially investigated whenever "stress" or "traumatic" events are thought to be relevant to any medical or neuropsychiatric disorder. The HPA axis is amenable to manipulations under a variety of circumstances, and its hierarchical and feedback organization is well documented in the literature. Thus, it is not surprising that a syndrome whose onset, symptomatology and course of illness are directly linked to traumatic events and life stressors would be most intensively investigated in relation to HPA function.

The HPA axis has several targets of potential dysfunction and includes the hypothalamus, pituitary and adrenal gland. All of these sites, along with their associated hormonal feedback mechanisms, have been extensively studied in PTSD. Despite apparent increased release of CRH [358, 359], current information suggests that PTSD patients exhibit a unique HPA profile marked by lower urinary and plasma cortisol levels, up-regulation of glucocorticoid receptors, and super-suppression to dexamethasone [359, 360]. Although not all studies have found lower urinary free cortisol levels [342], most evidence suggests that hypocortisolaemia characterizes many patients with PTSD [359, 360] and is putatively linked to an enhanced negative feedback of the HPA axis [328, 359].

The ultimate value of understanding these relationships in PTSD is extremely important both in terms of understanding the regulation of anxiety and stress mechanisms and in dissecting out the role of genetic, environmental and gene–environment interactions in the transmission of PTSD within families and across generations.

THE FUTURE

Historically, anxiety was largely viewed as a time-limited (i.e. cross-sectional), state-dependent expression of physiological arousal. It was understood that people could experience, depending on the particulars of the situation, a range of arousal-cognitive states from being lethargic and inattentive (at the low end), to being alert and attentive and, finally, to being hyperaroused and hypervigilant (at the upper end). It is generally viewed that most people move "across" this continuum of arousal-cognitive states, largely dependent upon the external circumstances. In fact, the ability of a person to rapidly adjust and match an appropriate arousal-cognitive state to the environmental context is highly adaptive in the broadest sense of human survival. It has also been generally appreciated that some individuals tend to fall, semi-independently of the particular circumstances, on the low end or the high end of the arousal-cognitive continuum. Thus, some people tend to have low or high "trait" anxiety.

Early in the study of anxiety disorders, some investigators tended to study *primarily* the biological mechanisms of arousal, concentrating on the anatomical and neurobiological systems that underlie the mediation of the full range of arousal states. Other research teams tended to study *primarily* the cognitive dimensions of human experience. More recent investigations have focused on the interplay between the neurobiological and cognitive dimensions of alarm, arousal and anxiety experiences. These attempts (i.e. to investigate interactive and interdependent biological and cognitive functions during "natural" and "induced" anxiety states) have led to a greater appreciation of how impossible, if not nonsensical, it is to assign *relative* importance to the brain or mind or body in the mediation of normal or abnormal anxiety states. Yet, attempts at making such relative distinctions have been highly productive both in advancing our knowledge about anxiety disorders and in the development of new drug and non-drug treatments.

Brain, mind and body—they are all important. Each may be more or less important in different individuals, or more or less critical at different times within the same individual; but in the end they are intimately entangled functions. From a clinical management perspective, integrative (e.g. bio-psychosocial) models are the best way to understand and treat anxiety disorders. Yet, from a research methodological perspective, studying "integrative" models or systems in humans and animals is extraordinarily complex. The scientific inquiry into and advancement of knowledge about anxiety disorders has progressed via cycles of "lumping" and "splitting" diagnostic categories [145], a process akin to our attempts to ascertain the *relative* importance of "nature" versus "nurture" in the onset and course of anxiety disorders. These attempts have been largely limited, not by the importance of the questions, but by the inadequacies of our research tools. Probably for the first time in the history of anxiety disorder research, we stand on the threshold of being able to seriously investigate integrative neurobiological systems and mind–body–brain functions.

What has made this possible is the human genome project. With the final completion of the human and mouse genome, we will have unprecedented opportunities to investigate genetic, environmental and gene–environmental interactions in humans and animal models of anxiety. The adequate performance of alarm, fear, anxiety and stress functions, themselves mediated by overlapping but different neuroanatomic and neurobiological systems [70], is equally critical for both animal and human "survival" as the performance of cardiac or pulmonary systems. With traditional research tools, advances in knowledge about how cardiovascular or pulmonary systems as opposed to the brain impacted living processes were more easily achieved.

However, new tools (e.g. microarrays and gene chips) open the door for the study of genes and gene–environment interactions in the regulation of brain-mediated anxiety–fear–stress–alarm responses. DNA array technology permits the study of parallel and possibly sequential expression of thousands of genes [21, 22]. As a result of this technology and gene chips, hundreds of new candidate genes for the anxiety or related stress-responsive disorders will be identified. It is theoretically possible that even the role of single-nucleotide polymorphisms on subtle subsets of emotions (e.g. alarm and fear), cognitions, reflexes (e.g. acoustic startle) and behaviours (inhibition, avoidance), which together form the multi-faceted basis of anxiety syndromes, will be amenable to investigation. After the identification of candidate genes, other novel techniques (e.g. virally mediated gene transfer) could be used in animal models to examine the short-term and long-term impact of up-regulation versus down-regulation of candidate genes in brain-specific regions at different stages of development (e.g. prepubertal versus pubertal) and stressful conditions.

While these approaches appear extraordinarily promising, they are still limited by the inability to obtain brain tissue in living humans. Furthermore, the study of gene and gene–environmental interactions in anxiety disorders remains several steps removed from identifying the relevant proteins associated with specific anxiety disorders or related traits (e.g. shyness, behavioural inhibition). Thus, even identifying a role for multiple genes or polymorphisms does not tell us how proteins mediate abnormalities in the anxiety–alarm–arousal–fear systems. Future research will focus on how genetic and genetic–environmental factors influence the production and interactions among "downstream" proteins in anatomic-specific brain regions (e.g. central nucleus of the amygdala versus bed nucleus of the stria terminalis [70]. It is likely that alterations in protein "activity", localization and/or structure will be relevant to the functions of alarm, anxiety and fear. Thousands of relevant proteins, beyond currently identified receptors, will become targets for drug discovery.

Future clinical research in humans and animals will combine new research methodologies (e.g. microarray gene chips and brain imaging technologies) with older tools—non-drug (e.g. sleep deprivation, phobic exposure) and chemical or neuroendocrine challenge (e.g. caffeine or CRH) techniques—to identify multi-locus genetic, functional proteomic and environmental factors critical in the regulation of anxiety–fear–alarm–arousal systems. Current diagnostic nomenclature, which is largely focused on phenomenology and longitudinal course, will ultimately be replaced by a classification scheme that reflects a more sophisticated understanding of the genetic and biopsychosocial causations of disturbances in anxiety–fear–alarm–arousal systems. As our knowledge about genetic-proteomic and biopsychosocial factors in anxiety–fear–alarm–arousal regulation increases, new treatments, both drug and non-drug, will shift from focusing on treatment toward focusing on prevention.

ACKNOWLEDGEMENTS

We gratefully acknowledge the secretarial and technical assistance of Debbie Fossano, MA.

REFERENCES

1. James W. (1890) *The Principles of Psychology*, Holt, Rinehart & Winston, New York.
2. James W. (1893) *Psychology*, Holt, Rinehart & Winston, New York.
3. Chambless D.L., Beck A.T., Gracely E.J., Grisham J.R. (2000) Relationship of cognitions to fear of somatic symptoms: a test of the cognitive theory of panic. *Depress. Anxiety*, **11**: 1–9.
4. McNally R.J. (1994) *Panic Disorder*, Guilford Press, New York.
5. Silverman W.K., Ginsburg G.S., Goedhart A.W. (1999) Factor structure of the childhood anxiety sensitivity index. *Behav. Res. Ther.*, **37**: 903–917.
6. Scott E.L., Heimberg R.G., Jack M.S. (2000) Anxiety sensitivity in social phobia: comparison between social phobics with and without panic attacks. *Depress. Anxiety*, **12**: 189–192.
7. Koszycki D., Bradwejn J. (2001) Anxiety sensitivity does not predict fearful responding to 35% carbon dioxide in patients with panic disorder. *Psychiatry Res.*, **101**: 137–143.
8. Jang K.L., Stein M.B., Taylor S., Livesley W.J. (1999) Gender differences in the etiology of anxiety sensitivity: a twin study. *J. Gend. Specif. Med.*, **2**: 39–44.
9. Cannon W.B. (1929) *Bodily Changes in Pain, Hunger, Fear, and Rage*, Appleton and Lang Century-Crofts, New York.
10. Cannon W.B. (1939) *The Wisdom of the Body*, 2nd ed., Norton, New York.
11. Selye H., Stone H. (1950) *On the Experimental Morphology of the Adrenal Cortex.* American Lecture Series in Endocrinology, 74, Thomas, Springfield.
12. Mason J.W. (1968) A review of psychoendocrine research on the sympathetic-adrenal medullary system. *Psychosom. Med.*, **30**: 631–653.
13. Uhde T.W., Nemiah J.C. (1988) Panic and generalized anxiety disorders. In *Comprehensive Textbook of Psychiatry*, 5th ed. (Eds H.I. Kaplan, B.J. Sadock), pp. 953–972, Williams and Wilkins, Baltimore.
14. Cohen M.E., White P.D. (1949) Life situations, emotions and neurocirculatory asthenia (anxiety neurosis, neuroasthenia, effort syndrome). *Res. Nerv. Ment. Dis.*, **29**: 832–869.
15. Klein D.F. (1964) Delineation of two drug-responsive anxiety syndromes. *Psychopharmacologia*, **5**: 397–408.
16. Klein D.F. (1981) Anxiety reconceptualized. In *Anxiety: New Research and Changing Concepts* (Eds D.F. Klein, J. Rabkin), pp. 235–263, Raven Press, New York.
17. Pitts F.N. Jr., McClure J.N. Jr. (1967) Lactate metabolism in anxiety neurosis. *N. Engl. J. Med.*, **277**: 1329–1336.

18. Lorberbaum J.P., Newman J.D., Dubno J.R., Horwitz A.R., Nahas Z., Teneback C.C., Bloomer C.W., Bohning D.E., Vincent D., Johnson M.R., *et al.* (1999) Feasibility of using fMRI to study mothers responding to infant cries. *Depress. Anxiety*, **10**: 99–104.
19. Posse S., Binkofski F., Schneider F., Gembris D., Frings W., Habel U., Salloum J.B., Mathiak K., Wiese S., Kiselev V. *et al.* (2001) A new approach to measure single-event related brain activity using real-time fMRI: feasibility of sensory, motor, and higher cognitive tasks. *Hum. Brain Mapp.*, **12**: 25–41.
20. Uhde T.W. (2000) Genetics and brain function: implications for the treatment of anxiety. *Biol. Psychiatry*, **48**: 1142–1143.
21. Watson S.J., Akil H. (1999) Gene chips and arrays revealed: a primer on their power and their uses. *Biol. Psychiatry*, **45**: 533–543.
22. Watson S.J., Meng F., Thompson R.C., Akil H. (2000) The "chip" as a specific tool. *Biol. Psychiatry*, **48**: 1147–1156.
23. Eaton W.W., Kessler R.C., Wittchen H.U., Magee W.J. (1994) Panic and panic disorder in the United States. *Am. J. Psychiatry*, **151**: 413–420.
24. Markowitz J.S., Weissman M.M., Ouelette R., Leik J. (1989) Quality of life in panic diosrder. *Arch. Gen. Psychiatry*, **46**: 984–992.
25. DuPont R.L., Rice D.P., Miller L.S., Shiraki S.S., Rowland C.R., Harwood H.J. (1996) Economic costs of anxiety disorders. *Depress. Anxiety*, **2**: 167–172.
26. Katerndahl D.A., Realini J.P. (1997) Use of health care services by persons with panic symptoms. *Psychiatr. Serv.*, **48**: 1027–1032.
27. Greenberg P.E., Sisitsky T., Kessler R.C., Finkelstein S.N., Berndt E.R., Davidson J.R., Ballenger J.C., Fyer A.J. (1999) The economic burden of anxiety disorders in the 1990s. *J. Clin. Psychiatry*, **60**: 427–435.
28. Sherbourne C.D., Wells K.B., Judd L.L. (1996) Functioning and wellbeing of patients with panic disorder. *Am. J. Psychiatry*, **153**: 213–218.
29. Mendlowicz M.V., Stein M.B. (2000) Quality of life in individuals with anxiety disorders. *Am. J. Psychiatry*, **157**: 669–682.
30. Weissman M.M., Klerman G.L., Markowitz J.S., Ovellette S. (1989) Suicidal ideation and suicide attempts in panic disorder and attacks. *N. Engl. J. Med.*, **321**: 1209–1218.
31. Crowe R.R., Noyes R., Pauls D.L., Slymen D. (1983) A family study of panic disorder. *Arch. Gen. Psychiatry*, **40**: 1065–1069.
32. Noyes R. Jr., Crowe R.R., Harris E.L., Hampa B.J., McChesney C.M., Chaudry D.R. (1986) Relationship between panic disorder and agoraphobia: a family study. *Arch. Gen. Psychiatry*, **43**: 227–232.
33. Mendlewicz J., Papdimitriou G., Wilmotte J. (1993) Family study of panic disorder: comparison with generalized anxiety disorder, major depression and normal subjects. *Psychiatr. Genet.*, **3**: 73–78.
34. Maier W., Lichtermann D., Minges J., Oehrlein A., Franke P. (1993) A controlled family study in panic disorder. *J. Psychiatr. Res.*, **27**(Suppl. 1): 79–87.
35. Weissman M.M., Wickramaratne P., Adams P.B., Lish J.D., Horwath E., Charney D., Woods S.W., Leeman E., Frosch E. (1993) The relationship between panic disorder and major depression: a new family study. *Arch. Gen. Psychiatry*, **50**: 767–780.
36. Fyer A.J, Mannuzza S., Chapman T.F., Martin L.Y., Klein D.F. (1995) Specificity in familial aggregation of phobic disorder and social phobia. *Arch. Gen. Psychiatry*, **52**: 564–573.
37. Fyer A.J., Mannuzza S., Chapman T., Lipsitz J., Martin L., Klein D. (1996) Panic disorder and social phobia; effect of comorbidity in family transmission. *Anxiety*, **2**: 173–178.

38. Togerson S. (1990) Twin studies in panic disorder. In *Neurobiology of Panic Disorder* (Ed. J.C. Ballenger), pp. 51–58, Liss, New York.

39. Hamilton S.P., Slager S.L., Helleby L., Heiman G.A., Klein D.F., Hodge S.E., Weissman M.M., Fyer A.J., Knowles J.A. (2001) No association or linkage between polymorphisms in the genes encoding cholecystokinin and the cholecystokinin B receptor and panic disorder. *Mol. Psychiatry*, **6**: 59–65.

40. Wang Z.W., Crowe R.R., Noyes R. Jr. (1992) Adrenergic receptor genes as a candidate gene for panic disorder: a linkage study. *Am. J. Psychiatry*, **149**: 470–474.

41. Crowe R.R., Wang Z., Noyes R. Jr., Albrecht B.E., Darlison M.G., Bailey M.E., Johnson K.J., Zoega T. (1997) Candidate gene study of eight GABAA receptor subunits in panic disorder. *Am. J. Psychiatry*, **154**: 1096–1100.

42. Deckert J., Catalano M., Syagailo Y.V., Bosi M., Okladnova O., Di Bella D., Nothen M.M., Maffei P., Franke P., Fritze J. *et al.* (1999) Excess of high activity of monoamine oxidase A gene promoter alleles in female patients with panic disorder. *Hum. Mol. Genet.*, **8**: 621–624.

43. Wang Z., Valdes J., Noyes R., Zoega T., Crowe R.R. (1998) Possible association of a cholecystokinin promoter polymorphism (CCK-36CT) with panic disorder. *Am. J. Med. Genet.*, **81**: 228–234.

44. Weissman M.M., Fyer A.J., Haghighi F., Heiman G., Deng Z., Hen R., Hodge S.E., Knowles J.A. (2000) Potential panic disorder syndrome: clinical and genetic linkage evidence. *Am. J. Med. Genet.*, **96**: 24–35.

45. Gelernter J., Bonvicini K., Page G., Woods S.W., Goddard A.W., Kruger S., Pauls D.L., Goodson S. (2001) Linkage genome scan for loci predisposing to panic disorder or agoraphobia. *Am. J. Med. Genet.* **105**: 548–557.

46. Smoller J.W., Tsuang M.T. (1998) Panic and phobic anxiety: defining phenotypes for genetic studies. *Am. J. Psychiatry*, **155**: 1152–1162.

47. Reiman E.M., Raichle M.E., Robins E., Butler F.K., Herscovitch P., Fox P., Perlmutter J. (1986) The application of positron emission tomography to the study of panic disorder. *Am. J. Psychiatry*, **143**: 469–477.

48. Nordahl T.E., Semple W.E., Gross M., Mellman T.A., Stein M.B., Goyer P., King A.C., Uhde T.W., Cohen R.M. (1990) Cerebral glucose metabolic differences in patients with panic disorder. *Neuropsychopharmacology*, **3**: 261–272.

49. Bisaga A., Katz J.L., Antonini A., Wright C.E., Margouleff C., Gorman J.M., Eidelberg D. (1998) Cerebral glucose metabolism in women with panic disorder. *Am. J. Psychiatry*, **155**: 1178–1183.

50. Stewart R.S., Devous M.D. Sr., Rush A.J., Lane L., Bonte F.J. (1988) Cerebral blood flow changes during sodium-lactate-induced panic attacks. *Am. J. Psychiatry*, **145**: 442–449.

51. Gorman J.M., Kent J.M., Sullivan G.M., Coplan J.D. (2000) Neuroanatomical hypothesis of panic disorder, revised. *Am. J. Psychiatry*, **157**: 493–505.

52. Woods S.W., Koster K., Krystal J.K., Smith E.O., Zubal I.G., Hoffer P.B., Charney D.S. (1988) Yohimbine alters regional cerebral blood flow in panic disorder. *Lancet*, **ii**: 678.

53. De Cristofaro M.T., Sessarego A., Pupi A., Biondi F., Faravelli C. (1993) Brain perfusion abnormalities in drug-naive, lactate-sensitive panic patients: a SPECT study. *Biol. Psychiatry*, **33**: 505–512.

54. Gorman J.M., Goetz R.R., Uy J., Ross D., Martinez J., Fyer A.J., Liebowitz M.R., Klein D.F. (1988) Hyperventilation occurs during lactate-induced panic. *J. Anxiety Disord.*, **2**: 193–202.

55. Ball S., Shekhar A. (1997) Basilar artery response to hyperventilation in panic disorder. *Am. J. Psychiatry*, **154**: 1603–1604.

56. Dager S.R., Strauss W.L., Marro K.I., Richards T.L., Metzger G.D., Artru A.A. (1995) Proton magnetic resonance spectroscopy investigation of hyperventilation in subjects with panic disorder and comparison subjects. *Am. J. Psychiatry*, **152**: 666–672.
57. Davis M. (1999) Functional neuroanatomy of anxiety and fear: a focus on the amygdala. In *Neurobiology of Mental Illness* (Eds D.S. Charney, E.J. Nestler, B.S. Bunney), pp. 463–473, Oxford University Press, New York.
58. LeDoux J.E., Iwata J., Cicchetti P., Reis D.J. (1988) Different projections of the central amygdaloid nucleus mediate autonomic and behavioral correlates of conditioned fear. *J. Neurosci.*, **8**: 2517–2529.
59. Davis M. (1992) The role of amygdala in fear and anxiety. *Annu. Rev. Neurosci.*, **15**: 353–375.
60. Redmond D.E. Jr. (1979) New and old evidence for the involvement of a brain norepinephrine system in anxiety. In *The Phenomenology and Treatment of Anxiety* (Ed. W.E. Fann), pp. 153–203, Spectrum Press, New York.
61. Redmond D.E. Jr., Huang Y.H. (1979) New evidence for a locus ceruleus connection with anxiety. *Life Sci.*, **25**: 2149–2162.
62. Gurguis G.N.M., Uhde T.W. (1990) Anxiety disorders: a review of neurotransmitter systems and new directions in research. In *Panic Disorders and Agoraphobia: A Guide for the Practitioner* (Eds J.R. Walker, G.N. Norton, C.A. Ross), pp. 433–469, Brooks/Cole Publishing Company, Pacific Grove.
63. Davis M. (1997) Neurobiology of fear responses: the role of amygdala. *J. Neuropsychiatry Clin. Neurosci.*, **9**: 382–402.
64. Uhde T.W., Tancer M.E., Rubinow D.R., Roscow D.B., Boulenger J.P., Vittone B., Gurguis G.N.M., Geraci M.F., Black B., Post R.M. (1992) Evidence for hypothalamo-growth dysfunction in panic disorder: profile of growth hormone (GH) responses to clonidine, yohimbine, caffeine, glucose, GRF, and TRH in panic disorder patients versus healthy volunteers. *Neuropsychopharmacology*, **6**: 101–118.
65. Lane R.D., Reiman E.M., Axelrod B., Yun L.S., Holmes A., Schwartz G.E. (1998) Neural correlates of levels of emotional awareness. Evidence of an interaction between emotion and attention in the anterior cingulated cortex. *J. Cogn. Neurosci.*, **10**: 525–535.
66. Charney D.S., Bremner J.D. (1999) The neurobiology of anxiety disorders. In *Neurobiology of Mental Illness* (Eds D.S. Charney, E.J. Nestler, B.S. Bunney), pp. 494–517, Oxford University Press, New York.
67. Hamner M.B., Lorberbaum J.P., George M.S. (1999) Potential role of the anterior cingulate cortex in PTSD: review and hypothesis. *Depress. Anxiety*, **9**: 1–14.
68. Dunn A.J., Berridge C.W. (1990) Physiological and behavioral responses to corticotropin-releasing factor administration: is CRF a mediator of anxiety or stress responses? *Brain Res. Rev.*, **15**: 71–100.
69. De Bellis M.D., Chrousos G.P., Dorn L.D., Burke L., Helmers K., Kling M.A., Trickett P.K., Putnam F.W. (1994) Hypothalamic–pituitary–adrenal axis dysregulation in sexually abused girls. *J. Clin. Endocrinol. Metab.*, **78**: 249–255.
70. Davis M. (1998) Are different parts of the extended amygdala involved in fear versus anxiety? *Biol. Psychiatry.*, **44**: 1239–1247.
71. Caldji C., Diorio J., Meaney M.J. (2000) Variations in maternal care in infancy regulate the development of stress reactivity. *Biol. Psychiatry*, **48**: 1164–1174.
72. Caldji C., Francis D., Sharma S., Plotsky P.M., Meaney M.J. (2000) The effects of early rearing environment on the development of $GABA_A$ and central benzodiazepine receptor levels and novelty-induced fearfulness in the rat. *Neuropsychopharmacology*, **22**: 219–229.

73. Bakshi V.P., Kalin N.H. (2000) Corticotropin-releasing hormone and animal models of anxiety: gene–environment interactions. *Biol. Psychiatry*, **48**: 1175–1198.
74. Liebowitz M.R., Fyer A.J., Gorman J.M., Dillon D., Appleby I.L., Levy G., Anderson S., Levitt M., Palij M., Davies S.O., Klein D.F. (1984) Lactate provocation of panic attacks. I. Clinical and behavioral findings. *Arch. Gen. Psychiatry*, **41**: 764–770.
75. Pohl R., Yeragani V.K., Balon R., Rainey J.M., Lycaki H., Ortiz A., Berchou R., Weinberg P. (1988) Isoproterenol-induced panic attacks. *Biol. Psychiatry*, **24**: 891–902.
76. Gorman J.M., Goetz R.R., Dillon D., Liebowitz M.R., Fyer A.J., Davies S., Klein D.F. (1990) Sodium D-lactate infusion of panic disorder patients. *Neuropsychopharmacology*, **3**: 181–189.
77. Fyer A.J., Gorman J.M., Liebowitz M.R., Levitt M., Danielson E., Martinez J., Klein D.F. (1984) Sodium lactate infusion, panic attacks, and ionized calcium. *Biol. Psychiatry.*, **19**: 1437–1447.
78. Gorman J.M., Cohen B.S., Liebowitz M.R., Fyer A.J., Ross D., Davies S.O., Klein D.F. (1986) Blood gas changes and hypophosphatemia in lactate-induced panic. *Arch. Gen. Psychiatry*, **43**: 1067–1071.
79. Mathew R.J., Wilson W.H., Tant S. (1989) Response to hypercarbia induced by acetazolamide in panic disorder patients. *Am. J. Psychiatry*, **146**: 996–1000.
80. Reiman E.M., Raichle M.E., Robins E., Mintun M.A., Fusselman M.J., Fox P.T., Price J.L., Hackman K.A. (1989) Neuroanatomical correlates of a lactate-induced anxiety attack. *Arch. Gen. Psychiatry*, **46**: 493–500.
81. Papp L.A., Gorman J.M. (1995) Respiratory neurobiology of panic. In *Panic Disorder: Clinical, Biological and Treatment Aspects* (Eds G.M. Asnis, H.M. van Pragg), pp. 255–275, Wiley, New York.
82. Sanderson W.C., Weltzer S. (1990) Five percent carbon dioxide challenge: valid analogue and marker of panic disorder? *Biol. Psychiatry*, **27**: 689–701.
83. Gorman J.M., Askanazi J., Liebowitz M.R., Fyer A.J., Stein J., Kinney J.M., Klein D.F. (1984) Response to hyperventilation in a group of patients with panic disorder. *Am. J. Psychiatry*, **141**: 857–861.
84. Gorman J.M., Fyer M.R., Goetz R., Askanazi J., Liebowitz M.R., Fyer A.J., Kinney J., Klein D.F. (1988) Ventilatory physiology of patients with panic disorder. *Arch. Gen. Psychiatry*, **45**: 31–39.
85. Gorman J.M., Papp L.A., Coplan J.D., Martinez J.M., Lennon S., Goetz R.R., Ross D., Klein D.F. (1994) Anxiogenic effects of CO_2 and hyperventilation in patients with panic disorder. *Am. J. Psychiatry*, **151**: 547–553.
86. Gorman J.M., Kent J., Martinez J., Browne S., Coplan J., Papp L.A. (2001) Physiological changes during carbon dioxide inhalation in patients with panic disorder, major depression, and premenstrual dysphoric disorder: evidence for a central fear mechanism. *Arch. Gen. Psychiatry*, **58**: 125–131.
87. Griez E., Lousberg H., van den Hout M.A., Zandbergen J. (1987) CO_2 vulnerability in panic disorder. *Psychiatry Res.*, **20**: 87–95.
88. Pain M.C.F., Biddle N., Tiller J.W.G. (1988) Panic disorder, the ventilatory response to carbon dioxide and respiratory variables. *Psychosom. Med.*, **50**: 541–548.
89. Perna G., Battaglia M., Garberi A., Arancio C., Bertani A., Bellodi L. (1994) Carbon dioxide/oxygen challenge test in panic disorder. *Psychiatry Res.*, **52**: 159–171.
90. Perna G., Gabriele A., Caldirola D., Bellodi L. (1995) Hypersensitivity to inhalation of carbon dioxide and panic attacks. *Psychiatry Res.*, **57**: 267–273.

91. Papp L.A., Martinez J.M., Klein D.F., Coplan J.D., Norman R.G., Cole R., de Jesus M.J., Ross D., Goetz R., Gorman J.M. (1997) Respiratory psychophysiology of panic disorder: three respiratory challenges in 98 subjects. *Am. J. Psychiatry*, **154**: 1557–1565.

92. Griez E., Zandbergen J., Pols H., Loof C.D. (1990) Response to 35% CO_2 as a marker of panic in severe anxiety. *Am. J. Psychiatry*, **145**: 796–797.

93. Harrington P.J., Schmidt N.B., Telch M.J. (1996) Prospective evaluation of panic potentiation following 35% CO_2 challenge in nonclinical subjects. *Am. J. Psychiatry*, **153**: 823–825.

94. Perna G., Bertani A., Arancio C., Ronchi P., Bellodi L. (1995) Laboratory response of patients with panic and obsessive-compulsive disorders to 35% CO_2 challenges. *Am. J. Psychiatry*, **152**: 85–89.

95. Perna G., Barbini B., Cocchi S., Bertani A., Gasperini M. (1995) 35% CO_2 challenge in panic and mood disorders. *J. Affect. Disord.*, **33**: 189–194.

96. Perna G., Bussi R., Allevi L., Bellodi L. (1999) Sensitivity to 35% carbon dioxide in patients with generalized anxiety disorder. *J. Clin. Psychiatry*, **60**: 379–384.

97. Verburg K., Klaassen T., Pols H., Griez E. (1998) Comorbid depressive disorder increases vulnerability to the 35% carbon dioxide (CO_2) challenge in panic disorder patients. *J. Affect Disord.*, **49**: 195–201.

98. Pols H., Zandbergen J., de Loof C., Griez E. (1991) Attenuation of carbon dioxide induced panic after clonazepam treatment. *Acta Psychiatr. Scand.*, **84**: 585–586.

99. Sanderson W.C., Weltzer S., Asnis G.M. (1994) Alprazolam blockade of CO_2 provoked panic in patients with panic disorder. *Am. J. Psychiatry*, **151**: 1220–1222.

100. Bertani A., Caldirola D., Bussi R., Bellodi L., Perna G. (2001) The 35% CO_2 hyperreactivity and clinical symptomatology in patients with panic disorder after 1 week of treatment with citalopram: an open study. *J. Clin. Psychopharmacol.*, **3**: 262–267.

101. Gorman J.M., Browne S.T., Papp L.A., Martinez J., Welkowitz L., Coplan J.D., Goetz R.R., Kent J., Klein D.F. (1997) Effect of antipanic treatment on response to carbon dioxide. *Biol. Psychiatry*, **42**: 982–991.

102. Klein D.F. (1993) False suffocation alarm, spontaneous panic attacks, and related conditions: an integrative hypothesis. *Arch. Gen. Psychiatry*, **50**: 306–317.

103. Carr D.B., Sheehan D.V. (1984) Panic anxiety: a new biological model. *J. Clin. Psychiatry*, **45**: 323–330.

104. Perna G., Cocchi S., Bertani A., Arancio C., Bellodi L. (1994) Pharmacologic effect of toloxatone on reactivity to the 35% carbon dioxide challenge: a single-blind, random, placebo-controlled study. *J. Clin. Psychopharmacol.*, **14**: 414–418.

105. Perna G., Cocchi S., Bertani A., Arancio C., Bellodi L. (1995) Sensitivity to 35% CO_2 in healthy first-degree relatives of patients with panic disorder. *Am. J. Psychiatry*, **152**: 623–625.

106. Coryell W., Arndt S. (1999) The 35% CO_2 inhalation procedure: test–retest reliability. *Biol. Psychiatry*, **45**: 923–927.

107. Nicole V.B., Griez E. (2000) Reactivity to a 35% CO_2 challenge in healthy first-degree relatives of patients with panic disorder. *Biol. Psychiatry*, **47**: 830–835.

108. Coryell W., Fyer A., Pine D., Martinez J., Arndt S. (2001) Aberrant respiratory sensitivity to CO_2 as a trait of familial panic disorder. *Biol. Psychiatry*, **49**: 582–587.

109. Sheehan D.V., Ballenger J., Jacobsen G. (1980) Treatment of endogenous anxiety with phobic, hysterical and hypochondriacal symptoms. *Arch. Gen. Psychiatry*, **37**; 51–59.
110. Uhde T.W., Roy-Byrne P.P., Gillin J.C., Mendelson W.D., Boulenger J.P., Vittone B.J., Post R.M. (1984) The sleep of patients with panic disorder. *Psychiatry Res.*, **12**: 251–259.
111. Uhde T.W. (1986) Treating panic and anxiety. *Psychiatr. Ann.*, **16**: 536–541.
112. Taylor C.B., Sheikh J., Agras W.S., Roth W.T., Margraf J., Ehlers A., Maddock R.J., Gossard D. (1986) Ambulatory heart rate changes in patients with panic attacks. *Am. J. Psychiatry*, **143**: 478–482.
113. Mellman T.A., Uhde T.W. (1987) Sleep in panic and generalized anxiety disorders. In *Neurobiological Aspects of Panic Disorder*, Vol. 5 (Ed. J.C. Ballenger), pp. 94–100, Liss, New York.
114. Hauri P.J., Friedman M., Ravaris C.L. (1989) Sleep in patients with spontaneous panic attacks. *Sleep*, **12**; 323–337.
115. Krystal J.H., Kosten T.R., Southwick S., Mason J.W., Perry B.D., Giller E.L. (1989) Neurobiological aspects of PTSD: review of clinical and preclinical studies. *Behav. Ther.*, **20**; 177–198.
116. Arriaga F., Paiva T., Matos-Pires A., Cavaglia F., Lara E., Bastos L. (1996) The sleep of non-depressed patients with panic disorder: a comparison with normal controls. *Acta Psychiatr. Scand.*, **93**: 191–194.
117. Craske M.G., Barlow D.H. (1989) Nocturnal panic. *J. Nerv. Ment. Dis.*, **177**: 160–167.
118. Mellman T.A., Uhde T.W. (1989) Sleep panic attacks: new clinical findings and theoretical implications. *Am. J. Psychiatry*, **146**; 1204–1207.
119. Mellman T.A., Uhde T.W. (1990) Patients with frequent sleep panic: clinical findings and response to medication treatment. *J. Clin. Psychiatry*, **51**; 513–516.
120. Stein M.B., Enns M.W., Kryger M.H. (1993) Sleep in non-depressed patients with panic disorder, II: Polysomnographic assessment of sleep architecture and sleep continuity. *J. Affect. Disord.*, **28**: 1–6.
121. Uhde T.W. (2000) The anxiety disorders. In *Principles and Practice of Sleep Medicine* (Eds M.H. Kryger, T. Roth, W.C. Dement), pp. 1123–1139, Saunders, Philadelphia.
122. Roy-Byrne P.P., Uhde T.W., Post R.M. (1986) Effects of one night's sleep deprivation on mood and behavior in panic disorder patients compared with depressed and normal controls. *Arch. Gen. Psychiatry*, **43**; 895–899.
123. Labbate L.A., Johnson M.R., Lydiard R.B., Brawman-Mintzer O., Emmanuel N., Crawford M., Kapp R., Ballenger J.C. (1997) Sleep deprivation in panic disorder and obsessive-compulsive disorder. *Can. J. Psychiatry*, **42**: 982–983.
124. Uhde T.W., Mellman T.A. (1987) Commentary on "Relaxation-induced panic (RIP): when resting isn't peaceful". *Integr. Psychiatry*, **5**: 101–104.
125. Uhde T.W. (1994) Anxiety and growth disturbance: is there a connection? A review of biological studies in social phobia. *J. Clin. Psychiatry*, **55**(Suppl. 6): 17–27.
126. Charney D.S., Heninger G.R., Breier A. (1984) Noradrenergic function in panic anxiety: effects of yohimbine in healthy subjects and patients with agoraphobia and panic disorder. *Arch. Gen. Psychiatry*, **41**: 751–763.
127. Nesse R.M., Cameron O.G., Curtis G.C., McCann D.S., Huber-Smith M.J. (1984) Adrenergic function in patients with panic anxiety. *Arch. Gen. Psychiatry*, **41**: 771–776.

128. Uhde T.W., Boulenger J.P., Post R.M., Siever L.J., Vittone B.J., Jimerson D.C., Roy-Byrne P.P. (1984) Fear and anxiety: relationship to noradrenergic function. *Psychopathology*, **17**: 18–23.
129. Charney D.S., Heninger G.R. (1986) Abnormal regulation of noradrenergic function in panic disorders: effect of clonidine in healthy subjects and patients with agoraphobia and panic diosrder. *Arch. Gen. Psychiatry*, **43**: 1042–1054.
130. Charney D.S., Innis R.B., Duman R.S., Woods S.W., Heninger G.R. (1989) Platelet alpha-2-receptor binding and adenylate cyclase activity in panic disorder. *Psychopharmacology*, **98**: 102–107.
131. Nutt D.J. (1989) Altered central alpha-2-adrenoceptor sensitivity in panic disorder. *Arch. Gen. Psychiatry*, **46**: 165–169.
132. Charney D.S., Woods S.W., Goodman W.K., Heninger G.R. (1987) Neurobiological mechanisms of panic anxiety: biochemical and behavioral correlates of yohimbine-induced panic attacks. *Am. J. Psychiatry*, **144**: 1030–1036.
133. Gurguis G.N.M., Uhde T.W. (1990) Plasma 3-methoxy-4-hydroxyphen-ylethylene glycol (MHPG) and growth hormone response to yohimbine in panic disorder patients and normal control. *Psychoneuroendocrinology*, **15**: 217–224.
134. Glazer W.M., Charney D.S., Heninger G.R. (1987) Noradrenergic function in schizophrenia. *Arch. Gen. Psychiatry*, **44**: 898–904.
135. Rasmussen S.A., Goodman W.K., Woods S.W., Heninger G.R., Charney D.S. (1987) Effects of yohimbine in obsessive-compulsive disorder. *Psychopharmacology*, **93**: 308–313.
136. Charney D.S., Woods S.W., Heninger G.R. (1989) Noradrenergic function in generalized anxiety disorder: effects of yohimbine in healthy subjects and patients with generalized anxiety disorder. *Psychiatry Res.*, **27**: 173–182.
137. Uhde T.W., Stein M.B., Vittone B.J., Boulenger J.P., Klein E.H., Mellman T.A. (1989) Behavioral and physiological effects of short-term and long-term clonidine administration in panic disorder. *Arch. Gen. Psychiatry*, **46**: 170–177.
138. Siever L.J., Uhde T.W. (1984) New studies and the perspectives on the noradrenergic receptor system in depression: effects of the alpha-2-adrenergic agonist clonidine. *Biol. Psychiatry*, **19**: 131–156.
139. Asnis G.M., van Praag H.M. (1995) The norepinephrine system in panic disorder. In *Panic Disorder: Clinical, Biological and Treatment Aspects* (Eds G.M. Asnis, H.M. van Praag), pp. 119–150, Wiley, New York.
140. Coplan J.D., Papp L.A., Martinez J., Pine D., Rosenblum L.A., Cooper T., Liebowitz M.R., Gorman J.M. (1995) Persistence of blunted human growth hormone response to clonidine in fluoxetine-treated patients with panic disorder. *Am. J. Psychiatry*, **152**: 619–622.
141. Margraf J., Ehlers A., Roth W.T. (1986) Sodium lactate infusions and panic attacks: a review and critique. *Psychosom. Med.*, **48**: 23–51.
142. Gorman J.M., Fyer M.R., Liebowitz M.R., Klein D.F. (1987) Pharmacologic provocation of panic attacks. In *Psychopharmacology: The Third Generation of Progress* (Ed. H.Y. Meltzer), pp. 985–998, Raven Press, New York.
143. Uhde T.W., Joffe R.T., Jimerson D.C., Post R.M. (1988) Normal urinary free cortisol and plasma MHPG in panic disorder: clinical and theoretical implication. *Biol. Psychiatry*, **23**: 575–585.
144. Uhde T.W., Tancer M.E. (1988) Chemical models of panic: a review and critique. In *Psychopharmacology of Anxiety* (Ed. P. Tyrer), pp. 110–113, Oxford University Press, Oxford.
145. Uhde T.W., Tancer M.E., Gurguis G.N.M. (1990) Chemical models of anxiety: evidence for diagnostic and neurotransmitter specificity. *Int. Rev. J. Psychiatry*, **2**: 367–384.

146. Uhde T.W. (1995) Caffeine-induced anxiety: an ideal chemical model of panic disorder? In *Panic Disorder: Clinical, Biological and Treatment Aspects* (Eds G.M. Asnis, H.M. van Praag), pp. 181–205, Wiley, New York.

147. Uhde T.W. (1998) Caffeine: practical facts for the psychiatrist. In *Anxiety: New Research Findings for the Clinician* (Ed. P.P. Roy-Byrne), pp. 73–98, American Psychiatric Press, Washington.

148. Greden J.F. (1974) Anxiety or caffeinism: a diagnostic dilemma. *Am. J. Psychiatry*, **131**: 1089–1092.

149. Uhde T.W. (1990) Caffeine provocation of panic: a focus on biological mechanisms. In *Neurobiology of Panic Disorder* (Ed. J.C. Ballenger), pp. 219–242, Liss, New York.

150. Victor B., Lubetsky M., Greden J. (1981) Somatic manifestation of caffeinism. *J. Clin. Psychiatry*, **42**: 185–188.

151. Winstead D.K. (1976) Coffee consumption among psychiatric inpatients. *Am. J. Psychiatry*, **133**: 1447–1450.

152. Boulenger J.-P., Patel J., Marnagos P.J. (1983) Effects of caffeine and theophylline on adenosine and benzodiazepine receptors in human brain. *Neurosci. Lett.*, **30**: 161.

153. Uhde T.W., Boulenger J.P., Vittone B., Jimerson D.C., Post R.M. (1984) Caffeine: relationship to human anxiety, plasma MHPG and cortisol. *Psychopharmacol. Bull.*, **20**: 426–430.

154. Lin A.S.-K., Uhde T.W., Slate S.O., McCann U.D. (1997) Effects of intravenous caffeine administered to healthy males during sleep. *Depress. Anxiety*, **5**: 21–28.

155. Charney D.S., Heninger G.R., Jatlow P.I. (1985) Increased anxiogenic effects of caffeine in panic disorder. *Arch. Gen. Psychiatry*, **42**: 233–243.

156. Apfeldorf W.J., Shear M.K. (1993) Caffeine potentiation of taste in panic disorder. *Biol. Psychiatry*, **33**: 217–219.

157. DeMet E., Stein M.K., Tran C., Chicz-DeMet A., Sangdahl C., Nelson J. (1989) Caffeine taste test for panic disorder: adenosine receptor supersensitivity. *Psychiatry Res.*, **30**: 231–242.

158. Tancer M.E., Stein M.B., Uhde T.W. (1994/1995) Lactic acid response to caffeine in panic disorders: comparison with social phobics and normal controls. *Depress. Anxiety*, **1**: 138–140.

159. Fredholm B.B., Persson C.G.A. (1982) Xanthine derivatives as adenosine receptor antagonists. *Eur. J. Pharmacol.*, **81**: 673–676.

160. Ledent C., Vaugeois J.M., Schiffmann S.N., Pedrazzini T., El Yacoubi M., Vanderhaeghen J.J., Costentin J., Heath J.K., Vassart G., Parmentier M. (1997) Aggressiveness, hypoalgesia and high blood pressure in mice lacking the adenosine A2a receptor. *Nature*, **388**: 674–678.

161. Florio C., Prezioso A., Papaioannou A., Vertua R. (1998) Adenosine A1 receptors modulate anxiety in CD1 mice. *Psychopharmacology*, **136**: 311–319.

162. El Yacoubi M., Ledent C., Parmentier M., Costentin J., Vaugeois J.M. (2000) The anxiogenic-like effect of caffeine in two experimental procedures measuring anxiety in the mouse is not shared by selective A(2A) adenosine receptor antagonists. *Psychopharmacology*, **148**: 153–163.

163. Stein M.B., Black B., Brown T.M., Uhde T.W. (1993) Lack of efficacy of the adenosine reuptake inhibitor dipyridamole in the treatment of anxiety disorders. *Biol. Psychiatry*, **33**: 647–650.

164. Targum S.D., Marshall L.E. (1989) Fenfluramine provocation of anxiety in patients with panic disorder. *Psychiatry Res.*, **28**: 295–306.

165. Coplan J.D., Gorman J.M., Klein D.F. (1992) Serotonin related functions in panic anxiety: a critical overview. *Neuropsychopharmacology*, **6**: 189–200.

166. Charney D.S., Heninger G.R. (1986) Serotonin function in panic disorder. The effects of intravenous tryptophan in healthy subjects and panic disorder patients before and after alprazolam treatment. *Arch. Gen. Psychiatry*, **43**: 1059–1065.
167. DenBoer J.A., Westenberg H.G.M. (1990) Behavioral, neuroendocrine and biochemical effects of 5-hydroxytryptophan administration in panic disorder. *Psychiatry Res.*, **31**: 367–378.
168. van Vliet I.M., Slaap B.R., Westenberg H.G., Den Boer J.A. (1996) Behavioral, neuroendocrine and biochemical effects of different doses of 5-HTP in panic disorder. *Eur. Neuropsychopharmacol.*, **6**: 103–110.
169. Goddard A.W., Sholomskas D.E., Walton K.E., Augeri F.M., Charney D.S., Heninger G.R., Goodman W.K., Price L.H. (1994) Effects of tryptophan depletion in panic disorder. *Biol. Psychiatry*, **36**: 775–777.
170. Lewis D.A., Noyes R. Jr., Coryell W., Clancy J. (1985) Tritiated imipramine binding to platelets is decreased in patients with agoraphobia. *Psychiatry Res.*, **16**: 1–9.
171. Uhde T.W., Berrettini W.H., Roy-Byrne P.P., Boulenger J.P., Post R.M. (1987) Platelet [³H]imipramine binding in patients with panic disorder. *Biol. Psychiatry*, **22**: 52–58.
172. Maguire K.P., Norman T.R., Apostolopoulos M., Judd F.K., Burrows G.D. (1995) Platelet [³H]paroxetine binding in panic disorder. *J. Affect. Disord.*, **33**: 117–122.
173. Stein M.B., Delany S.M., Charteir M.J., Kroft C.D., Hazen A.L. (1995) [³H] paroxetine binding to platelets of patients with social phobia: comparison to patients with panic disorder and healthy volunteers. *Biol. Psychiatry*, **37**: 224–228.
174. Marazziti D., Rossi A., Dell'Osso L., Palego L., Placidi G.P., Giannaccini G., Lucacchini A., Cassano G.B. (1999) Decreased platelet 3H-paroxetine binding in untreated panic disorder patients. *Life Sci.*, **65**: 2735–2741.
175. Lesch K.P., Weismann M., Hoh A., Muller T., Disselkamp-Tietze J., Osterheider M., Schulte H.M. (1992) 5-HT 1A receptor effector system responsivity in panic disorder. *Psychopharmacology*, **106**: 111–117.
176. Julius D. (1998) Serotonin receptor knockouts: a moody subject. *Proc. Natl. Acad. Sci. USA*, **95**: 15 153–15 154.
177. Menard J., Treit D. (1999) Effects of centrally administered anxiolytic compounds in animal models of anxiety. *Neurosci. Biobehav. Rev.*, **23**: 591–613.
178. Gross C., Santarelli L., Brunner D., Zhuang X., Hen R. (2000) Altered fear circuits in 5HT$_{1A}$ receptor KO mice. *Biol. Psychiatry*, **48**: 1157–1163.
179. Uhde T.W., Boulenger J.P., Siever L.J., DuPont R.L., Post R.M. (1982) Animal models of anxiety: implications for research in humans. *Psychopharmacol. Bull.*, **18**: 47–52.
180. Parks C.L., Robinson P.S., Sibille E., Shenk T., Toth M. (1998) Increased anxiety of mice lacking the serotonin A receptor. *Proc. Natl. Acad. Sci. USA*, **95**: 10 734–10 739.
181. Heisler L.K., Chu H.M., Brennan T.J., Danao J.A., Bajwa P., Parsons L.H., Tecott L.H. (1998) Elevated anxiety and antidepressant-like responses in serotonin 5-HT1A receptor mutant mice. *Proc. Natl. Acad. Sci. USA*, **95**: 15 049–15 054.
182. Ramboz S., Oosting R., Amara D.A., Kung H.F., Blier P., Mendelsohn M., Mann J.J., Brunner D., Hen R. (1998) Serotonin receptor 1A knockout: an animal model of anxiety-related disorder. *Proc. Natl. Acad. Sci. USA*, **95**: 14 476–14 481.

183. Slade T., Andrews G. (2001) DSM-IV and ICD-10 generalized anxiety disorder: discrepant diagnoses and associated disability. *Soc. Psychiatry Psychiatr. Epidemiol.*, **36**: 45–51.
184. Wolff M., Alsobrook J.P. II, Pauls D.L. (2000) Genetic aspects of obsessive-compulsive disorder. *Psychiatr. Clin. North Am.*, **23**: 535–544.
185. Leckman J.F., Zhang H., Alsobrook J.P., Pauls D.L. (2001) Symptom dimensions in obsessive-compulsive disorder: toward quantitative phenotypes. *Am. J. Med. Genet.*, **105**: 28–30.
186. Zorumski C.F., Isenberg K.E. (1991) Insights into the structure and function of GABA-benzodiazepine receptors: ion channels and psychiatry. *Am. J. Psychiatry*, **148**: 162–173.
187. Smith T.A. (2001) Type A gamma-aminobutyric acid (GABAA) receptor subunits and benzodiazepine binding: significance to clinical syndromes and their treatment. *Br. J. Biomed. Sci.*, **58**: 111–121.
188. Nutt D.J., Glue P., Lawson C., Wilson S. (1990) Flumazenil provocation of panic attacks. Evidence for altered benzodiazepine receptor sensitivity in panic disorder. *Arch. Gen. Psychiatry*, **47**: 917–925.
189. Woods S.W., Charney D.S., Silver J.M., Krystal J.H., Heninger G.R. (1991) Behavioral, biochemical, and cardiovascular responses to the benzodiazepine receptor antagonist flumazenil in panic disorder. *Psychiatry Res.*, **36**: 115–127.
190. Strohle A., Kellner M., Yassouridis A., Holsboer F., Wiedemann K. (1998) Effect of flumazenil in lactate-sensitive patients with panic disorder. *Am. J. Psychiatry*, **155**: 610–612.
191. Coupland N.J., Bell C., Potokar J.P., Dorkins E., Nutt D.J. (2000) Flumazenil challenge in social phobia. *Depress. Anxiety*, **11**: 27–30.
192. Bernik M.A., Gorenstein C., Vieira Filho A.H. (1998) Stressful reactions and panic attacks induced by flumazenil in chronic benzodiazepine users. *J. Psychopharmacol.*, **12**: 146–150.
193. Sand P., Kavvadias D., Feineis D., Riederer P., Schreier P., Kleinschnitz M., Czygan F.C., Abou-Mandour A., Bringmann G., Beckmann H. (2000) Naturally occurring benzodiazepines: current status of research and clinical implications. *Eur. Arch. Psychiatry Clin. Neurosci.*, **250**: 194–202.
194. Sand P., Kleinschnitz M., Vogel P., Kavvadias D., Schreier P., Riederer P. (2001) Naturally occurring benzodiazepines may codetermine chronotypes. *J. Neural Transm.*, **108**: 747–753.
195. Adamec R.E. (2000) Evidence that long-lasting potentiation in limbic circuits mediating defensive behaviour in the right hemisphere underlies pharmacological stressor (FG-7142) induced lasting increases in anxiety-like behaviour: role of benzodiazepine receptors. *J. Psychopharmacol.*, **14**: 307–322.
196. Disney A., Calford M.B. (2001) Neurosteroids mediate habituation and tonic inhibition in the auditory midbrain. *J. Neurophysiol.*, **86**: 1052–1056.
197. Smith J.B. (2000) Specificity of effects of chronically administered diazepam on the responding of rats under two different spaced-responding schedules. *Behav. Pharmacol.*, **11**: 45–55.
198. Kuikka J.T., Pitkanen A., Lepola U., Partanen K., Vainio P., Bergstrom K.A., Wieler H.J., Kaiser K.P., Mittelbach L., Koponen H. et al. (1995) Abnormal regional benzodiazepine receptor uptake in the prefrontal cortex in patients with panic disorder. *Nucl. Med. Commun.*, **16**: 273–280.
199. Kaschka W., Feistel H., Ebert D. (1995) Reduced benzodiazepine receptor binding in panic disorders measured by iomazenil SPECT. *J. Psychiatr. Res.*, **29**: 427–434.

200. Malizia A.L., Cunningham V.J., Bell C.J., Liddle P.F., Jones T., Nutt D.J. (1998) Decreased brain GABA(A)-benzodiazepine receptor binding in panic disorder: preliminary results from a quantitative PET study. *Arch. Gen. Psychiatry*, **55**: 715–720.

201. Bremner J.D., Innis R.B., White T., Fujita M., Silbersweig D., Goddard A.W., Staib L., Stern E., Cappiello A., Woods S. *et al.* (2000) SPECT [I-123]iomazenil measurement of the benzodiazepine receptor in panic disorder. *Biol. Psychiatry*, **47**: 96–106.

202. Roy-Byrne P.P., Cowley D.S., Greenblatt D.J., Shader R.I., Hammer D. (1990) Reduced benzodiazepine sensitivity in panic disorder. *Arch. Gen. Psychiatry*, **47**: 534–538.

203. Roy-Byrne P., Wingerson D.K., Radant A., Greenblatt D.J., Cowley D.S. (1996) Reduced benzodiazepine sensitivity in patients with panic disorder: comparison with patients with obsessive-compulsive disorder and normal subjects. *Am. J. Psychiatry*, **153**: 1444–1449.

204. Lydiard R.B., Ballenger J.C., Laraia M.T., Fossey M.D., Beinfeld M.C. (1992) CSF cholecystokinin concentrations in patients with panic disorder and in normal comparison subjects. *Am. J. Psychiatry*, **149**: 691–693.

205. Brambilla F., Bellodi L., Perna G., Garberi A., Panerai A., Sacerdote P. (1993) Lymphocyte cholecystokinin concentrations in panic disorder. *Am. J. Psychiatry*, **150**: 1111–1113.

206. Abelson J.L., Nesse R.M. (1994) Pentagastrin infusions in patients with panic disorder. I. Symptoms and cardiovascular responses. *Biol. Psychiatry*, **39**; 465–466.

207. Bradwejn J., Koszycki D. (1994) The cholecystokinin hypothesis of anxiety and panic disorder. *Ann. N.Y. Acad. Sci.*, **713**: 273–282.

208. McCann U.D., Morgan C.M., Geraci M., Slate S.O., Murphy D.L., Post R.M. (1997) Effects of the 5-HT3 antagonist, ondansetron, on the behavioral and physiological effects of pentagastrin in patients with panic disorder and social phobia. *Neuropsychopharmacology*, **17**: 360–369.

209. McCann U.D., Slate S.O., Geraci M., Roscow-Terrill D., Uhde T.W. (1997) A comparison of the effects of intravenous pentagastrin on patients with social phobia, panic disorder and healthy controls. *Neuropsychopharmacology*, **16**: 229–237.

210. Van Megen H.F., Westenberg H.G., den Boer J.A., Haigh J.R., Traub M. (1994) Pentagastrin induced panic attacks: enhanced sensitivity in panic disorder patients. *Psychopharmacology*, **114**: 449–455.

211. Bradwejn J., Koszycki D., Couetoux du Tertre A., van Megen H., den Boer J., Westenberg H. (1994) The panicogenic effects of cholecystokinin-tetrapeptide are antagonized by L-365,260, a central cholecystokinin receptor antagonist, in patients with panic disorder. *Arch. Gen. Psychiatry*, **51**: 486–493.

212. Bradwejn J., Koszycki D., Paradis M., Reece P., Hinton J., Sedman A. (1995) Effect of CI-988 on cholecystokinin tetrapeptide-induced panic symptoms in healthy volunteers. *Biol. Psychiatry*, **38**: 742–746.

213. Bradwejn J., Koszycki D. (1994) Imipramine antagonism of the panicogenic effects of cholecystokinin tetrapeptide in panic disorder. *Am. J. Psychiatry*, **151**: 261–263.

214. Le Melledo J.M., Bradwejn J., Koszycki D., Bichet D.G., Bellavance F. (1998) The role of the beta-noradrenergic system in cholecystokinin-tetrapeptide-induced panic symptoms. *Biol. Psychiatry*, **44**: 364–366.

215. Kramer M.S., Cutler N.R., Ballenger J.C., Patterson W.M., Mendels J., Chenault A., Shrivastava R., Matzura-Wolfe D., Lines C., Reines S. (1995) A placebo-

controlled trial of L-365,260, a CCKB antagonist, in panic disorder. *Biol. Psychiatry*, **37**: 462–466.

216. Cowley D.S., Adams J.B., Pyke R.E., Cook J., Zaccharias P., Wingerson D., Roy-Byrne P.P. (1996) Effect of CI-988, a cholecystokinin-B receptor antagonist, on lactate-induced panic. *Biol. Psychiatry*, **40**: 550–552.

217. Pande A.C., Greiner M., Adams J.B., Lydiard R.B., Pierce M.W. (1999) Placebo-controlled trial of the CCK-B antagonist, CI-988, in panic disorder. *Biol. Psychiatry*, **46**: 860–862.

218. deMontigny C. (1989) Cholecystokinin tetrapeptide induces panic-like attacks in healthy volunteers: preliminary findings. *Arch. Gen. Psychiatry*, **46**: 511–517.

219. McCann U.D., Slate S.O., Geraci M., Uhde T.W. (1994/1995) Peptides and anxiety: a dose–response evaluation of pentagastrin in healthy volunteers. *Depress. Anxiety*, **1**: 258–267.

220. de Leeuw A.S., den Boer J.A., Slaap B.R., Westenberg H.G. (1996) Pentagastrin has panic-inducing properties in obsessive-compulsive disorder. *Psychopharmacology*, **126**: 339–344.

221. Abelson J.L., Liberzon I. (1999) Dose response of adrenocorticotropin and cortisol to the CCK-B agonist pentagastrin. *Neuropsychopharmacology*, **21**: 485–494.

222. Goldstein S., Halbreich U., Asnis G., Endicott J., Alvir J. (1987) The hypothalamic–pituitary–adrenal system in panic disorder. *Am. J. Psychiatry*, **144**: 1320–1323.

223. Holsboer F., von Bardeleben U., Buller R., Heuser I., Steiger A. (1987) Stimulation response to corticotropin-releasing hormone (CRH) in patients with depression, alcoholism and panic disorder. *Horm. Metab. Res.* **16**(Suppl.): 80–88.

224. Kathol R.G., Noyes R. Jr., Lopez A.L., Reich J.H. (1988) Relationship of urinary free cortisol levels in patients with panic disorder to symptoms of depression and agoraphobia. *Psychiatry Res.*, **24**: 211–221.

225. Abelson J.L., Curtis G.C. (1996) Hypothalamic–pituitary–adrenal axis in panic disorder: 24-hour secretion of corticotrophin and cortisol. *Arch. Gen. Psychiatry*, **53**: 323–331.

226. Stein M.B., Uhde T.W. (1990) Panic disorder and major depression: life-time relationship and biological markers. In *Clinical Aspects of Panic Disorder* (Ed. J.C. Ballenger), pp. 151–168, Liss, New York.

227. Roy-Byrne P.P., Uhde T.W., Post R.M., Gallucci W., Chrousos G.P., Gold P.W. (1986) The corticotropin-releasing hormone stimulation test in patients with panic disorder. *Am. J. Psychiatry*, **143**: 896–899.

228. Curtis G.C., Abelson J.L., Gold P.W. (1997) Adrenocorticotropic hormone and cortisol responses to corticotropin-releasing hormone: changes in panic disorder and effects of alprazolam treatment. *Biol. Psychiatry*, **41**: 76–85.

229. Klein E., Zohar J., Geraci F., Murphy D.L., Uhde T.W. (1991) Anxiogenic effects of m-CPP in patients with panic disorder: comparison to caffeine's anxiogenic effects. *Biol. Psychiatry*, **30**: 973–984.

230. Gurguis G.N., Vittone B.J., Uhde T.W. (1997) Behavioral, sympathetic and adrenocortical responses to yohimbine in panic disorder patients and normal controls. *Psychiatry Res.*, **71**: 27–39.

231. Seier F.E., Kellner M., Yassouridis A., Heese R., Strian F., Wiedemann K. (1997) Autonomic reactivity and hormonal secretion in lactate-induced panic attacks. *Am. J. Physiol.*, **272**: H2630–H2638.

232. Sinha S.S., Coplan J.D., Pine D.S., Martinez J.A., Klein D.F., Gorman J.M. (1999) Panic induced by carbon dioxide inhalation and lack of hypothalamic-pituitary-adrenal axis activation. *Psychiatry Res.*, **86**: 93–98.

233. Uhde T.W., Malloy L.C., Slate S.O. (1992) Fearful behavior, body size and serum IGF-1 levels in nervous and normal pointer dogs. *Pharmacol. Biochem. Behav.*, **43**: 263–269.

234. Uhde T.W., Malloy L.C., Benson B.B. (1994) Growth hormone response to clonidine in the nervous pointer dog model of anxiety. *Depress. Anxiety*, **1**: 45–49.

235. Rasmussen S.A., Eisen J.L. (1990) Epidemiology of obsessive-compulsive disorder. *J. Clin. Psychiatry*, **51**(Suppl. 2): 10–13.

236. Koran L.M. (2000) Quality of life in obsessive-compulsive disorder. *Psychiatr. Clin. North Am.*, **23**: 509–517.

237. Black D.W., Noyes R. Jr., Goldstein R.B., Blum N. (1992) A family study of obsessive-compulsive disorder. *Arch. Gen. Psychiatry*, **49**: 362–368.

238. Pauls D.L., Alsobrook J.P., Goodman W., Rasmussen S., Leckman J.F. (1995) A family study of obsessive-compulsive disorder. *Am. J. Psychiatry*, **152**: 76–84.

239. Jonnal A.H., Gardner C.O., Prescott C.A., Kendler K.S. (2000) Obsessive and compulsive symptoms in a general population sample of female twins. *Am. J. Med. Genet.*, **96**: 791–796.

240. Santangelo S.L., Pauls D.L., Lavori P.W., Goldstein J.M., Faraone S.V., Tsuang M.T. (1996) Assessing risk for the Tourette spectrum of disorders among first-degree relatives of probands with Tourette syndrome. *Am. J. Med. Genet.*, **67**: 107–116.

241. Bienvenu O.J., Samuels J.F., Riddle M.A., Hoehn-Saric R., Liang K.Y., Cullen B.A., Grados M.A., Nestadt G. (2000) The relationship of obsessive-compulsive disorder to possible spectrum disorders: results from a family study. *Biol. Psychiatry*, **48**: 287–293.

242. Nicolini H., Cruz C., Camarena B., Orozco B., Kennedy J.L., King N., Weissbecker K., de la Fuente J.R., Sidenberg D. (1996) DRD2, DRD3 and 5HT2A receptor genes polymorphisms in obsessive-compulsive disorder. *Mol. Psychiatry*, **1**: 461–465.

243. Karayiorgou M., Altemus M., Galke B.L., Goldman D., Murphy D.L., Ott J., Gogos J.A. (1997) Genotype determining low catechol-O-methyltransferase activity as a risk factor for obsessive-compulsive disorder. *Proc. Natl. Acad. Sci. USA*, **94**: 4572–4575.

244. Billett E.A., Richter M.A., Sam F., Swinson R.P., Dai X.Y., King N., Badri F., Sasaki T., Buchanan J.A., Kennedy J.L. (1998) Investigation of dopamine system genes in obsessive-compulsive disorder. *Psychiatr. Genet.*, **8**: 163–169.

245. Cavallini M.C., Di Bella D., Catalano M., Bellodi L. (2000) An association study between 5-HTTLPR polymorphism, COMT polymorphism, and Tourette's syndrome. *Psychiatry Res.*, **97**: 93–100

246. Frisch A., Michaelovsky E., Rockah R., Amir I., Hermesh H., Laor N., Fuchs C., Zohar J., Lerer B., Buniak S.F. *et al.* (2000) Association between obsessive-compulsive disorder and polymorphisms of genes encoding components of the serotonergic and dopaminergic pathways. *Eur. Neuropsychopharmacol.*, **10**: 205–209.

247. Bengel D., Greenberg B.D., Cora-Locatelli G., Altemus M., Heils A., Li Q., Murphy D.L. (1999) Association of the serotonin transporter promoter regulatory region polymorphism and obsessive-compulsive disorder. *Mol. Psychiatry*, **4**: 463–466.

248. Schindler K.M., Richter M.A., Kennedy J.L., Pato M.T., Pato C.N. (2000) Association between homozygosity at the COMT gene locus and obsessive compulsive disorder. *Am. J. Med. Genet.*, **96**: 721–724.

249. Luxenberg J.S., Swedo S.E., Flament M.F., Friedland R.P., Rapoport J., Rapoport S.I. (1998) Neuroanatomical abnormalities in obsessive-compulsive disorder detected with quantitative X-ray computed tomography. *Am. J. Psychiatry*, **145**: 1089–1093.
250. Robinson D., Wu H., Munne R.A., Ashtari M., Alvir J.M., Lerner G., Koreen A., Cole K., Bogerts B. (1995) Reduced caudate nucleus volume in obsessive-compulsive disorder. *Arch. Gen. Psychiatry*, **52**: 393–398.
251. Kellner C.H., Jolley R.R., Holgate R.C., Austin L., Lydiard R.B., Laraia M., Ballenger J.C. (1991) Brain MRI in obsessive-compulsive disorder. *Psychiatry Res.*, **36**: 45–49.
252. Scarone S., Colombo C., Livian S., Abbruzzese M., Ronchi P., Locatelli M., Scotti G., Smeraldi E. (1992) Increased right caudate nucleus size in obsessive-compulsive disorder: detection with magnetic resonance imaging. *Psychiatry Res.*, **45**: 115–121.
253. Baxter L.R. (1999) Functional imaging of brain systems mediating obsessive-compulsive disorder. In *Neurobiology of Mental Illness* (Eds D.S. Charney, E.J. Nestler, B.S. Bunney), pp. 534–547, Oxford University Press, New York.
254. Saxena S., Rauch S.L. (2000) Functional neuroimaging and the neuroanatomy of obsessive-compulsive disorder. *Psychiatr. Clin. North Am.*, **23**: 563–586.
255. Benkelfat C., Nordahl T.E., Semple W.E., King A.C., Murphy D.L., Cohen R.M. (1990) Local cerebral glucose metabolic rates in obsessive-compulsive disorder. Patients treated with clomipramine. *Arch. Gen. Psychiatry*, **47**: 840–848.
256. Baxter L.R. (1992) Neuroimaging studies of obsessive-compulsive disorder. *Psychiatr. Clin. North Am.*, **15**: 871–884.
257. Swedo S.E., Pietrini P., Leonard H.L., Schapiro M.B., Rettew D.C., Goldberger E.L., Rapoport S.I., Rapoport J.L., Grady C.L. (1992) Cerebral glucose metabolism in childhood-onset obsessive-compulsive disorder. Revisualization during pharmacotherapy. *Arch. Gen. Psychiatry*, **49**: 690–694.
258. Schwartz J.M., Stoessel P.W., Baxter L.R. Jr., Martin K.M., Phelps M.E. (1996) Systematic changes in cerebral glucose metabolic rate after successful behavior modification treatment of obsessive-compulsive disorder. *Arch. Gen. Psychiatry*, **53**: 109–113.
259. Saxena S., Brody A.L., Maidment K.M., Dunkin J.J., Colgan M., Alborzian S., Phelps M.E., Baxter L.R. Jr. (1999) Localized orbitofrontal and subcortical metabolic changes and predictors of response to paroxetine treatment in obsessive-compulsive disorder. *Neuropsychopharmacology*, **21**: 683–693.
260. Hoehn-Saric R., Pearlson G.D., Harris G.J., Machlin S.R., Camargo E.E. (1991) Effects of fluoxetine on regional cerebral blood flow in obsessive-compulsive patients. *Am. J. Psychiatry*, **148**: 1243–1245.
261. Rubin R.T., Ananth J., Villanueva-Meyer J., Trajmar P.G., Mena I. (1995) Regional 133xenon cerebral blood flow and cerebral 99mTc-HMPAO uptake in patients with obsessive-compulsive disorder before and during treatment. *Biol. Psychiatry*, **38**: 429–437.
262. Zohar J., Insel T.R., Berman K.F., Foa E.B., Hill J.L., Weinberger D.R. (1989) Anxiety and cerebral blood flow during behavioral challenge: dissociation of central from peripheral and subjective measures. *Arch. Gen. Psychiatry*, **46**: 505–510.
263. McGuire P.K., Bench C.J., Frith C.D., Marks I.M., Frackowiak R.S., Dolan R.J. (1994) Functional anatomy of obsessive-compulsive phenomena. *Br. J. Psychiatry*, **164**: 459–468.
264. Rauch S.L., Jenike M.A., Alpert N.M., Baer L., Breiter H.C., Savage C.R., Fischman A.J. (1994) Regional cerebral blood flow measured during

symptom provocation in obsessive-compulsive disorder using oxygen 15-labeled carbon dioxide and positron emission tomography. *Arch. Gen. Psychiatry*, **51**: 62–70.
265. Hollander E., Prohovnik I., Stein D.J. (1995) Increased cerebral blood flow during m-CPP exacerbation of obsessive-compulsive disorder. *J. Neuropsychiatry Clin. Neurosci.*, **7**: 485–490.
266. Breiter H.C., Rauch S.L., Kwong K.K., Baker J.R., Weisskoff R.M., Kennedy D.N., Kendrick A.D., Davis T.L., Jiang A., Cohen M.S. *et al.* (1996) Functional magnetic resonance imaging of symptom provocation in obsessive-compulsive disorder. *Arch. Gen. Psychiatry*, **53**: 595–606.
267. Cottraux J., Gerard D., Cinotti L., Froment J.C., Deiber M.P., Le Bars D., Galy G., Millet P., Labbe C., Lavenne F. *et al.* (1996) A controlled positron emission tomography study of obsessive and neutral auditory stimulation in obsessive-compulsive disorder with checking rituals. *Psychiatry Res.*, **60**: 101–112.
268. Insel T.R. (1998) Obsessive-compulsive disorder: a neuroethological perspective. *Psychopharmacol. Bull.*, **24**: 365–369.
269. Rapoport J.L., Wise S.P. (1988) Obsessive-compulsive disorder: is it a basal ganglia dysfunction? *Psychopharmacol. Bull.*, **24**: 380–384.
270. Modell J.G., Mountz J.M., Curtis G.C., Greden J.F. (1989) Neurophysiologic dysfunction in basal ganglia/limbic striatal and thalamocortical circuits as a pathogenetic mechanism of obsessive-compulsive disorder. *J. Neuropsychiatry Clin. Neurosci.*, **1**: 27–36.
271. Insel T.R. (1992) Toward a neuroanatomy of obsessive-compulsive disorder. *Arch. Gen. Psychiatry*, **49**: 739–744.
272. Cheyette S.R., Cummings J.L. (1995) Encephalitis lethargica: lessons for contemporary neuropsychiatry. *J. Neuropsychiatry Clin. Neurosci.*, **7**: 125–134.
273. Insel T.R., Gillin J.C., Moore A., Mendelson W.B., Loewenstein R.J., Murphy D.L. (1982) The sleep of patients with obsessive-compulsive disorder. *Arch. Gen. Psychiatry*, **39**: 1372–1377.
274. Hohagen F., Lis S., Krieger S., Winkelmann G., Riemann D., Fritsch-Montero R., Rey E., Aldenhoff J., Berger M. (1994) Sleep EEG of patients with obsessive-compulsive disorder. *Eur. Arch. Psychiatry Clin. Neurosci.*, **243**: 273–278.
275. Robinson D., Walsleben J., Pollack S., Lerner G. (1998) Nocturnal polysomnography in obsessive-compulsive disorder. *Psychiatry Res.*, **80**: 257–263.
276. Huwig-Poppe C., Voderholzer U., Backhaus J., Riemann D., Konig A., Hohagen F. (1999) The tryptophan depletion test. Impact on sleep in healthy subjects and patients with obsessive-compulsive disorder. *Adv. Exp. Med. Biol.*, **467**: 35–42.
277. Klaassen T., Riedel W.J., Deutz N.E., van Someren A., van Praag H.M. (1999) Specificity of the tryptophan depletion method. *Psychopharmacology*, **141**: 279–286.
278. Joffe R.T., Swinson R.P. (1988) Total sleep deprivation in patients with obsessive-compulsive disorder. *Acta. Psychiatr. Scand.*, **77**: 483–487.
279. Rosenberg D.R., Hanna G.L. (2000) Genetic and imaging strategies in obsessive-compulsive disorder: potential implications for treatment development. *Biol. Psychiatry*, **48**: 1210–1222.
280. Insel T.R., Mueller E.A., Alterman I., Linnoila M., Murphy D.L. (1985) Obsessive-compulsive disorder and serotonin: is there a connection? *Biol. Psychiatry*, **20**: 1174–1188.
281. Thoren P., Asberg M., Bertilsson L., Mellstrom B., Sjoqvist F., Traskman L. (1980) Clomipramine treatment of obsessive-compulsive disorder. II. Biochemical aspects. *Arch. Gen. Psychiatry*, **37**: 1289–1294.

282. Leckman J.F., Goodman W.K., Anderson G.M., Riddle M.A., Chappell P.B., McSwiggan-Hardin M.T., McDougle C.J., Scahill L.D., Ort S.I., Pauls D.L. *et al.* (1995) Cerebrospinal fluid biogenic amines in obsessive compulsive disorder, Tourette's syndrome, and healthy controls. *Neuropsychopharmacology*, **12**: 73–86.

283. Zohar J., Mueller E.A., Insel T.R., Zohar-Kadouch R.C., Murphy D.L. (1987) Serotonergic responsivity in obsessive-compulsive disorder. Comparison of patients and healthy controls. *Arch. Gen. Psychiatry*, **44**: 946–951.

284. Hollander E., DeCaria C.M., Nitescu A., Gully R., Suckow R.F., Cooper T.B., Gorman J.M., Klein D.F., Liebowitz M.R. (1992) Serotonergic function in obsessive-compulsive disorder. Behavioral and neuroendocrine responses to oral m-chlorophenylpiperazine and fenfluramine in patients and healthy volunteers. *Arch. Gen. Psychiatry*, **49**: 21–28.

285. Pigott T.A., Hill J.L., Grady T.A., L'Heureux F., Bernstein S., Rubenstein C.S., Murphy D.L. (1993) A comparison of the behavioral effects of oral versus intravenous mCPP administration in OCD patients and the effect of metergoline prior to i.v. mCPP. *Biol. Psychiatry*, **33**: 3–14.

286. Goodman W.K., McDougle C.J., Price L.H., Barr L.C., Hills O.F., Caplik J.F., Charney D.S., Heninger G.R. (1995) m-Chlorophenylpiperazine in patients with obsessive-compulsive disorder: absence of symptom exacerbation. *Biol. Psychiatry*, **38**: 138–149.

287. Smeraldi E., Diaferia G., Erzegovesi S., Lucca A., Bellodi L., Moja E.A. (1996) Tryptophan depletion in obsessive-compulsive patients. *Biol. Psychiatry*, **40**: 398–402.

288. Hollander E., DeCaria C., Gully R., Nitescu A., Suckow R.F., Gorman J.M., Klein D.F., Liebowitz M.R. (1991) Effects of chronic fluoxetine treatment on behavioral and neuroendocrine responses to meta-chlorophenylpiperazine in obsessive-compulsive disorder. *Psychiatry Res.*, **36**: 1–17.

289. Zohar J., Insel T.R., Zohar-Kadouch R.C., Hill J.L., Murphy D.L. (1988) Serotonergic responsivity in obsessive-compulsive disorder. Effects of chronic clomipramine treatment. *Arch. Gen. Psychiatry*, **45**: 167–172.

290. Keuler D.J., Altemus M., Michelson D., Greenberg B., Murphy D.L. (1996) Behavioral effects of naloxone infusion in obsessive-compulsive disorder. *Biol. Psychiatry*, **40**: 154–156.

291. Leckman J.F., Goodman W.K., North W.G., Chappell P.B., Price L.H., Pauls D.L., Anderson G.M., Riddle M.A., McDougle C.J., Barr L.C. (1994) The role of central oxytocin in obsessive-compulsive disorder and related normal behavior. *Psychoneuroendocrinology*, **19**: 723–749.

292. Altemus M., Pigott T., Kalogeras K.T., Demitrack M., Dubbert B., Murphy D.L., Gold P.W. (1992) Abnormalities in the regulation of vasopressin and corticotropin releasing factor secretion in obsessive-compulsive disorder. *Arch. Gen. Psychiatry*, **49**: 9–20.

293. Neziroglu F., Anemone R., Yaryura-Tobias G.A. (1992) Onset of obsessive-compulsive disorder in pregnancy. *Am. J. Psychiatry*, **149**: 947–950.

294. Swedo S.E. (1994) Sydenham's chorea: a model for childhood autoimmune neuropsychiatric disorders (clinical conference). *JAMA*, **272**: 1788–1791.

295. Swedo S.E., Leonard H.L., Kiessling L. (1994) Speculations on antineuronal antibody-mediated neuropsychiatric disorders of childhood. *Pediatrics*, **93**: 323–326.

296. Swedo S.E., Leonard H.L., Mittleman B.B., Allen A.J., Rapoport J.L., Dow S.P., Kanter M.E., Chapman F., Zabriskie J. (1997) Identification of children with pediatric autoimmune neuropsychiatric disorders associated with streptococ-

cal infections by a marker associated with rheumatic fever. *Am. J. Psychiatry*, **154**: 110–112.

297. Swedo S.E., Leonard H.L., Garvey M., Mittleman B., Allen A.J., Perlmutter S., Lougee L., Dow S., Zamkoff J., Dubbert B.K. (1998) Pediatric autoimmune neuropsychiatric disorders associated with streptococcal infections: clinical description of the first 50 cases. *Am. J. Psychiatry*, **155**: 264–271.

298. Peterson B.S., Leckman J.F., Tucker D., Scahill L., Staib L., Zhang H., King R., Cohen D.J., Gore J.C., Lombroso P. (2000) Preliminary findings of antistreptococcal antibody titers and basal ganglia volumes in tic, obsessive-compulsive, and attention deficit/hyperactivity disorders. *Arch. Gen. Psychiatry*, **57**: 364–372.

299. Murphy T.K., Goodman W.K., Fudge M.W., Williams R.C., Ayoub E.M., Dalal M., Lewis M.H., Zabriskie J.B. (1997) B lymphocyte antigen D8/17: a peripheral marker for childhood-onset obsessive-compulsive disorder and Tourette's syndrome? *Am. J. Psychiatry*, **154**: 402–407.

300. Perlmutter S.J., Leitman S.F., Garvey M.A., Hamburger S., Feldman E., Leonard H.L., Swedo S.E. (1999) Therapeutic plasma exchange and intravenous immunoglobulin for obsessive-compulsive disorder and tic disorders in childhood. *Lancet*, **354**: 1153–1158.

301. Garvey M.A., Perlmutter S.J., Allen A.J., Hamburger S., Lougee L., Leonard H.L., Witowski M.E., Dubbert B., Swedo S.E. (1999) A pilot study of penicillin prophylaxis for neuropsychiatric exacerbations triggered by streptococcal infections. *Biol. Psychiatry*, **45**: 1564–1571.

302. Kessler R.C., Sonnega A., Bromet E., Hughes M., Nelson C.B. (1995) Posttraumatic stress disorder in the National Comorbidity Survey. *Arch. Gen. Psychiatry*, **52**: 1048–1060.

303. Yehuda R., Schmeidler J., Giller E.L. Jr., Siever L.J., Binders-Brynes K. (1998) Relationship between posttraumatic stress disorder characteristics of Holocaust survivors and their adult offspring. *Am. J. Psychiatry*, **155**: 841–843.

304. True W.R., Rice J., Eisen S.A., Heath A.C., Goldberg J., Lyons M.J., Nowak J. (1993) A twin study of genetic and environmental contributions to liability for posttraumatic stress symptoms. *Arch. Gen. Psychiatry*, **50**: 257–264.

305. Xian H., Chantarujikapong S.I., Scherrer J.F., Eisen S.A., Lyons M.J., Goldberg J., Tsuang M., True W.R. (2000) Genetic and environmental influences on posttraumatic stress disorder, alcohol and drug dependence in twin pairs. *Drug Alcohol Depend.*, **61**: 95–102.

306. Robinson J.L., Kagan J., Reznick J.S., Corley R. (1992) The heritability of inhibited and uninhibited behavior: a twin study. *Dev. Psychol.*, **28**: 1030–1037.

307. Lyons M.J., Goldberg J., Eisen S.A., True W., Tsuang M.T., Meyer J.M., Henderson W.G. (1993) Do genes influence exposure to trauma? A twin study of combat. *Am. J. Med. Genet.* **48**: 22–27.

308. Farmer A., Redman K., Harris T., Mahmood A., Sadler S., McGuffin P. (2001) Sensation-seeking, life events and depression. The Cardiff Depression Study. *Br. J. Psychiatry*, **78**: 549–552.

309. Miles D.R., van den Bree M.B., Gupman A.E., Newlin D.B., Glantz M.D., Pickens R.W. (2001) A twin study on sensation seeking, risk taking behavior and marijuana use. *Drug Alcohol Depend.*, **62**: 57–68.

310. Comings D.E., Muhleman D., Gysin R. (1996) Dopamine D2 receptor (DRD2) gene and susceptibility to posttraumatic stress disorder: a study and replication. *Biol. Psychiatry*, **40**: 368–372.

311. Gelernter J., Southwick S., Goodson S., Morgan A., Nagy L., Charney D.S. (1999) No association between D_2 dopamine receptor (DRD2) "A" system

alleles, or DRD2 haplotypes, and posttraumatic stress disorder. *Biol. Psychiatry*, 620–625.

312. Radant A., Tsuang D., Peskind E.R., McFall M., Raskind W. (2001) Biological markers and diagnostic accuracy in the genetics of posttraumatic stress disorder. *Psychiatry Res.*, 102: 203–215.

313. Bremner J.D., Randall P., Scott T.M., Bronen R.A., Seibyl J.P., Southwick S.M., Delaney R.C., McCarthy G., Charney D.S., Innis R.B. (1995) MRI-based measurement of hippocampal volume in patients with combat-related posttraumatic stress disorder. *Am. J. Psychiatry*, 152: 973–981.

314. Bremner J.D., Randall P., Vermetten E., Staib L., Bronen R.A., Mazure C., Capelli S., McCarthy G., Innis R.B., Charney D.S. (1997) Magnetic resonance imaging-based measurement of hippocampal volume in posttraumatic stress disorder related to childhood physical and sexual abuse—a preliminary report. *Biol. Psychiatry*, 41: 23–32.

315. Stein M.B., Koverola C., Hanna C., Torchia M.G., McClarty B. (1997) Hippocampal volume in women victimized by childhood sexual abuse. *Psychol. Med.*, 27: 951–960.

316. Gurvits T.V., Shenton M.E., Hokama H., Ohta H., Lasko N.B., Gilbertson M.W., Orr S.P., Kikinis R., Jolesz F.A., McCarley R.W. *et al.* (1996) Magnetic resonance imaging study of hippocampal volume in chronic, combat-related posttraumatic stress disorder. *Biol. Psychiatry*, 40: 1091–1099.

317. Bremner J.D., Innis R.B., Ng C.K., Staib L.H., Salomon R.M., Bronen R.A., Duncan J., Southwick S.M., Krystal J.H., Rich D. *et al.* (1997) Positron emission tomography measurement of cerebral metabolic correlates of yohimbine administration in combat-related posttraumatic stress disorder. *Arch. Gen. Psychiatry*, 54: 246–254.

318. Shin L.M., Kosslyn S.M., McNally R.J., Alpert N.M., Thompson W.L., Rauch S.L., Macklin M.L., Pitman R.K. (1997) Visual imagery and perception in posttraumatic stress disorder. A positron emission tomographic investigation. *Arch. Gen. Psychiatry*, 54: 233–241.

319. Semple W.E., Goyer P.F., McCormick R., Compton-Toth B., Morris E., Donovan B., Muswick G., Nelson D., Garnett M.L., Sharkoff J. *et al.* (1996) Attention and regional cerebral blood flow in posttraumatic stress disorder patients with substance abuse histories. *Psychiatry Res.*, 67: 17–28.

320. Bremner J.D., Staib L.H., Kaloupek D., Southwick S.M., Soufer R., Charney D.S. (1999) Neural correlates of exposure to traumatic pictures and sound in Vietnam combat veterans with and without posttraumatic stress disorder: a positron emission tomography study. *Biol. Psychiatry*, 45: 806–816.

321. LeDoux J. (1998) Fear and the brain: where have we been, and where are we going? *Biol. Psychiatry*, 44: 1229–1238.

322. Liberzon I., Taylor S.F., Amdur R., Jung T.D., Chamberlain K.R., Minoshima S., Koeppe R.A., Fig L.M. (1999) Brain activation in PTSD in response to trauma-related stimuli. *Biol. Psychiatry*, 45: 817–826.

323. Zola-Morgan S., Squire L.R. (1990) The neuropsychology of memory. Parallel findings in humans and nonhuman primates. *Ann. N.Y. Acad. Sci.*, 608: 434–456

324. Zola-Morgan S., Squire L.R. (1993) Neuroanatomy of memory. *Annu. Rev. Neurosci.*, 16: 547–63.

325. Squire L.R., Zola-Morgan S. (1991) The medial temporal lobe memory system. *Science*, 253: 1380–1386.

326. Charles G., Hansenne M., Ansseau M., Pitchot W., Machowski R., Schittecatte M., Wilmotte J. (1995) P300 in post traumatic stress disorder. *Neuropsychobiology*, **32**: 72–74.
327. Morgan C., Grillon C. (1999) Abnormal mismatch negativity in women with sexual assault-related posttraumatic stress disorder. *Biol. Psychiatry*, **45**: 827–832.
328. Newport D.J., Nemeroff C.B. (2000) Neurobiology of posttraumatic stress disorder. *Curr. Opin. Neurobiol.*, **10**: 211–218.
329. Skinner R.D., Rasco L.M., Fitzgerald J., Karson C.N., Matthew M., Williams D.K., Garcia-Rill E. (1999) Reduced sensory gating of the P1 potential in rape victims and combat veterans with posttraumatic stress disorder. *Depress. Anxiety*, **9**: 122–30.
330. Stein M.B., Hanna C., Koverola C., Torchia M., McClarty B. (1997) Structural brain changes in PTSD. Does trauma alter neuroanatomy? *Ann. N.Y. Acad. Sci.*, **821**: 76–82.
331. Sachinvala N., von Scotti H., McGuire M., Fairbanks L., Bakst K., Brown N. (2000) Memory, attention, function, and mood among patients with chronic posttraumatic stress disorder. *J. Nerv. Ment. Dis.*, **188**: 818–23.
332. Gilbertson M.W., Gurvits T.V., Lasko N.B., Orr S.P., Pitman R.K. (2001) Multivariate assessment of explicit memory function in combat veterans with posttraumatic stress disorder. *J. Traumatic Stress.*, **14**: 413–32.
333. Orr S.P. (1997) Psychophysiologic reactivity to trauma-related imagery in PTSD. Diagnostic and theoretical implications of recent findings. *Ann. N.Y. Acad. Sci.*, **821**: 114–124.
334. Orr S.P., Lasko N.B., Metzger L.J., Berry N.J., Ahern C.E., Pitman R.K. (1997) Psychophysiologic assessment of PTSD in adult females sexually abused during childhood. *Ann. N.Y. Acad. Sci.*, **821**: 491–3.
335. Southwick S.M., Bremner J.D., Rasmusson A., Morgan C.A. III, Arnsten A., Charney D.S. (1999) Role of norepinephrine in the pathophysiology and treatment of posttraumatic stress disorder. *Biol. Psychiatry*, **46**: 1192–1204.
336. Ross R.J., Ball W.A., Sullivan K.A., Caroff S.N. (1989) Sleep disturbance as the hallmark of posttraumatic stress disorder. *Am. J. Psychiatry*, **146**: 697–707.
337. Hurwitz T.D., Mahowald M.W., Kuskowski M., Engdahl B.E. (1988) Polysomnographic sleep is not clinically impaired in Vietnam combat veterans with chronic posttraumatic stress disorder. *Biol. Psychiatry*, **44**: 1066–1073.
338. Mellman T.A. (1997) Psychobiology of sleep disturbance in posttraumatic stress disorder. *Ann. N.Y. Acad. Sci.*, **821**: 142–149.
339. Engdahl B.E., Eberly R.E., Hurwitz T.D., Mahowald M.W., Blake J. (2000) Sleep in a community sample of elderly war veterans with and without posttraumatic stress disorder. *Biol. Psychiatry*, **47**: 520–525.
340. Ross R.J., Ball W.A., Dinges D.F., Kribbs N.B., Morrison A.R., Silver S.M., Mulvaney F.D. (1994) Rapid eye movement sleep disturbance in posttraumatic stress disorder. *Biol. Psychiatry*, **35**: 195–202.
341. Dow B.M., Kelsoe J.R. Jr., Gillin J.C. (1996) Sleep and dreams in Vietnam PTSD and depression. *Biol. Psychiatry*, **39**: 42–50.
342. De Bellis M.D., Baum A.S., Birmaher B., Keshavan MS., Eccard C.H., Boring A.M., Jenkins F.J., Ryan N.D. (1999) A.E. Bennett Research Award. Developmental traumatology. Part I: Biological stress systems. *Biol. Psychiatry*, **45**: 1259–1270.
343. Kosten T.R., Mason J.W., Giller E.L., Ostroff R.B., Harkness L. (1987) Sustained urinary norepinephrine and epinephrine elevation in post-traumatic stress disorder. *Psychoneuroendocrinology*, **12**: 13–20.

344. Yehuda R., Southwick S., Giller E.L., Ma X., Mason J.W. (1992) Urinary cat-echolamine excretion and severity of PTSD symptoms in Vietnam combat veterans. *J. Nerv. Ment. Dis.*, **180**: 321–325.

345. Perry B.D., Southwick S.M., Yehuda R., Giller E.L. (1990) Adrenergic receptor regulation in posttraumatic stress disorder. In *Biological Assessment and Treatment of Post-traumatic Stress Disorder* (Ed. E.L. Giller), pp. 87–114, American Psychiatric Press, Washington.

346. Perry B.D. (1994) Neurobiological sequelae of childhood trauma: PTSD in children. In *Catecholamine Function in Post-traumatic Stress Disorder: Emerging Concepts* (Ed. M. Murburg), pp. 233–256, American Psychiatric Press, Washington.

347. Pitman R.K., Orr S.P., Forgue D.F., Altman B., de Jong J.B., Herz L.R. (1990) Psychophysiologic responses to combat imagery of Vietnam veterans with posttraumatic stress disorder versus other anxiety disorders. *J. Abnorm. Psychol.*, **99**: 49–54.

348. McFall M.E., Veith R.C., Murburg M.M. (1992) Basal sympathoadrenal function in posttraumatic distress disorder. *Biol. Psychiatry*, **31**: 1050–1056.

349. Mellman T.A., Kumar A., Kulick-Bell R., Kumar M., Nolan B. (1995) Nocturnal/daytime urine noradrenergic measures and sleep in combat-related PTSD. *Biol. Psychiatry*, **38**: 174–179.

350. Blanchard E.B., Kolb L.C., Prins A., Gates S., McCoy G.C. (1991) Changes in plasma norepinephrine to combat-related stimuli among Vietnam veterans with posttraumatic stress disorder. *J. Nerv. Ment. Dis.*, **179**: 371–373.

351. Liberzon I., Abelson J.L., Flagel S.B., Raz J., Young E.A. (1999) Neuroendocrine and psychophysiologic responses in PTSD: a symptom provocation study. *Neuropsychopharmacology*, **21**: 40–50.

352. Southwick S.M., Krystal J.H., Morgan C.A., Johnson D., Nagy L.M., Nicolaou A., Heninger G.R., Charney D.S. (1993) Abnormal noradrenergic function in posttraumatic stress disorder. *Arch. Gen. Psychiatry*, **50**: 266–74.

353. Southwick S.M., Yehuda R., Morgan C.A III. (1995) Clinical studies of neurotransmitter alterations in post-traumatic stress disorder. In *Neurobiological and Clinical Consequences of Stress: From Normal Adaptation to Post Traumatic Stress Disorder* (Eds M.J. Freidman, D.S. Charney, A.Y. Deutsch), pp. 335–350, Lippincott-Raven, Philadelphia.

354. Spivak B., Vered Y., Graff E., Blum I., Mester R., Weizman A. (1999) Low platelet-poor plasma concentrations of serotonin in patients with combat-related posttraumatic stress disorder. *Biol. Psychiatry*, **45**: 840–845.

355. Maes M., Lin A.H., Verkerk R., Delmeire L., Van Gastel A., Van der Planken M., Scharpe S. (1999) Serotonergic and noradrenergic markers of post-traumatic stress disorder with and without major depression. *Neuropsychopharmacology*, **20**: 188–197.

356. Davis L.L., Clark D.M., Kramer G.L., Moeller F.G., Petty F. (1999) D-Fenfluramine challenge in posttraumatic stress disorder. *Biol. Psychiatry*, **45**: 928–930.

357. Southwick S.M., Krystal J.H., Bremner J.D., Morgan C.A. III, Nicolaou A.L., Nagy L.M., Johnson D.R., Heninger G.R., Charney D.S. (1997) Noradrenergic and serotonergic function in posttraumatic stress disorder. *Arch. Gen. Psychiatry*, **54**: 749–758.

358. Baker D.G., West S.A., Nicholson W.E., Ekhator N.N., Kasckow J.W., Hill K.K., Bruce A.B., Orth D.N., Geracioti T.D. Jr. (1999) Serial CSF corticotropin-releasing hormone levels and adrenocortical activity in combat veterans with posttraumatic stress disorder. *Am. J. Psychiatry*, **156**: 585–588.

359. Yehuda R. (2000) Biology of posttraumatic stress disorder. *J. Clin. Psychiatry*, **61**(Suppl. 7): 14–21.
360. Yehuda R. (2001) Are glucocortoids responsible for putative hippocampal damage in PTSD? How and when to decide. *Hippocampus*, **11**: 85–89.

9

Biological Research on Dementias

Simon Lovestone

Departments of Old Age Psychiatry and Neuroscience, Institute of Psychiatry, De Crespigny Park, London SE5 8AF, United Kingdom

INTRODUCTION

In 1907, Alois Alzheimer described in the brain of a middle-aged woman the plaques and tangles that have provided the focus for all subsequent research on the dementias. These lesions, visualized by silver staining, also occur in the brains of old people with dementia, and this realization, known before Alzheimer but rediscovered in the modern age in the 1960s [1], was one of the most important steps forward in care of the elderly, as it turned senility from an unfortunate but seemingly inevitable, and hence ignored, consequence of ageing, into a disease process. From this followed medical and other services, the establishment of the lay societies and subsequent increasing recognition by the general public, support for carers and the ever-improving recognition and treatment of cognitive decline in late life. Thus, the first and still the most dramatic consequence of biological research in the dementias is to have put dementia on the public, political and medical map. Other consequences arriving in recent years is the first specific treatments, but the real goal of biological research is treatments that will be preventative or curative—disease-modifying, in other words. It is a testament to the speed of processes in the molecular sciences that such treatments are now on the horizon.

NEUROPATHOLOGY

Neuropathology of Alzheimer's Disease

The two cardinal lesions of Alzheimer's disease (AD) are plaques and tangles. Plaques are extracellular structures consisting of a core of fibrillar

Psychiatry as a Neuroscience. Edited by Juan José López-Ibor, Wolfgang Gaebel, Mario Maj and Norman Sartorius. © 2002 John Wiley & Sons Ltd.

protein in a β-pleated sheet structure surrounded by neuritic change, these neurites containing highly phosphorylated tau protein. The core of the plaque consists of amyloid (Aβ), itself a peptide derived from the amyloid precursor protein (APP). Using antibodies against this protein, a new class of plaques was discovered—the diffuse plaque [2]. Diffuse plaques, which are not visualized with silver staining, are probably a precursor of the matured cored plaques. As all people with Down's syndrome suffer from AD pathology early in life, neuropathological examination of Down's syndrome brain reveals the sequence of events in AD pathology. Such studies confirmed that diffuse plaques evolve to cored, matured, neuritic plaques [3]. These studies, and others in normal and AD brains, also suggested that plaque formation preceded other forms of neuropathology [4–6]. However, not all lesions are equal. It is possible, for example, that plaques are more readily cleared from brain than other lesions such as neurofibrillary tangles, and hence, in any one particular brain, lesion density may represent lesion preservation as much as lesion occurrence. The same difficulty arises when trying to determine which lesion accounts for the clinical appearance of dementia. The majority of studies find a greater correlation of cognitive loss with neurofibrillary tangle formation than with plaque number [7–11], although some have suggested a correlation between amyloid load and cognitive loss [12, 13]. The problem with these studies is that the assessment of cognitive loss precedes (fairly obviously) the neuropathological examination, sometimes by some considerable period, and in between clinical and pathological assessments the more soluble lesions may be preferentially cleared from brain.

The second characteristic lesion of AD is the neurofibrillary tangles. These are intraneuronal inclusions that occur first in the transentorhinal cortex, spread to the hippocampus and from there spread further to cortical structures, but never to cerebellum. The typical and apparently consistent pattern of spread of neurofibrillary tangles suggests an intimate relationship with the disease pathogenesis, in contrast to the distribution of amyloid plaques, which appears more random and occurs in areas of the brain apparently clinically unaffected, such as cerebellum [14]. Neurofibrillary tangles are flame-shaped as they occur in pyramidal neurons, where they fill cytoplasm and eventually lead to the demise of the neuron, leaving a "ghost" or "tombstone" tangle. Tangles are composed of the microtubule-associated protein tau, which is aggregated into highly insoluble and highly phosphorylated polymers [15]. Unlike the case with plaques, there is a direct correlation between tangles and cognitive loss, although, as noted above, this may be biased because of their insolubility [15]. Careful study of large numbers of brains reveals the probable evolution of the tangle; the initial signs of pathology are the accumulation of highly phosphorylated tau in cytoplasm before actual tangle formation, which in turn is followed by the spread of the pathology [16]. This progression has been described in six stages (the Braak staging); the first few stages are clinically silent and precede dementia by many years [17].

Other lesions also occur in the AD brain, including granulovacuolar degeneration and Hirano bodies. The molecular origin of these is largely unknown. Amyloid deposition and tau aggregation also both occur at sites other than the plaque and tangle. Thus, amyloid is deposited in vessel walls as congophilic angiopathy, and tau aggregation occurs in the neurites of mature plaques and in wispy neuropil threads that are probably remnants of degenerating axons.

The Lewy Body—Linking Subcortical and Cortical Neurodegeneration

The Lewy body was discovered first in the early 1900s and then again in the 1970s [18]. Lewy was a colleague of Alzheimer and described round inclusion bodies in the substantia nigra in Parkinson's disease (PD). With haematoxylin and eosin staining, these pink inclusions are readily visible in the pigmented nigral neurons, but they were unrecognizable in cortex, where they also occur, until the use of ubiquitin antibodies. Ubiquitin is a protein that targets other proteins for degradation by the proteosome; many inclusion bodies are ubiquitinated, Lewy bodies being no exception. With the "discovery" of Lewy bodies in the cortex, the clinical history of these patients revealed a "new" disease—"dementia with Lewy bodies" (DLB), characterized by fluctuating confusion, parkinsonism and visual hallucinations [19]. In truth, there is a large overlap with other disorders, in particular AD, as patients with autosomal dominant (and hence not nosologically confused) AD also have Lewy bodies [20–22] and the vast majority of DLB patients also have AD changes [23]. Nonetheless, DLB does have clinical and neurochemical differences to AD [24], and some patients with DLB have no AD changes [25, 26], demonstrating that the Lewy body is a sufficient condition for dementia.

Synucleinopathy, Taupathy and Amyloidopathy: A New Classification Of Neurodegeneration

The core of the Lewy body is a fibrillar protein now known to be synuclein [27]. This protein is also deposited in the glial inclusions of multi-system atrophy [28], and a new classification of the neurodegenerative disorders has been suggested, with multiple system atrophy (MSA), DLB and PD as the synucleinopathies [29]. Other disorders, such as progressive supranuclear palsy (PSP) and the frontal lobe dementias, such as that associated with parkinsonism and Pick's disease itself, have inclusion bodies that contain tau. These include the eponymous Pick body itself, but also other neuronal inclusions that are similar to the tangle of AD and glial lesions [30]. These tau-positive pathologies have been grouped as the tauopathies. The amyloidopathies include those disorders with extracellular β-pleated sheet, congophilic amyloid deposits. Such disorders include the rare British familial dementia, where the amyloid is formed from a peptide derived from the novel gene BRI (named after *Brit*ain), and the spongiform encephalopathies, including Creutzfeld–Jacob disease, where the prion protein forms an amyloid plaque. AD has some characteristics of all three neurodegenerative disorders: it could be classified as an amyloidopathy or a tauopathy or, as Lewy bodies also occur in some cases of AD, as a synucleinopathy as well.

The insight highlighted by this new classification is that there are pathologies held in common between apparently very different dementias—PD and DLB, frontotemporal dementia with Parkinson's disease (FTDP) and PSP, for example. The different phenotype results in some instances from different neuroanatomical location of the lesions (PD and DLB being the obvious example, with the cortical pathology of DLB associated with "cortical" symptoms such as hallucinations and dementia and the subcortical pathology of PD associated with subcortical motor clinical signs). The challenge for the future is twofold: firstly, to determine whether there are common pathogeneses or whether these lesions are simply the final common product of diverse pathological pathways and, secondly, and more speculatively, to determine whether there might be common therapeutic approaches. "One drug, many disorders" is the possibility exciting many in the field, not least the pharmaceutical industry.

NEUROCHEMISTRY

The Cholinergic Hypothesis

The drugs currently available for treating the core symptoms of AD—the acetyl cholinesterase inhibitors—were developed as a direct consequence of work in the 1960s and 1970s that led to the cholinergic hypothesis of AD [31]. There are two broad lines of evidence underpinning this hypothesis. Firstly, lesions in the cholinergic system in animals, induced by chemical or surgical means, and chemical inhibition of cholinergic neurotransmission in man, result in cognitive deficits, and, secondly, post-mortem studies in AD suggest a predominant cholinergic neuron loss [32–34].

Post-mortem studies in AD found neuronal loss to be particularly pronounced in the cholinergic nucleus basalis of Meynert [35], this cell loss being accompanied by, and therefore likely to be caused by, neurofibrillary tangle formation [36, 37]. Markers of cholinergic activity, including acetyl-cholinesterase [38, 39] and choline acetyltransferase [40], were shown to be reduced in AD brain. However, the cholinergic receptors were not so clearly disrupted. In AD brain, extensive loss of cholinergic fibres is not accompanied by loss of muscarinic receptor binding activity [41], although differential loss of M_2 muscarinic receptors may occur [42]. Indeed, one in situ hybridization study suggested that muscarinic receptor gene message was up-regulated in AD, possibly in response to loss of cholinergic activity [43]. This finding is important: it suggested that correction of the cholinergic loss was a useful aim as the remaining neurons are likely to be responsive.

The hypothesis has stood the test of time, in that it has resulted in the development of efficacious compounds [44]. Moreover, it has recently received some adaptation and extension, with suggestions that the cholinergic deficit may not just be a consequence but may also be involved in the molecular pathogenesis and spread of AD [44], and with the additional suggestion that the cholinergic deficit might underlie some of the behavioural and psychological symptoms of dementia (BPSD) [45]. Furthermore, some evidence in favour of the cholinergic hypothesis comes from studies comparing neurotransmitter loss in different dementias, suggesting therefore a certain specificity to the hypothesis. In frontal lobe dementia, for example, there is loss of serotonin receptors and α-amino-3-hydroxy-4-isoxazole propionic acid (AMPA) receptors from both temporal and frontal lobes [46]. On the other hand, the cholinergic loss in DLB is even greater than that in AD [47, 48].

Other Neurotransmitter Loss

The cholinergic hypothesis, as it was first developed, is clearly too simplistic. In fact, many neurotransmitter lesions in animals result in cognitive deficits, and the complexity of the relationship between neurochemistry and cognition is considerable and increasingly revealed by more sophisticated experimentation. Secondly, the neurotransmitter loss in AD is not confined to cholinergic neurons but also involves noradrenergic, serotonergic and other neurons. A review of over 250 post-mortem studies suggested the order of loss of neurochemical function to be first cholinergic system, then serotonergic system, followed by excitatory amino acids and the GABAergic system, with little change in dopaminergic fibres [49]. Finally, these studies all suffer from the intrinsic problems of post-mortem investigations— changes due to post-mortem delay and the inability to examine any state other than the final end-point of disease. As markers of cholinergic activity for use in functional imaging are developed (see, for example, [50]), it will be interesting to examine the sequential and early functional neurochemical changes as they occur.

Neurochemistry and the Clinical Features of AD

There is some evidence that loss of different neurotransmitter systems contributes to the diverse phenotype of AD. Loss of noradrenergic neurons in the locus coeruleus and decreased markers of noradrenergic activity have been found to be more pronounced in those with depression and dementia than in non-depressed AD patients at post mortem [39, 51, 52]. However, these are difficult studies for a number of reasons, and not all find the same result [53]. The findings in respect of serotonergic loss are even less consistent. For example, depressed AD patients may show decreased neuronal counts in dorsal raphe nucleus [54] and decreased markers of serotonergic activity [52, 54], but other studies fail to replicate these findings [55, 56]. Decreased serotonergic activity measures have also been reported in psychosis in AD [57].

The cholinergic system itself might be responsible for more than cognitive loss in AD. This was first suggested by the evidence that the cholinergic system is particularly depleted in DLB (a disorder characterized by psychotic features and fluctuating confusion in addition to parkinsonism) and by the observation that, in man, antimuscarinic drugs alter consciousness and induce hallucinations [58]. It follows that the cholinergic system might be responsible for some of the BPSD in AD and related dementias [45]. This has been subsequently supported by evidence suggesting that muscarinic agonists might be antipsychotic in animal models [59] and that acetylcholinesterase inhibitors might reduce BPSD in AD [60].

GENETICS

Autosomal Dominant Neurodegeneration

If it was neurochemistry that led to the development of symptomatic treatments for AD, and it is epidemiology that seeks preventative strategies, then it is molecular biology and genetics that will lead to the development of disease-modifying treatments. No less than a cure is the goal, and it is an extraordinary testament to the power of molecular medicine that such a vision seems only optimistic and not ridiculous. The first real signs of progress came with the biochemical characterization of the amyloid peptide, and its parent protein, the APP, which forms the core of the neuritic plaque [61]. However, it was the finding that the gene coding for APP on chromosome 21 was mutated in some families with autosomal dominant AD that really proved the fundamental role of this protein in the aetiopathogenesis of AD. A similar train of events was repeated a decade later, when the gene coding for the protein that forms the other lesion of AD, neurofibrillary tangles, was also found to be mutated in some forms of autosomal dominant dementia. In both instances it was biochemistry that identified the protein and genetics that proved the aetiology.

Mutations in APP are a rare cause of autosomal dominant early-onset AD and are also responsible for another rare disorder—hereditary cerebral haemorrhage with amyloidosis, Dutch type. As the gene is carried on chromosome 21, trisomy APP is also probably the reason why people with Down's syndrome suffer from AD at an early age. The mutations cluster at three main positions: on both the amino and carboxy termini of the amyloid peptide, and also in the middle of the peptide itself [62–64]. The position of these mutations strongly suggests that the mutations alter the processing of the resulting protein, and studies in cells and animals (discussed below) have confirmed this. The processing of APP is also altered by the presenilin proteins, the genes for which (PS-1 and PS-2) are also associated with early-onset familial AD [65]. PS-1 mutations are the most frequent cause of the still rare autosomal dominant AD, whereas mutations in PS-2 are found most frequently in the Volga German people, a genetically relatively isolated group now living in the USA [66].

The second main class of dementias to be associated with a single gene are the frontal lobe dementias. At a consensus conference, a series of families with a similar phenotype were grouped together as having the frontotemporal degeneration with Parkinson's disease linked to chromosome 17 (FTDP-17) [67]. As the tau gene is on chromosome 17, and as these disorders, like AD, have tau-positive inclusions, this gene was a prime candidate and it was no surprise when mutations were found in a family with the condition [68]. Subsequently, mutations in the same gene have also been associated with Pick's disease [69, 70] and with progressive subcortical gliosis [71], and polymorphic variation in the gene with PSP [72, 73]. Mutations in the tau gene are of two main types: missense mutations in the coding region and intronic mutations that disrupt splicing of the gene, leading to altered expression of the resulting protein, disrupting the normal balance between the different isoforms of the protein [74].

There are now numerous different neurodegenerative disorders identified that have rare autosomal dominant variants, including the triplet repeat disorders such as Huntington's disease (HD), other amyloid conditions such as British familial dementia, and the spongiform encephalopathies like Creutzfeldt–Jacob disease caused by mutations in the prion gene. The description of the single-gene dementias is very nearly complete. There are some families with autosomal dominant inheritance with unidentified mutations, possibly in as yet unknown genes, but these are now very few indeed. The understanding of the role of amyloid and tau that has followed, and the clinical consequences that flow from these discoveries, are discussed below.

Genotype-Phenotype Correlation

In some autosomal dominant neurodegenerative disorders, different mutations give rise to the same clinical and neuropathological phenotype (PS-1 and APP mutations causing AD, for example). In others, mutations in the same gene give rise to completely different phenotypes—disorders that were previously considered entirely different (tau mutations causing frontotemporal dementia and progressive subcortical gliosis, for example). The relationship between genotype and phenotype is not necessarily straightforward even in the single-gene disorders. The 144-bp insertion in the prion protein gene, for example, has given rise to multiple phenotypes even in a single family, including AD, HD, PD, myoclonic epilepsy, atypical dementia, Pick's disease, Creutzfeldt–Jakob disease and Gerstmann–Straussler syndrome [75]. This implies that some other event, either environmental, developmental or genetic, must be influencing the phenotypic expression of the gene mutation. A similar phenomenon is seen in HD, where early psychotic features appear to segregate in some families [76, 77] and a family-based study demonstrates that this is not due to the HD gene itself, but to some other, presumably genetic, factor [32]. A similar family-based study in AD also demonstrated some sharing of phenotype in siblings not due to any known genetic factor [78], and the age at onset tends to be similar within families, suggesting a genotypic–phenotypic correlation.

These findings from diverse neurodegenerative disorders demonstrate that not only are there genes causing autosomal disorders, but there are also other genetic factors that influence the phenotypic expression of these single genes. An intriguing possibility follows from these observations: it is possible that the genetic factors that interact with the major disease-causing genes, and indeed the genes that influence complex multi-factorial disease like late-onset AD, could be the same genes that underlie the genetics of other neuropsychiatric diseases. Thus, the HD and AD studies cited above suggest a genetic factor that lowers the vulnerability to psychotic experiences, such that those individuals within a family that carry the HD or AD genes become psychotic. These psychosis-vulnerability genes might be the same as those that influence schizophrenia. The same may be true for whatever gene it is that causes depression to be shared in families with AD [78–80].

Clinical Genetics of Late-Onset AD

The genetic contribution to late-life disorders is intrinsically difficult to estimate due to attrition by other causes. Typically, 10–30% of subjects with AD have a positive family history, but this figure is entirely dependent upon the age of the relatives—the older the relatives, the more likely they are to have AD, the strongest risk factor for which is age itself [81]. A series of clinical genetic studies attempted to overcome this problem by determining the incidence of AD in relatives by age. These studies all found a cumulative incidence of around 50% or more [82], considerably greater than that expected from incidence and prevalence figures in the general population. It has been pointed out that this, and the concordance rates in twins, is compatible with a small number of genes of large effect (approaching autosomal dominance) or a large number of genes of small effect [83, 84].

There have been two general approaches to discovering the genes that are responsible for this risk: by association and by linkage. In general terms, the former has greater power and studies are relatively easier to conduct. However, the problem with association studies is one of lack of reproducibility. Whether because of sample population stratification or because of intrinsic statistical artefact, the single biggest outcome of the association studies has been a series of false positive findings. At the time of writing, there are more than 30 genes positively associated with AD in well-conducted studies that have not been reproduced in other, equally well-conducted studies. The possible statistical reason for such a disappointing outcome is that, although some studies control for multiple testing within a study, none control for multiple testing between studies, and given the hundreds of candidate genes analysed it is not surprising that false positives are so frequently encountered.

Genes Associated with Late-Onset AD

There remains only one gene unequivocally associated with late-onset AD: apolipoprotein E (APOE). A single gene codes for the three commonly encountered protein isoforms that can be distinguished by electrophoretic isofocusing—apolipoprotein E2, E3 and E4. These three isoforms result from a cysteine/arginine change at two positions in the APOE gene (112 and 158), giving rise to the three common alleles (APOEε2, ε3 and ε4). The APOE protein is part of the normal regulation of lipid transport and metabolism, and the polymorphic variation in the APOE gene is associated with variation in serum cholesterol levels (lower in APOEε2 [85]) and with risk of cardiac disease (higher in APOEε4 [86]). Previously, late-onset AD had been linked to chromosome 19, near the locus of the myotonic dystrophy gene and the APOE-APOCII complex [87], and the Duke group, then leaders in the genetics of myotonic dystrophy, demonstrated association with the APOE gene [88, 89]. In marked contrast to all the other genes putatively associated with AD before and since, this finding was very rapidly replicated in small European, American and Japanese populations [90–97] and then with large epidemiologically based samples from diverse ethnic groups.

There is absolutely no doubt whatsoever that APOE modifies risk of AD, with APOE4 increasing and APOE2 decreasing risk. Less clear is by how much risk is altered, although the consensus appears to be two- to four-fold for the APOE4/* heterozygotic condition and up to 10-fold for the rare APOE4/4 homozygotes. In addition, although there appears to be no population that is free from APOE-influenced risk, the effect size does differ between populations and may be lower in some black and Hispanic populations [98–101]. Although some of these studies were performed in the genetically heterogeneous African-American population, the effect of APOE on African peoples is not yet known. Furthermore, there is very considerable genetic heterogeneity even within African countries (the distinct ethnic and cultural groups within Nigeria for example). This is important, as some African populations (for example the Khoi-San people of Northern Africa) have amongst the highest APOE4 frequency in the world; if their risk is as high as that of white people who have been examined, then as the health care of the countries in which they live improves, they will suffer disproportionately more AD than the currently industrialized nations (and, alongside this, less ability to pay for it). It is possible that the variation in incidence in AD across the world is itself partially due to variation between populations in APOE4 frequency.

The biology of APOE and its relationship to AD is discussed below, but a number of studies have tried to examine how APOE works through phenotype-genotype correlations. Most studies find no correlation between speed of decline and APOE genotype [102–106], although a higher rate of decline in those with [107, 108], and without [109] an ε4 allele has also been found in some studies. If APOE does influence the rate of progression, it must be a small effect, and this is also true for any effect on the non-cognitive phenomenology of AD [110, 111]. Correlation is found with the neuropathology, in particular with plaque formation, suggesting a relationship with amyloid processing [112–114]. In line with this, APOE does not appear to be a risk factor for FTD—a disorder with tangles but not plaques [115, 116]. The clearest association, however, is with age of onset. Within the late-life age range, APOE4 tends to bring forward and APOE2 delays the age of onset, leading to the suggestion that APOE influences "when, not if" an individual suffers from AD [117].

No other genes are unequivocally associated with AD. However, of the other candidate genes for association with AD, three deserve mention. α_2–macroglobulin (α2M) was an excellent candidate, not least because it is a ligand for the APOE receptors and hence might be in competition with APOE [118]. Early studies found an association, others replicated the association, but still others failed to repeat the finding; the conclusion of all this remains uncertain, but it is unlikely that α2M has a significant role to play in the genetic aetiology of AD. Polymorphic variations separate to the main genetic finding in all the unequivocal "AD genes", including APP, the presenilins, tau and APOE, are good candidates, and variation in all of these genes has been linked in some but not all studies with late-onset AD. Of this group, perhaps an intronic polymorphism in the PS-1 gene is the best studied [119], but given the disparate findings it is by no means certain that this is a risk factor for AD. Finally, variation in the gene encoding angiotensin-converting enzyme (ACE) may be associated with hypertension (although this too is disputed) and, as cardiac risk factors are associated with AD, then ACE might be a risk gene for AD. Three independent populations all provided association with AD [120], a finding repeated in some but not all studies [121–124]. A meta-analysis supports the association, leaving this gene the most likely "second" gene of risk in AD [123].

Chromosomes Linked to Late-Onset AD

The pattern of the candidate gene studies is clear and disappointing: a biologically good candidate is associated with AD in a study, repeated in another, not repeated in yet another, and a meta-analysis is equivocal, weakly positive and often disputed. A more robust but very considerably more taxing approach is to examine for regions associated with AD by linkage. Given that parents of people with late-onset AD are not available for study, linkage studies are limited to sibling pairs, of which a number have been reported. These studies have been made possible by the availability of dense marker coverage across the genome and will be considerably enhanced by the production of single nucleotide polymorphism (SNP) maps that will shortly result from the human genome mapping project.

The sibling pair genome scans thus far reported have found a number of regions linked to AD. These include the APOE locus on chromosome 19, a locus on chromosome 21 that might or might not be APP and a locus on chromosome 12 that might or might not be α2M or another APOE receptor (LRP) [125–127]. However, the most interesting region is one on chromosome 10q. Not only has this been linked to AD in a two-stage sibling pair genome scan and a replication study, but it has also been linked to variation in serum amyloid levels in families [128–130]. This very strongly suggests a gene on the region that increases risk of AD by altering APP metabolism. One candidate close to the region is insulin-degrading enzyme (IDE). This intriguing gene is already a candidate as it has been demonstrated that the IDE protein not only degrades insulin but also amyloid [131]. It remains to be seen whether in fact this is another false lead in the difficult genetics of late-onset AD.

Clinical Implications of Molecular Genetics of AD

From a clinical perspective, the early-onset familial dementias and the late-onset dementias (whether familial or not) are entirely different disorders. For early-onset familial autosomal dominant AD, the genetic advances have enabled predictive and diagnostic testing. Diagnostic testing means that, among individuals with clinical dementia and with an autosomal dominant pedigree, the majority can receive a definitive differential diagnosis. Molecular genetic testing will distinguish between frontal lobe dementias, familial spongiform encephalopathies and familial AD, all of which can be clinically difficult to distinguish. However, it should be noted that even diagnostic testing is not without problems [132, 133]. Finding a mutation known to cause disease cannot be used to aid early diagnosis, as even people harbouring the mutation can have other disorders, such as depression, that can mimic the early stages of dementia. A similar situation occurs in HD, where a positive test does not help to determine whether mild symptoms are due to anxiety or the start of the HD itself. Only a clinical examination can do this. Also there are, if not ethical, then difficult personal issues that flow from performing a molecular diagnostic test. Although the diagnosis of familial AD may have been made and explained to the family, and although finding a mutation in the affected person does not alter the risk suffered by the family (which remains 50% for first-degree relatives), there is something so final and firm about a "gene test" that experience suggests it raises considerable anxieties in families. It also raises new issues as predictive testing becomes a possibility for relatives.

Predictive testing involves testing a currently unaffected person to determine his or her risk of suffering the condition. This has been most worked through for HD, where predictive testing has been performed since the gene was discovered, where a protocol is widely observed internationally and where the problems are recognized and have been addressed. These problems include the certainty that the gene being tested for is the correct one—a problem even more acute for the dementias than for HD. As there are many gene mutations which give rise to similar disorders (phenocopies), it is absolutely mandatory to first determine which mutation occurs in a particular family by testing an affected person first. Other issues encountered in the course of predictive testing include the risk of depression and other adverse events in those tested, the difficult ethical problem of those at 25% risk (grandparent affected, parent not tested and below the age of onset), issues regarding competency and testing of minors and the problem of non-penetrance. This latter problem is particularly acute in AD, where some of the genes are demonstrably not fully penetrant, making the advice given on the basis of a genetic test necessarily cautious. Because of these diverse and difficult issues, all people contemplating genetic testing should be extensively counselled following the HD protocols [134–136] beforehand, and this counselling and the actual laboratory analysis should preferably be performed within the context of medical genetic services and not research groups (although of course often the two are synonymous).

The situation for late-onset AD is even more problematical. For APOE variation, possession of the ε4 allele is not necessary to develop AD, and, equally, not having the ε4 allele offers only relative protection. This means that possession of an ε4 allele only modestly alters risk and this risk is itself age-dependent. A series of consensus groups are unanimous in their view that there is no role for predictive testing or even risk-counselling using the APOE genotype [137–139]. There may be a role, however, for APOE genotyping as part of the diagnostic work-up. A large post-mortem study demonstrated an increase in specificity of diagnosis (at the expense of sensitivity) by adding APOE genotype to clinical diagnosis [140]. However, this study had a lower accuracy of clinical diagnosis compared to other post-mortem studies and relatively few non-AD dementias. As in some studies APOE variation is associated with both DLB and vascular dementia, then it seems unlikely that genotyping will have a major role in diagnosis. In the UK, a consensus group finds no clinical role for APOE genotyping [138], and in the USA, community based studies do not find evidence in favour of diagnostic testing [141]. Finally, a role for APOE in pharmacogenetics has been widely flagged as a possible development. Pharmacogenetics has been heralded as a means of delivering therapies to those genetically determined to be responsive—targeting effectivity. In an early study, those carrying the APOEε4 allele were found to be less responsive to an acetylcholinesterase inhibitor, but subsequent studies have failed to replicate this [142–144]. There is little, therefore, to suggest that APOE genotyping will help to identify responders from non-responders in dementia therapy, but nevertheless considerable hope remains that this will become possible, if not using APOE, then using some other gene.

MOLECULAR BIOLOGY

The Amyloid Cascade Hypothesis

The discovery of mutations in the APP paved the way for the development of the amyloid cascade hypothesis, the most enduring central hypothesis of AD pathogenesis, which has been, somewhat ironically, strengthened by the discovery that mutations in tau can be a cause of related dementias. Restated many times in somewhat differing forms, the amyloid cascade hypothesis postulates a central and early role for amyloid in the pathogenesis of AD, with all other neuropathological features following from amyloid formation [145]. Originally the formation of amyloid and the generation of plaques were taken to be synonymous, but more recently one variation in the hypothesis accommodates the possibility that it might be intracellular amyloid that is the aetiopathogenetic element, and not the extracellular plaque, which may in fact be a true epiphenomenon [146]. The tau mutations add to the hypothesis as they finally put to rest the debate about which came first, plaque or tangle. In AD, mutations in APP or PS-1/2 give rise to plaques and tangles, but in FTDP-17 mutations in tau give rise to tangles only. If one cause gives rise to two consequences but another gives rise to only one, then it is assumed that this latter cause and consequence are secondary to the former. This is classically how biochemical pathways were elucidated—if inhibiting one enzyme prevents the formation of two substances, but inhibiting a second enzyme gives rise to only one of these substances, it is assumed that the second enzyme is indeed "downstream" of the first. As an APP mutation gives plaques and tangles but a tau mutation give tangles only, it follows that plaques are biochemically "upstream" of tangles. The caveat is that this applies to these autosomal dominant conditions. It remains possible—indeed some evidence suggests likely—that in late-onset AD an entirely different initiating event gives rise to both plaques and tangles. Nonetheless, the autosomal dominant dementias fully substantiate the amyloid cascade and back up the original neuropathological evidence, particularly from Down's syndrome, finding formation of plaques in younger brain and plaques and tangles in older brain.

Metabolism of APP

The amyloid peptide ($A\beta$) deposited in plaques in AD is a 39- to 42-amino-acid derivative of APP that has a tendency to self-aggregate into fibrils [147]. The longer forms of the peptide $A\beta42$ are less common but more fibrillogenic than the less common $A\beta40$ peptide. However, both peptides are normally produced in brain and peripherally, and it is likely therefore that AD results from the relative production of total Aβ or the relative proportion of Aβ42 to Aβ40 rather than the specific abnormal production of Aβ42 [148]. APP itself is a ubiquitous type 1 integral membrane protein with a large extracellular domain and a shorter intracellular carboxy terminus, the function of which is not known, although its very ubiquity and evolutionary conservation suggest a fundamental "housekeeping" role and its intracellular location and topology suggest a role in cell–cell communication or tethering.

The mutations in APP associated with disease almost perfectly mirror the known cleavage sites in the protein. Three secretases were suggested by analysis of the metabolic products of APP: α-, β- and γ-secretase. The mutations are close to each of these sites, strongly suggesting that they might alter the metabolism of the protein. This has now been repeatedly proven in fibroblasts from patients, in transfected cells and in animal models [149, 150]. The Swedish mutation (a double mutation at position 670/671) at the amino end of the Aβ moiety, near the β-secretase site, increases total Aβ levels [151], while the London mutation at the carboxy terminus, near the γ-secretase site, alters the ratio of Aβ42/Aβ40 [152, 153]. It is the γ-secretase site that is variable, allowing the generation of Aβ40 or Aβ42. Interestingly, the Flemish mutation at position 692 produces an AD-like phenotype and generates increased total Aβ, whereas the Dutch mutation at 693 is associated with an entirely different disease (hereditary cerebral haemorrhage with amyloidosis, Dutch type) and does not alter Aβ42 or total Aβ levels, but might increase the fibrillogenicity of the peptide [154, 155].

The Aβ itself is generated by sequential activity of β-secretase and γ-secretase. Metabolism by α-secretase, on the other hand, cleaves in the centre of the amyloid moiety and hence cannot generate Aβ. These two routes have been dubbed amyloidogenic and non-amyloidogenic metabolism, and it follows that inhibition of the former or promotion of the latter might be therapeutic. Some evidence in transfected non-neuronal cell lines suggests a direct relationship between the two metabolic routes—promotion of α-secretase activity reducing the generation of amyloid [156]. However, other experiments in neurons did not find a direct and reciprocal relationship [157]. Whilst any individual molecule of APP must go down one route or the other, it is almost certainly the case that the majority of APP molecules go down neither but are degraded, as are most proteins, by the proteosome.

Progress has been made in identifying all three secretases. β-secretase has been identified and named BACE (for β-site APP cleaving enzyme) [158]. This enzyme is present at high levels in brain, in neurons more than in glia, and is a membrane-bound aspartyl protease, the locus for which is 11q23.3.

The protein is present in both golgi complexes and endosomes, both putative metabolic locations of APP, and overexpression and inhibition studies
both demonstrate activity at the β-secretase site. A homologue of BACE
(BACE2) has been identified, and this enzyme also cleaves APP, but at a
different site, and is not present at high levels in brain, arguing against a role
in AD [159, 160].

The γ-secretase enzyme is likely either to be presenilin or very closely
associated biochemically with presenilin. The two PS genes (PS-1 and PS-2)
are both associated with early-onset autosomal dominant AD, and the proteins derived from these genes are highly homologous eight-pass transmembrane proteins [65]. These are normally cleaved within the large
extracellular loop, and the functional protein probably results from hetero-
dimeric association of the two cleaved products. Following the discovery of
these genes, transgenic knock-out mice lacking PS-1 were generated. This is
lethal to the developing foetus, which displays very severe skeletal and
neurodevelopmental abnormalities [161], highly reminiscent of those that
also result in mice lacking the Notch gene [162]. Like APP, Notch codes for a
single-pass membrane-bound protein which has a metabolic cleavage site
buried within the membrane (similar to the γ-secretase site). This suggested
that PS-1 might be regulating γ-secretase cleavage of APP and of notch, and
in cell models PS-1 was indeed shown to regulate notch cleavage [163].
Studies on neurons from the embryonically lethal PS-1 knock-out mice
showed highly diminished γ-secretase cleavage of APP, despite preserved
β-secretase activity [164], and similar experiments on neurons from double
knock-out mice lacking PS-1 and PS-2 demonstrated complete absence of γ-
secretase activity [165]. PS-1 is associated closely with a protein nicastrin
(named after Nicastra, the home of a family suffering from one of the
earliest reported autosomal dominant ADs) and either PS-1 alone or PS-1/
nicastrin complexes possess γ-secretase activity [166].

The α-secretase has not been identified, but because of its known properties has been placed in a family of enzymes that includes, for example, ACE
secretase [167]. These enzymes (including α-secretase) all respond to protein
kinase C (PKC), and basal levels of activity are increased following activation of PKC [168]. As PKC is a second messenger to many neurotransmitters, the effect of neurotransmission on APP metabolism has been examined.
The muscarinic cholinergic receptors M_1 and M_3 are both coupled to PKC,
and muscarinic agonists increase the generation of α-secretase-cleaved
products (known as sAPPα for secreted, α-secretase-cleaved APP) in cells,
including neurons [168, 169]. It follows that muscarinic agonists or any
compound that increases muscarinic activity (including the acetylcholinesterase inhibitors) should increase sAPPα. In line with this, cholinesterase
inhibitors have been shown to increase this non-amyloidogenic metabolism
[170–172], and in man muscarinic agonists increase sAPPα in cerebrospinal

fluid [173]. It remains to be seen whether this is accompanied by a reduction in Aβ.

Tau and the Formation of Tangles

The second main pathology of AD is the neurofibrillary tangle. These flame-shaped inclusions are composed of fibrils that under the electron micro-scope are shown to be formed from paired helical filaments (PHF). These structures, and other straight filaments, are found not only in tangles, but also in the neurites surrounding plaques and in neuropil threads—wispy structures probably representing decaying axons. The PHF are themselves formed from abnormal aggregates of highly phosphorylated tau protein [174, 175]. Tau is a microtubule-associated protein, normally found predom-inantly in axons and which functions to stabilize the polymers of tubulin that make up microtubules. In mitotic cells, microtubules function in intra-cellular transport and also in guiding the chromosomes to their respective daughter cells. In postmitotic neurons, this normal function is lost and microtubules have a role in transport only. In axons they form relative straight structures parallel with the axon itself and, together with neurofila-ments, transport the protein machinery required at the synapse from the cell body.

It is not surprising that such an important function should be tightly regulated, and in mammalian neurons this regulation is achieved through both phosphorylation and alternative splicing [176]. Highly phosphorylated tau does not bind to or stabilize microtubules as well as non-phosphorylated tau, and tau isoforms with three microtubule binding domains do not bind microtubules as tightly as tau with four binding domains. Both of these regulatory processes are altered in development and both show signs of disruption in dementia. In the developing brain, it is probably necessary to have relatively unstable and flexible microtubules as the axons find their final destinations, and in line with this in foetuses the tau is highly phos-phorylated and the three-repeat isoforms are predominantly expressed. In adult brain, tau is also phosphorylated, but relatively less than in foetal brain. The regulation of tau phosphorylation may be associated with some of the plasticity characteristics of the mature neuron. In AD brain, the PHF-tau that aggregates in tangles is very highly and stably phosphorylated [176]. Some evidence suggests that, in normal brain, accumulation of highly phosphorylated but non-aggregated tau precedes PHF formation and is one of the earliest signs of the developing pathology in the entorhinal cortex and hippocampus [16]. Other authors suggest that tau phosphorylation follows rather than precedes aggregation, which may be precipitated by abnormal proteolysis [177].

The kinases responsible for the phosphorylation of tau have been actively sought. In vitro many kinases, particularly those in the proline-directed kinase family, phosphorylate tau, but two kinases in brain, named tau protein kinase I and II (TPKI and TPKII), were responsible for the most avid tau phosphorylation activity [178, 179]. In cells, one enzyme—glycogen synthase kinase 3 (GSK-3)—had the most obvious tau-kinase activity [180, 181]. When TPKI was identified, it was realized that it and GSK-3β were one and the same [182], and most of the evidence now points to GSK-3 as being the predominant physiological kinase in neurons. The GSK-3 homologue in *Drosophila* is named *shaggy* and lithium treatment of flies results in a phenotype similar to that of *shaggy* mutants [183]. As predicted from this observation, lithium turns out to be a relatively specific and potent GSK-3 inhibitor, and studies in neurons and transfected cells have demonstrated that lithium reduces tau phosphorylation and increases tau binding to microtubules [184–186]. There has been some speculation as to whether the action of lithium on GSK-3 is responsible for its therapeutic action in affective disorder, and it is noteworthy that effects of lithium on tau can be observed in cell models within the therapeutic range [187]. However, whether the action of GSK is responsible for lithium therapeutic or toxic action remains to be seen. GSK-3 is also inhibited as a consequence of insulin signalling, and tau phosphorylation in neurons is reduced by insulin [188]. This is of interest, as diabetes and insulin resistance syndrome are both linked to AD [189], and insulin also increases non-amyloidogenic metabolism [190]. These findings suggest a common link between APP metabolism and tau phosphorylation through a signalling cascade shown to be associated with AD, thus linking molecular biology and epidemiology.

Whilst it was known for many years that tau was the basic component of tangles, it was disputed whether this was an epiphenomenon or primary to aetiopathogenesis. The debate was silenced by the finding of mutations in tau in FTDP-17, then in other related disorders [69, 70, 191, 192]. The mutations are of two main types—splice site and missense. The splice site mutations alter the relative ratio of the isoforms of tau containing three and four microtubule-binding domains [193]. The consequences of this are not fully understood, but as one or other isoform can predominate in the inclusions in different diseases, and as the ratio is tightly controlled in development, it is assumed that the relative proportion expressed is critical to normal tau function in microtubule binding. The missense mutations have diverse effects and have been shown to alter tau aggregation, tau phosphorylation, but most consistently tau function in binding microtubules and promoting microtubule extension in vitro and in vivo [194].

One hypothesis that emerges from these findings is that any disruption of the normal microtubule–tau association (increased phosphorylation, mutation in the binding region, alteration in the isoform ratio) results in increased free cytoplasmic tau. In vitro tau can be made to self-aggregate into PHF, and it follows therefore that any event that increases free cytoplasmic tau might result in increased tau aggregation. Transgenic mice have been generated that overexpress mutated tau, and these show a neurodegeneration phenotype similar to that of the FTDP-17 [195]. However, mice overexpressing normal tau also develop inclusions and a neurodegeneration phenotype [196], rather suggesting that the critical factor is not the mutation per se but the increased cytoplasmic unbound tau that can then self-aggregate.

APOE: Proven Association, Unknown Mechanism

There have been a number of different approaches to understanding the mechanism underlying the association between APOE and AD, and none can yet be fully accepted or rejected. These approaches can be categorized into those suggesting a remote effect via altered rates of vascular disease, those suggesting altered neuronal vulnerability and those postulating an APOE interaction with plaques or with tangles. Some evidence suggested that vascular disease might underlie the association, but a prospective study found that the risk of AD given particular APOE genotypes was not altered taking into account diverse signs of cardiac risk. Altered local cholesterol transport in brain, resulting in altered neuronal vulnerability, is a strong hypothesis, but difficult to address directly. Some evidence suggests that altered cholesterol levels in the brain may directly give rise to plaque formation.

Evidence linking APOE to plaques is moderately robust, in that transgenic mice expressing the APP gene carrying the mutation for AD develop plaques early, but when crossed with APOE knock-out mice develop plaques late [197]. In addition, the Aβ load is greater in individuals with the APOEε4/* genotype [198]. Finally, in vitro APOE protein binds Aβ [199] but this evidence is not strong and may depend upon the preparation of APOE protein used.

The first suggestion that an interaction between tau and APOE might underlie the observed association came when it was shown that APOE3, in contrast to APOE4, bound to tau in vitro avidly [200]. Subsequently it was shown that another microtubule-associated protein, MAP2c, also bound APOE, again with a similar isoform-specific avidity [201]. These findings led to the hypothesis that the strong binding of APOE3 to tau would reduce the availability of tau from phosphorylation [202].

The most convincing evidence that APOE might alter the neuronal cytoskeleton came from Nathan *et al.* [203], who demonstrated that purified human APOE3 increased neuritic extension and decreased branching in rabbit dorsal root ganglions, whilst APOE4 decreased both extension and branching, and subsequently it was shown that APOE4 induced microtubule collapse alongside neurite morphology changes [204]. These data suggest an APOE isoform-specific effect on neurite outgrowth and microtubule stability in cells, although whether this has relevance for the microtubule collapse seen in AD remains to be seen.

Molecular Relationship Between Plaques and Tangles

The relationship between plaques and tangles has been hotly contested. The amyloid cascade hypothesis predicts that tangles follow from plaque formation, but going against that is the observation that accumulation of highly phosphorylated tau is one of the earliest signs of pathology, occurring decades before dementia, the observation that normal neurons and amyloid plaques can co-exist side by side, and the finding that plaques and tangles do not always occur in the same neuroanatomical location, plaques occurring in the cerebellum, for example, which is never affected by tangles and remains apparently otherwise intact during the course of the disease. As discussed above, however, the finding of tau mutations has lent support to the cascade hypothesis, and therefore there must be a link between the two pathologies.

Aβ is undoubtedly toxic to cells in culture and when injected directly into cortex [205]. One result of this toxicity, at least in some studies, is an increase in tau phosphorylation [206]. This tau phosphorylation and the toxicity of amyloid can be prevented by GSK-3 antisense treatment and by lithium, strongly suggesting that amyloid triggers (probably indirectly) an increase in GSK-3 activity which in turn results in an increase in tau phosphorylation and hence neuronal death [207–209]. An alternative suggestion is that both tau phosphorylation and APP metabolism are linked through some third-party event, the most obvious candidate being PKC. As discussed above, PKC activation in turn stimulates α-secretase and non-amyloidogenic metabolism of APP. The activity of GSK-3 is inhibited by PKC, and so activation of PKC would be expected to increase non-amyloidogenic metabolism and decrease tau phosphorylation. This has now been demonstrated using muscarinic agonists in parallel experiments where, as predicted, both sAPPα is increased and tau phosphorylation is decreased. This has obvious and direct implications for treatment [210]. However, it also has some implications for understanding pathology. One of the most interesting adaptations of the amyloid cascade hypothesis suggests that the disease process spreads in neuroanatomical pathways because the death of a neuron results in less neurotransmission to the recipient neuron, and if the original, now dying, neuron was a cholinergic neuron then this would result in less muscarinic stimulation. It would follow that non-amyloidogenic metabolism in the recipient neuron would fall, and tau phosphorylation would increase, resulting in dissociation from the microtubules, functional loss and then actual loss of that neuron too. In turn, its recipient neuron would have less cholinergic input, resulting in a spread of pathology not in geographical relationships but along neuronal pathways. Thus the amyloid cascade and the cholinergic hypotheses are brought together [44].

CONCLUSIONS

As well as being the most durable hypothesis to explain the molecular and neuropathological findings in AD, the amyloid cascade hypothesis can be used to predict likely disease-modifying targets. The most obvious target is the generation of amyloid itself. If this can be prevented, or attenuated, then it is very likely that the disease process would be halted. Inhibiting γ-secretase activity might be problematical, as γ-secretase inhibitors would also be expected to inhibit the maturation of notch and thus might have adverse consequences on haematopoiesis amongst other processes. Inhibitors of BACE have already been identified and are being very intensively studied as potential disease-modifying agents. Increasing the activity of α-secretase via PKC is a definite alternative strategy, although the caveat remains that it has not yet been proven that this will result in a decrease in amyloid itself. Nonetheless, the great advantage of this strategy is that compounds that increase PKC activity are tried and tested and in the shape of cholinergic-enhancing compounds (cholinesterase inhibitors for example) are already in use in the target population. Furthermore, these compounds have also been shown to reduce tau phosphorylation, thus "hitting" the disease process at two sites simultaneously. An alternative approach to tackling amyloid is to prevent fibrillogenesis of the amyloid peptide or to dissemble early aggregates before plaque formation. Compounds seeking to achieve this are in generation.

Agents to prevent amyloid formation will be useful in AD but not the frontotemporal dementias, whereas anti-tau aggregation strategies would be active in both types of disorder. Tau aggregation itself is a site for potential therapeutic intervention, as is tau phosphorylation. Lithium is a relatively toxic GSK-3 inhibitor, but other less toxic GSK-3 inhibitors might be of some practical use in AD. Given that GSK-3 is inhibited by lithium, these compounds will be of considerable interest as potential agents in affective disorders as well.

However, beyond all question, the most exciting development is a highly novel approach using immunological clearance of amyloid plaques. It was a highly surprising finding that peripheral administration of passive and active immunization against amyloid not only stopped further development of amyloid plaques in transgenic animals, but also cleared existing plaques in mature transgenic animals and, most remarkably, reversed the acquired cognitive deficit that occurred in some of these animals [211, 212]. The importance of this finding is difficult to overestimate. If these findings are replicated, safely, in man, the first truly disease-modifying treatment would have resulted for this devastating condition and the challenge would then be our ability to deliver it to those most in need.

REFERENCES

1. Blessed G., Tomlinson B.E., Roth M. (1968) The association between quantitative measures of dementia and of senile change in the cerebral grey matter of elderly subjects. *Br. J. Psychiatry*, **114**: 797–811.
2. Yamaguchi H., Hirai S., Morimatsu M., Shoji M., Harigaya Y. (1988) Diffuse type of senile plaques in the brains of Alzheimer-type dementia. *Acta Neuropathol. (Berl.)*, **77**: 113–119.
3. Mann D.M., Brown A., Prinja D., Davies C.A., Landon M., Masters C.L., Beyreuthers K. (1989) An analysis of the morphology of senile plaques in Down's syndrome patients of different ages using immunocytochemical and lectin histochemical techniques. *Neuropathol. Appl. Neurobiol.*, **15**: 317–329.
4. Braak H., Braak E. (1990) Neurofibrillary changes confined to the entorhinal region and an abundance of cortical amyloid in cases of presenile and senile dementia. *Acta Neuropathol. (Berl.)*, **80**: 479–486.
5. Delaere P., Duyckaerts C., Brion J.P., Poulain V., Hauw J.J. (1989) Tau, paired helical filaments and amyloid in the neocortex: a morphometric study of 15 cases with graded intellectual status in aging and senile dementia of Alzheimer type. *Acta Neuropathol. (Berl.)*, **77**: 645–653.
6. Thal D.R., Rüb U., Schultz C., Sassin I., Ghebremedhin E., Del Tredici K., Braak E., Braak H. (2000) Sequence of Aβ-protein deposition in the human medial temporal lobe. *J. Neuropathol. Exp. Neurol.*, **59**: 733–748.
7. Berg L., McKeel D.W. Jr., Miller J.P., Baty J., Morris J.C. (1993) Neuropathological indexes of Alzheimer's disease in demented and nondemented persons aged 80 years and older. *Arch. Neurol.*, **50**: 349–358.
8. Dickson D.W., Crystal H.A., Bevona C., Honer W., Vincent I., Davies P. (1995) Correlations of synaptic and pathological markers with cognition of the elderly. *Neurobiol. Aging*, **16**: 285–298.
9. Haroutunian V., Purohit D.P., Perl D.P., Marin D., Khan K., Lantz M., Davis K.L., Mohs R.C. (1999) Neurofibrillary tangles in nondemented elderly subjects and mild Alzheimer disease. *Arch. Neurol.*, **56**: 713–718.
10. Nagy Z., Esiri M.M., Jobst K.A., Morris J.H., King E.M., McDonald B., Litchfield S., Smith A., Barnetson L., Smith A.D. (1995) Relative roles of plaques and tangles in the dementia of Alzheimer's disease: correlations using three sets of neuropathological criteria. *Dementia*, **6**: 21–31.
11. Bierer L.M., Hof P.R., Purohit D.P., Carlin L., Schmeidler J., Davis K.L., Perl D.P. (1995) Neocortical neurofibrillary tangles correlate with dementia severity in Alzheimer's disease. *Arch. Neurol.*, **52**: 81–88.

12. Näslund J., Haroutunian V., Mohs R., Davis K.L., Davies P., Greengard P., Buxbaum J.D. (2000) Correlation between elevated levels of amyloid β-peptide in the brain and cognitive decline. *JAMA*, **283**: 1571–1577.
13. Cummings B.J., Cotman C.W. (1995) Image analysis of β-amyloid load in Alzheimer's disease and relation to dementia severity. *Lancet*, **346**: 1524–1528.
14. Larner A.J. (1997) The cerebellum in Alzheimer's disease. *Dementia*, **8**: 203–209.
15. Lovestone S., Anderton B.H. (1992) Cytoskeletal abnormalities in Alzheimer's disease. *Curr. Opin. Neurol. Neurosurg.*, **5**: 883–888.
16. Braak E., Braak H., Mandelkow E-M. (1994) A sequence of cytoskeleton changes related to the formation of neurofibrillary tangles and neuropil threads. *Acta Neuropathol. (Berl.)*, **87**: 554–567.
17. Braak H., Braak E. (1998) Evolution of neuronal changes in the course of Alzheimer's disease. *J. Neural Transm.*, **105**(Suppl. 53): 127–140.
18. Kosaka K., Yoshimura M., Ikeda K., Budka H. (1984) Diffuse type of Lewy body disease: progressive dementia with abundant cortical Lewy bodies and senile changes of varying degree—a new disease? *Clin. Neuropathol.*, **3**: 185–192.
19. McKeith I.G., Galasko D., Kosaka K., Perry E.K., Dickson D.W., Hansen L.A., Salmon D.P., Lowe J., Mirra S.S., Byrne E.J. *et al.* (1996) Consensus guidelines for the clinical and pathologic diagnosis of dementia with Lewy bodies (DLB): Report of the consortium on DLB international workshop. *Neurology*, **47**: 1113–1124.
20. Halliday G., Brooks W., Arthur H., Creasey H., Broe G.A. (1997) Further evidence for an association between a mutation in the APP gene and Lewy body formation. *Neurosci. Lett.*, **227**: 49–52.
21. Masliah E., Saitoh T. (1994) Lewy bodies, Alzheimer pathology and APP mutation. *Neurosci. Lett.*, **180**: 292–293.
22. Rosenberg C.K., Pericak-Vance M.A., Saunders A.M., Gilbert J.R., Gaskell P.C., Hulette C.M. (2000) Lewy body and Alzheimer pathology in a family with the amyloid-β precursor protein APP717 gene mutation. *Acta Neuropathol. (Berl.)*, **100**: 145–152.
23. Gearing M., Lynn M., Mirra S.S. (1999) Neurofibrillary pathology in Alzheimer disease with Lewy bodies—two subgroups. *Arch. Neurol.*, **56**: 203–208.
24. Perry E.K., Marshall E., Perry R.H., Irving D., Smith C.J., Blessed G., Fairbairn A.F. (1990) Cholinergic and dopaminergic activities in senile dementia of Lewy body type. *Alzheimer Dis. Assoc. Disord.*, **4**: 87–95.
25. Strong C., Anderton B.H., Perry R.H., Perry E.K., Ince P.G., Lovestone S. (1995) Hyperphosphorylated tau in senile dementia with Lewy bodies and Alzheimer's disease: evidence that the disorders are distinct. *Alzheimer Dis. Assoc. Disord.*, **9**: 218–222.
26. Harrington C.R., Perry R.H., Perry E.K., Hurt J., McKeith I.G., Roth M., Wischik C.M. (1994) Senile dementia of Lewy body type and Alzheimer type are biochemically distinct in terms of paired helical filaments and hyperphosphorylated tau protein. *Dementia*, **5**: 215–228.
27. Spillantini M.G., Schmidt M.L., Lee V.M., Trojanowski J.Q., Jakes R., Goedert M. (1997) Alpha-synuclein in Lewy bodies. *Nature*, **388**: 839–840.
28. Dickson D.W., Liu W.K., Hardy J., Farrer M., Mehta N., Uitti R., Mark M., Zimmerman T., Golbe L., Sage J. *et al.* (1999) Widespread alterations of α-synuclein in multiple system atrophy. *Am. J. Pathol.*, **155**: 1241–1251.
29. Duda J.E., Lee V.M.Y., Trojanowski J.Q. (2000) Neuropathology of synuclein aggregates: new insights into mechanisms of neurodegenerative diseases. *J. Neurosci. Res.*, **61**: 121–127.

30. Buée L., Delacourte A. (1999) Comparative biochemistry of tau in progressive supranuclear palsy, corticobasal degeneration, FTDP-17 and Pick's disease. *Brain Pathol.*, **9**: 681–693.

31. Coyle J.T., Price D.L., DeLong M.R. (1983) Alzheimer's disease: a disorder of cortical cholinergic innervation. *Science*, **219**: 1184–1190.

32. Drachman D.A., Leavitt J. (1974) Human memory and the cholinergic system. *Arch. Neurol.*, **30**: 113–121.

33. Fibiger H.C. (1991) Cholinergic mechanisms in learning, memory and dementia: a review of recent evidence. *Trends Neurosci.*, **14**: 220–223.

34. Davies P., Maloney A.J.F. (1976) Selective loss of central cholinergic neurones in Alzheimer's disease. *Lancet*, **2**: 1403–1406.

35. Wilcock G.K., Esiri M.M., Bowen D.M., Smith C.C. (1983) The nucleus basalis in Alzheimer's disease: cell counts and cortical biochemistry. *Neuropathol. Appl. Neurobiol.*, **9**: 175–179.

36. Saper C.B., German D.C., White C.L. (1985) Neuronal pathology in the nucleus basalis and associated cell groups in senile dementia of the Alzheimer's type: possible role in cell loss. *Neurology*, **35**: 1089–1095.

37. Rasool C.G., Svendsen C.N., Selkoe D.J. (1986) Neurofibrillary degeneration of cholinergic and noncholinergic neurons of the basal forebrain in Alzheimer's disease. *Ann. Neurol.*, **20**: 482–488.

38. Neary D., Snowden J.S., Mann D.M., Bowen D.M., Sims N.R., Northen B., Yates P.O., Davison A.N. (1986) Alzheimer's disease: a correlative study. *J. Neurol. Neurosurg. Psychiatry*, **49**: 229–237.

39. Bondareff W., Mountjoy C.Q., Roth M., Rossor M.N., Iversen L.L., Reynolds G.P., Hauser D.L. (1987) Neuronal degeneration in locus ceruleus and cortical correlates of Alzheimer disease. *Alzheimer Dis. Assoc. Disord.*, **1**: 256–262.

40. Tago H., McGeer P.L., McGeer E.G. (1987) Acetylcholinesterase fibers and the development of senile plaques. *Brain Res.*, **406**: 363–369.

41. Smith C.J., Perry E.K., Perry R.H., Candy J.M., Johnson M., Bonham J.R., Dick D.J., Fairbairn A., Blessed G., Birdsall N.J. (1988) Muscarinic cholinergic receptor subtypes in hippocampus in human cognitive disorders. *J. Neurochem.*, **50**: 847–856.

42. Quirion R., Aubert I., Lapchak P.A., Schaum R.P., Teolis S., Gauthier S., Araujo D.M. (1989) Muscarinic receptor subtypes in human neurodegenerative disorders: focus on Alzheimer's disease. *Trends Pharmacol. Sci.*, **Suppl.**: 80–84.

43. Harrison P.J., Barton A.J., Najlerahim A., McDonald B., Pearson R.C. (1991) Increased muscarinic receptor messenger RNA in Alzheimer's disease temporal cortex demonstrated by in situ hybridization histochemistry. *Brain Res. Mol. Brain Res.*, **9**: 15–21.

44. Francis P.T., Palmer A.M., Snape M., Wilcock G.K. (1999) The cholinergic hypothesis of Alzheimer's disease: a review of progress. *J. Neurol. Neurosurg. Psychiatry*, **66**: 137–147.

45. Cummings J.L., Back C. (1998) The cholinergic hypothesis of neuropsychiatric symptoms in Alzheimer's disease. *Am. J. Geriatr. Psychiatry*, **6**: S64–78.

46. Procter A.W., Qurne M., Francis P.T. (1999) Neurochemical features of frontotemporal dementia. *Dement. Geriatr. Cogn. Disord.*, **10**(Suppl. 1): 80–84.

47. Lippa C.F., Smith T.W., Perry E. (1999) Dementia with Lewy bodies: choline acetyltransferase parallels nucleus basalis pathology. *J. Neural Transm.*, **106**: 525–535.

48. Perry E.K., Haroutunian V., Davis K.L., Levy R., Lantos P., Eagger S., Honavar M., Dean A., Griffiths M., McKeith I.G. *et al.* (1994) Neocortical cholinergic

activities differentiate Lewy body dementia from classical Alzheimer's disease. *Neuroreport*, **5**: 747–749.

49. Gsell W., Strein I., Riederer P. (1996) The neurochemistry of Alzheimer type, vascular type and mixed type dementias compared. *J. Neural Transm.*, **103** (Suppl. 47): 73–101.

50. Carson R.E., Kiesewetter D.O., Jagoda E., Der M.G., Herscovitch P., Eckelman W.C. (1998) Muscarinic cholinergic receptor measurements with [^{18}F]FP-TZTP: control and competition studies. *J. Cereb. Blood Flow Metab.*, **18**: 1130–1142.

51. Palmer A.M., DeKosky S.T. (1993) Monoamine neurons in aging and Alzheimer's disease. *J. Neural Transm.*, **91**: 135–159.

52. Zubenko G.S., Moossy J., Kopp U. (1990) Neurochemical correlates of major depression in primary dementia. *Arch. Neurol.*, **47**: 209–214.

53. Hoogendijk W.J.G., Sommer I.E.C., Pool C.W., Kamphorst W., Hofman M.A., Eikelenboom P., Swaab D.F. (1999) Lack of association between depression and loss of neurons in the locus coeruleus in Alzheimer disease. *Arch. Gen. Psychiatry*, **56**: 45–51.

54. Zubenko G.S., Moossy J. (1988) Major depression in primary dementia. Clinical and neuropathologic correlates. *Arch. Neurol.*, **45**: 1182–1186.

55. Lawlor B.A., Ryan T.M., Bierer L.M., Schmeidler J., Haroutunian V., Mohs R., Davis K.L. (1995) Lack of association between clinical symptoms and postmortem indices of brain serotonin function in Alzheimer's disease. *Biol. Psychiatry*, **37**: 895–896.

56. Halliday G.M., McCann H.L., Pamphlett R., Brooks W.S., Creasey H., McCusker E., Cotton R.G.H., Broe G.A., Harper C.G. (1992) Brain stem serotonin-synthesizing neurons in Alzheimer's disease: a clinicopathological correlation. *Acta Neuropathol.(Berl.)*, **84**: 638–650.

57. Zubenko G.S., Moossy J., Martinez A.J., Rao G., Claassen D., Rosen J., Kopp U. (1991) Neuropathologic and neurochemical correlates of psychosis in primary dementia. *Arch. Neurol.*, **48**: 619–624.

58. Perry E.K., Perry R.H. (1995) Acetylcholine and hallucinations: disease-related compared to drug-induced alterations in human consciousness. *Brain Cogn.*, **28**: 240–258.

59. Shannon H.E., Rasmussen K., Bymaster F.P., Hart J.C., Peters S.C., Swedberg M.D.B., Jeppesen L., Sheardown M.J., Sauerberg P., Fink-Jensen A. (2000) Xanomeline, an M_1/M_4 preferring muscarinic cholinergic receptor agonist, produces antipsychotic-like activity in rats and mice. *Schizophr. Res.*, **42**: 249–259.

60. Farlow M.R., Cyrus P.A. (2000) Metrifonate therapy in Alzheimer's disease: a pooled analysis of four randomized, double-blind, placebo-controlled trials. *Dementia*, **11**: 202–211.

61. Glenner G.G., Wong C.W. (1984) Alzheimer's disease: initial report of the purification and characterization of a novel cerebrovascular amyloid protein. *Biochem. Biophys. Res. Commun.*, **120**: 885–890.

62. St. George-Hyslop P.H. (2000) Molecular genetics of Alzheimer's disease. *Biol. Psychiatry*, **47**: 183–199.

63. Clark R.F., Goate A.M. (1993) Molecular genetics of Alzheimer's disease. *Arch. Neurol.*, **50**: 1164–1172.

64. Mullan M., Crawford F. (1994) The molecular genetics of Alzheimer's disease. *Mol. Neurobiol.*, **9**: 15–22.

65. Da Silva H.A.R., Patel A.J. (1997) Presenilins and early-onset familial Alzheimer's disease. *Neuroreport*, **8**: I-XII.

66. Bird T.D., Lampe T.H., Nemens E.J., Miner G.W., Sumi S.M., Schellenberg G.D. (1988) Familial Alzheimer's disease in American descendants of the Volga Germans: probable genetic founder effect. *Ann. Neurol.*, **23**: 25–31.

67. Foster N.L., Wilhelmsen K., Sima A.A., Jones M.Z., D'Amato C.J., Gilman S. (1997) Frontotemporal dementia and parkinsonism linked to chromosome 17: a consensus conference. *Ann. Neurol.*, **41**: 706–715.

68. Goedert M., Crowther R.A., Spillantini M. (1998) Tau mutations cause fronto-temporal dementias. *Neuron*, **21**: 955–958.

69. Rizzini C., Goedert M., Hodges J.R., Smith M.J., Jakes R., Hills R., Xuereb J.H., Crowther R.A., Spillantini M.G. (2000) *Tau* gene mutation K257T causes a tauopathy similar to Pick's disease. *J. Neuropathol. Exp. Neurol.*, **59**: 990–1001.

70. Murrell J.R., Spillantini M.G., Zolo P., Guazzelli M., Smith M.J., Hasegawa M., Redi F., Crowther R.A., Pietrini P., Ghetti B. *et al.* (1999) Tau gene mutation G389R causes a tauopathy with abundant Pick body-like inclusions and axonal deposits. *J. Neuropathol. Exp. Neurol.*, **58**: 1207–1226.

71. Goedert M., Spillantini M.G., Crowther R.A., Chen S.G., Parchi P., Tabaton M., Lanska D.J., Markesbery W.R., Wilhelmsen K.C., Dickson D.W. *et al.* (1999) Tau gene mutation in familial progressive subcortical gliosis. *Nature Med.*, **5**: 454–457.

72. Baker M., Litvan I., Houlden H., Adamson J., Dickson D., Perez-Tur J., Hardy J., Lynch T., Bigio E., Hutton M. (1999) Association of an extended haplotype in the tau gene with progressive supranuclear palsy. *Hum. Mol. Genet.*, **8**: 711–715.

73. Higgins J.J., Golbe L.I., De Biase A., Jankovic J., Factor S.A., Adler R.L. (2000) An extended 5′-tau susceptibility haplotype in progressive supranuclear palsy. *Neurology*, **55**: 1364–1367.

74. Van Slegtenhorst M., Lewis J., Hutton M. (2000) The molecular genetics of the tauopathies. *Exp. Gerontol.*, **35**: 461–471.

75. Collinge J., Brown J., Hardy J., Mullan M., Rossor M.N., Baker H., Crow T.J., Lofthouse R., Poulter M., Ridley R. *et al.* (1992) Inherited prion disease with 144 base pair gene insertion. 2. Clinical and pathological features. *Brain*, **115**: 687–710.

76. Lovestone S., Hodgson S., Sham P., Differ A.M., Levy R. (1996) Familial psychiatric presentation of Huntington's disease. *J. Med. Genet.*, **33**: 128–131.

77. Tsuang D., DiGiacomo L., Lipe H., Bird T.D. (1998) Familial aggregation of schizophrenia-like symptoms in Huntington's disease. *Am. J. Med. Genet.*, **81**: 323–327.

78. Tunstall N., Owen M.J., Williams J., Rice F., Carty S., Lillystone S., Fraser L., Kehoe P., Neill D., Rudrasingham V. *et al.* (2000) Familial influence on variation in age of onset and behavioural phenotype in Alzheimer's disease. *Br. J. Psychiatry*, **176**: 156–159.

79. Lyketsos C.G., Tune L.E., Pearlson G., Steele C. (1996) Major depression in Alzheimer's disease. An interaction between gender and family history. *Psychosomatics*, **37**: 380–384.

80. Pearlson G.D., Ross C.A., Lohr W.D., Rovner B.W., Chase G.A., Folstein M.F. (1990) Association between family history of affective disorder and the depressive syndrome of Alzheimer's disease. *Am. J. Psychiatry*, **147**: 452–456.

81. Breitner J.C., Murphy E.A., Silverman J.M., Mohs R.C., Davis K.L. (1988) Age-dependent expression of familial risk in Alzheimer's disease. *Am. J. Epidemiol.*, **128**: 536–548.

82. Korten A.E., Jorm A.F., Henderson A.S., Broe G.A., Creasey H., McCusker E. (1993) Assessing the risk of Alzheimer's disease in first-degree relatives of Alzheimer's disease cases. *Psychol. Med.*, **23**: 915–923.

83. Breitner J.C.S., Murphy E.A. (1992) Twin studies of Alzheimer disease: II. Some predictions under a genetic model. *Am. J. Med. Genet.*, **44**: 628–634.
84. Breitner J.C.S. (1994) Genetic factors. In *Dementia* (Eds A. Burns, R. Levy), pp. 281–292), Chapman and Hall, London.
85. Lehtinen S., Lehtimäki T., Sisto T., Salenius J.-P., Nikkilä M., Jokela H., Koivula T., Ebeling F., Ehnholm C. (1995) Apolipoprotein E polymorphism, serum lipids, myocardial infarction and severity of angiographically verified coronary artery disease in men and women. *Atherosclerosis*, **114**: 83–91.
86. Van der Cammen T.J.M., Verschoor C.J., Van Loon C.P.M., van Harskamp F., De Koning I., Schudel W.J., Slooter A.J.C, Van Broeckhoven C., van Duijn C.M. (1998) Risk of left ventricular dysfunction in patients with probable Alzheimer's disease with APOE*4 allele. *J. Am. Geriatr. Soc.*, **46**: 962–967.
87. Pericak-Vance M.A., Bebout J.L., Gaskell P.C.J., Yamaoka L.H., Hung W.Y., Alberts M.J., Walker A.P., Bartlett R.J., Haynes C.A., Welsh K.A. *et al.* (1991) Linkage studies in familial Alzheimer disease: evidence for chromosome 19 linkage. *Am. J. Hum. Genet.*, **48**: 1034–1050.
88. Corder E.H., Saunders A.M., Strittmatter W.J., Schmechel D.E., Gaskell P.C., Small G.W., Roses A.D., Haines J.L., Pericak-Vance M.A. (1993) Gene dose of apolipoprotein E type 4 allele and the risk of Alzheimer's disease in late onset families. *Science*, **261**: 921–923.
89. Saunders A.M., Strittmatter W.J., Schmechel D., St. George-Hyslop P.H., Pericak-Vance M.A., Joo S.H., Rosi B.L., Gusella J.F., Crapper-MacLachlan D.R., Alberts M.J. *et al.* (1993) Association of apolipoprotein E allele ε4 with late-onset familial and sporadic Alzheimer's disease. *Neurology*, **43**: 1467–1472.
90. Anwar N., Lovestone S., Cheetham M.E., Levy R., Powell J.F. (1993) Apolipoprotein E-ε4 allele and Alzheimer's disease. *Lancet*, **342**: 1308–1309.
91. Borgaonkar D.S., Schmidt L.C., Martin S.E., Kanzer M.D., Edelsohn L., Growdon J., Farrer L.A. (1993) Linkage of late-onset Alzheimer's disease with apolipoprotein E type 4 on chromosome 19. *Lancet*, **342**: 625–625.
92. Czech C., Mönning U., Tienari P.J., Hartmann T., Masters C., Beyreuther K., Förstl H. (1993) Apolipoprotein E-ε4 allele and Alzheimer's disease. *Lancet*, **342**: 1309–1310.
93. Houlden H., Crook R., Duff K., Collinge J., Roques P., Rossor M., Hardy J. (1993) Confirmation that the apolipoprotein E4 allele is associated with late onset, familial Alzheimer's disease. *Neurodegeneration*, **2**: 283–286.
94. Lucotte G., David F., Visvikis S., Leininger-Müller B., Siest G., Babron M.C., Couderc R. (1993) Apolipoprotein E-ε4 allele and Alzheimer's disease. *Lancet*, **342**: 1309–1309.
95. Mayeux R., Stern Y., Ottman R., Tatemichi T.K., Tang M.-X., Maestre G., Ngai C., Tycko B., Ginsberg H. (1993) The apolipoprotein ε4 allele in patients with Alzheimer's disease. *Ann. Neurol.*, **34**: 752–754.
96. Noguchi S., Murakami K., Yamada N. (1993) Apolipoprotein E genotype and Alzheimer's disease. *Lancet*, **342**: 737–737.
97. Poirier J., Davignon J., Bouthillier D., Kogan S., Bertrand P., Gauthier S. (1993) Apolipoprotein E polymorphism and Alzheimer's disease. *Lancet*, **342**: 697–699.
98. Farrer L.A., Cupples L.A., Haines J.L., Hyman B., Kukull W.A., Mayeux R., Myers R.H., Pericak-Vance M.A., Risch N., van Duijn C.M. (1997) Effects of age, sex, and ethnicity on the association between apolipoprotein E genotype and Alzheimer disease—a meta-analysis. *JAMA*, **278**: 1349–1356.

99. Hendrie H.C., Hall K.S., Hui S., Unverzagt F.W., Yu C.E., Lahiri D.K., Sahota A., Farlow M., Musick B., Class C.A. *et al.* (1995) Apolipoprotein E genotypes and Alzheimer's disease in a community study of elderly African Americans. *Ann. Neurol.*, **37**: 118–120.

100. Osuntokun B.O., Sahota A., Ogunniyi A.O., Gureje O., Baiyewu O., Adeyinka A., Oluwole S.O., Komolafe O., Hall K.S., Unverzagt F.W. *et al.* (1995) Lack of an association between apolipoprotein E ε4 and Alzheimer's disease in elderly Nigerians. *Ann. Neurol.*, **38**: 463–465.

101. Sahota A., Yang M., Gao S.J., Hui S.L., Baiyewu O., Gureje O., Oluwole S., Ogunniyi A., Hall K.S., Hendrie H.C. (1997) Apolipoprotein E-associated risk for Alzheimer's disease in the African-American population is genotype dependent. *Ann. Neurol.*, **42**: 659–661.

102. Weiner M.F., Vega G., Risser R.C., Honig L.S., Cullum C.M., Crumpacker D., Rosenberg R.N. (1999) Apolipoprotein Eε4, other risk factors, and course of Alzheimer's disease. *Biol. Psychiatry*, **45**: 633–638.

103. Dal Forno G., Rasmusson X., Brandt J., Carson K.A., Brookmeyer R., Troncoso J., Kawas C.H. (1996) Apolipoprotein E genotype and rate of decline in probable Alzheimer's disease. *Arch. Neurol.*, **53**: 345–350.

104. Gomez-Isla T., West H.L., Rebeck G.W., Harr S.D., Growdon J.H., Locascio J.J., Perls T.T., Lipsitz L.A., Hyman B.T. (1996) Clinical and pathological correlates of apolipoprotein E ε4 in Alzheimer's disease. *Ann. Neurol.*, **39**: 62–70.

105. Kurz A., Egensperger R., Haupt M., Lautenschlager N., Romero B., Graeber M.B., Müller U. (1996) Apolipoprotein E ε4 allele, cognitive decline, and deterioration of everyday performance in Alzheimer's disease. *Neurology*, **47**: 440–443.

106. Sarochan M., Förstl H., Sattel H., Zerfass R., Czech C., Beyreuther K. (1996) Apolipoprotein E genotype does not promote the clinical progression of manifest Alzheimer's disease. *Dementia*, **7**: 120–120.

107. Kanai M., Shizuka M., Urakami K., Matsubara E., Harigaya Y., Okamoto K., Shoji M. (1999) Apolipoprotein E4 accelerates dementia and increases cerebrospinal fluid tau levels in Alzheimer's disease. *Neurosci. Lett.*, **267**: 65–68.

108. Craft S., Teri L., Edland S.D., Kukull W.A., Schellenberg G., McCormick W.C., Bowen J.D., Larson E.B. (1998) Accelerated decline in apolipoprotein E-ε4 homozygotes with Alzheimer's disease. *Neurology*, **51**: 149–153.

109. Stern Y., Brandt J., Albert M., Jacobs D.M., Liu X.H., Bell K., Marder K., Sano M., Albert S., Castenada C.D. *et al.* (1997) The absence of an apolipoprotein ε4 allele is associated with a more aggressive form of Alzheimer's disease. *Ann. Neurol.*, **41**: 615–620.

110. Cacabelos R., Rodríguez B., Carrera C., Beyer K., Lao J.I., Sellers M.A. (1997) Behavioral changes associated with different apolipoprotein E genotypes in dementia. *Alzheimer Dis. Assoc. Disord.*, **11**(Suppl. 4): S27–S34.

111. Holmes C., Levy R., McLoughlin D.M., Powell J.F., Lovestone S. (1996) Apolipoprotein E and the clinical features of late onset Alzheimer's disease. *J. Neurol. Neurosurg. Psychiatry*, **61**: 580–583.

112. Berr C., Hauw J.-J., Delaère P., Duyckaerts C., Amouyel P. (1994) Apolipoprotein E allele ε4 is linked to increased deposition of the amyloid β-peptide (A-β) in cases with or without Alzheimer's disease. *Neurosci. Lett.*, **178**: 221–224.

113. Polvikoski T., Sulkava R., Haltia M., Kainulainen K., Vuorio A., Verkkoniemi A., Niinistö L., Halonen P., Kontula K. (1995) Apolipoprotein E, dementia, and cortical deposition of β-amyloid protein. *N. Engl. J. Med.*, **333**: 1242–1247.

114. März W., Scharnagl H., Kirça M., Bohl J., Gross W., Ohm T.G. (1996) Apolipoprotein E polymorphism is associated with both senile plaque load and Alzheimer-type neurofibrillary tangle formation. *Ann. N.Y. Acad. Sci.*, **777**: 276–280.

115. Minthon L., Hesse C., Sjögren M., Englund E., Gustafson L., Blennow K. (1997) The apolipoprotein E ε4 allele frequency is normal in fronto-temporal dementia, but correlates with age at onset of disease. *Neurosci. Lett.*, **226**: 65–67.

116. Houlden H., Rizzu P., Stevens M., de Knijff P., van Duijn C.M., Van Swieten J.C., Heutink P., Perez-Tur J., Thomas V., Baker M. *et al.* (1999) Apolipoprotein E genotype does not affect the age of onset of dementia in families with defined tau mutations. *Neurosci. Lett.*, **260**: 193–195.

117. Meyer M.R., Tschanz J.T., Norton M.C., Welsh-Bohmer K.A., Steffens D.C., Wyse B.W., Breitner J.C.S. (1998) APOE genotype predicts when—not whether—one is predisposed to develop Alzheimer disease. *Nature Genet.*, **19**: 321–322.

118. Hyman B.T., Strickland D.K., Rebeck G.W. (1994) Alpha 2-macroglobulin receptor/low density lipoprotein receptor-related protein. Relationship to apolipoprotein E and role in Alzheimer disease senile plaques. *Ann. N.Y. Acad. Sci.*, **737**: 88–95.

119. Wragg M., Hutton M., Talbot C., Busfield F., Han S.W., Lendon C., Clark R.F., Morris J.C., Edwards D., Goate A. *et al.* (1996) Genetic association between intronic polymorphism in presenilin-1 gene and late-onset Alzheimer's disease. *Lancet*, **347**: 509–512.

120. Kehoe P.G., Russ C., McIlroy S., Williams H., Holmans P., Holmes C., Liolitsa D., Vahidassr D., Powell J., McGleenon B. *et al.* (1999) Variation in DCP1, encoding ACE, is associated with susceptibility to Alzheimer disease. *Nature Genet.*, **21**: 71–72.

121. Crawford F., Abdullah L., Schinka J., Suo Z., Gold M., Duara R., Mullan M. (2000) Gender-specific association of the angiotensin converting enzyme gene with Alzheimer's disease. *Neurosci. Lett.*, **280**: 215–219.

122. Farrer L.A., Sherbatich T., Keryanov S.A., Korovaitseva G.I., Rogaeva E.A., Petruk S., Premkumar S., Moliaka Y., Song Y.Q., Pei Y. *et al.* (2000) Association between angiotensin-converting enzyme and Alzheimer disease. *Arch. Neurol.*, **57**: 210–214.

123. Narain Y., Yip A., Murphy T., Brayne C., Easton D., Evans J.G., Xuereb J., Cairns N., Esiri M.M., Furlong R.A. *et al.* (2000) The ACE gene and Alzheimer's disease susceptibility. *J. Med. Genet.*, **37**: 695–697.

124. Hu J., Miyatake F., Aizu Y., Nakagawa H., Nakamura S., Tamaoka A., Takahash R., Urakami K., Shoji M. (1999) Angiotensin-converting enzyme genotype is associated with Alzheimer disease in the Japanese population. *Neurosci. Lett.*, **277**: 65–67.

125. Kehoe P., Wavrant-De Vrieze F., Crook R., Wu W.S., Holmans P., Fenton I., Spurlock G., Norton N., Williams H., Williams N., *et al.* (1999) A full genome scan for late onset Alzheimer's disease. *Hum. Mol. Genet.*, **8**: 237–245.

126. Zubenko G.S., Hughes H.B., Stiffler J.S., Hurtt M.R., Kaplan B.B. (1998) A genome survey for novel Alzheimer disease risk loci: results at 10-cM resolution. *Genomics*, **50**: 121–128.

127. Pericak-Vance M.A., Bass M.P., Yamaoka L.H., Gaskell P.C., Scott W.K., Terwedow H.A., Menold M.M., Conneally P.M., Small G.W., Vance J.M. *et al.* (1997) Complete genomic screen in late-onset familial Alzheimer disease— evidence for a new locus on chromosome 12. *JAMA*, **278**: 1237–1241.

128. Bertram L., Blacker D., Mullin K., Keeney D., Jones J., Basu S., Yhu S., McInnis M.G., Go R.C., Vekrellis K., Selkoe D.J., Saunders A.J., Tanzi R.E. (2000) Evidence for genetic linkage of Alzheimer's disease to chromosome 10q. *Science*, **290**: 2302–2303.

129. Ertekin-Taner N., Graff-Radford N., Younkin L.H., Eckman C., Baker M., Adamson J., Ronald J., Blangero J., Hutton M., Younkin S.G. (2000) Linkage of plasma Aβ42 to a quantitative locus on chromosome 10 in late-onset Alzheimer's disease pedigrees. *Science*, **290**: 2303–2304.

130. Myers A., Holmans P., Marshall H., Kwon J., Meyer D., Ramic D., Shears S., Booth J., DeVrieze F.W., Crook R. *et al.* (2000) Susceptibility locus for Alzheimer's disease on chromosome 10. *Science*, **290**: 2304–2305.

131. Qiu W.Q., Walsh D.M., Ye Z., Vekrellis K., Zhang J.M., Podlisny M.B., Rosner M.R., Safavi A., Hersh L.B., Selkoe D.J. (1998) Insulin-degrading enzyme regulates extracellular levels of amyloid β-protein by degradation. *J. Biol. Chem.*, **273**: 32730–32738.

132. Scourfield J., Soldan J., Gray J., Houlihan G., Harper P.S. (1997) Huntington's disease: psychiatric practice in molecular genetic prediction and diagnosis. *Br. J. Psychiatry*, **170**: 146–149.

133. Tyler A., Morris M., Lazarou L., Meredith L., Myring J., Harper P. (1992) Presymptomatic testing for Huntington's disease in Wales 1987–90. *Br. J. Psychiatry*, **161**: 481–488.

134. European Community Huntington's Disease Collaborative Study Group (1993) Ethical and social issues in presymptomatic testing for Huntington's disease: a European Community collaborative study. *J. Med. Genet.*, **30**: 1028–1035.

135. Simpson S.A., Harding A.E. (1993) Predictive testing for Huntington's disease: after the gene. The United Kingdom Huntington's Disease Prediction Consortium. *J. Med. Genet.*, **30**: 1036–1038.

136. Simpson S.A., Besson J., Alexander D., Allan K., Johnston A.W. (1992) One hundred requests for predictive testing for Huntington's disease. *Clin. Genet.*, **41**: 326–330.

137. Farrer L.A., Brin M.F., Elsas L., Goate A., Kennedy J., Mayeux R., Myers R.H., Reilly P., Risch N.J. (1995) Statement on use of apolipoprotein E testing for Alzheimer disease. *JAMA*, **274**: 1627–1629.

138. Tunstall N., Lovestone S. (1999) UK Alzheimer's disease genetics consortium. *Int. J. Geriatr. Psychiatry*, **14**: 789–791.

139. Medical and Scientific Committee ADI, Brodaty H., Conneally M., Gauthier S., Jennings C., Lennox A., Lovestone S. (1996) Consensus statement on predictive testing. *Alzheimer Dis. Assoc. Disord.*, **9**: 182–187.

140. Mayeux R., Saunders A.M., Shea S., Mirra S., Evans D., Roses A.D., Hyman B.T., Crain B., Tang M.X., Phelps C.H. (1998) Utility of the apolipoprotein E genotype in the diagnosis of Alzheimer's disease. Alzheimer's Disease Centers Consortium on apolipoprotein E and Alzheimer's disease. *N. Engl. J. Med.*, **338**: 506–511.

141. Tsuang D., Larson E.B., Bowen J., McCormick W., Teri L., Nochlin D., Leverenz J.B., Peskind E.R., Lim A., Raskind M.A. *et al.* (1999) The utility of apolipoprotein E genotyping in the diagnosis of Alzheimer disease in a community-based case series. *Arch. Neurol.*, **56**: 1489–1495.

142. Poirier J., Delisle M.C., Quirion R., Aubert I., Farlow M., Lahiri D., Hui S., Bertrand P., Nalbantoglu J., Gilfix B.M. *et al.* (1995) Apolipoprotein E4 allele as a predictor of cholinergic deficits and treatment outcome in Alzheimer disease. *Proc. Natl. Acad. Sci. USA*, **92**: 12260–12264.

143. Raskind M.A., Peskind E.R., Wessel T., Yuan W. (2000) Galantamine in AD: a 6-month randomized, placebo-controlled trial with a 6-month extension. *Neurology*, **54**: 2261–2268.

144. Rigaud A.S., Traykov L., Caputo L., Guelfi M.C., Latour F., Couderc R., Moulin F., de Rotrou J., Forette F., Boller F. (2000) The apolipoprotein E epsilon4 allele and the response to tacrine therapy in Alzheimer's disease. *Eur. J. Neurol.*, **7**: 255–258.

145. Hardy J.A., Higgins G.A. (1992) Alzheimer's disease: the amyloid cascade hypothesis. *Science*, **256**: 184–185.

146. Wilson C.A., Doms R.W., Lee V.M.Y. (1999) Intracellular APP processing and Aβ production in Alzheimer disease. *J. Neuropathol. Exp. Neurol.*, **58**: 787–794.

147. Selkoe D.J. (1999) Translating cell biology into therapeutic advances in Alzheimer's disease. *Nature*, **399**(Suppl): A23-A31.

148. Iwatsubo T., Odaka A., Suzuki N., Mizusawa H., Nukina N., Ihara Y. (1994) Visualization of Aβ42(43) and Aβ40 in senile plaques with end-specific Aβ monoclonals: evidence that an initially deposited species is Aβ42(43). *Neuron*, **13**: 45–53.

149. Borchelt D.R., Thinakaran G., Eckman C.B., Lee M.K., Davenport F., Ratovitsky T., Prada C.M., Kim G., Seekins S., Yager D. *et al.* (1996) Familial Alzheimer's disease-linked presenilin 1 variants elevate Aβ1-42/1-40 ratio in vitro and in vivo. *Neuron*, **17**: 1005–1013.

150. Price D.L., Sisodia S.S. (1998) Mutant genes in familial Alzheimer's disease and transgenic models. *Annu. Rev. Neurosci.*, **21**: 479–505.

151. Johnston J., O'Neill C., Lannfelt L., Winblad B., Cowburn R.F. (1994) The significance of the Swedish APP670/671 mutation for the development of Alzheimer's disease amyloidosis. *Neurochem. Int.*, **25**: 73–80.

152. Storey E., Cappai R. (1999) The amyloid precursor protein of Alzheimer's disease and the Aβ peptide. *Neuropathol. Appl. Neurobiol.*, **25**: 81–97.

153. Haass C., Selkoe D.J. (1993) Cellular processing of β-amyloid precursor protein and the genesis of amyloid β-peptide. *Cell*, **75**: 1039–1042.

154. Felsenstein K.M., Lewis-Higgins L. (1993) Processing of the β-amyloid precursor protein carrying the familial, Dutch-type, and a novel recombinant C-terminal mutation. *Neurosci. Lett.*, **152**: 185–189.

155. Watson D.J., Selkoe D.J., Teplow D.B. (1999) Effects of the amyloid precursor protein Glu^{693} → Gln "Dutch" mutation on the production and stability of amyloid β-protein. *Biochem. J.*, **340**: 703–709.

156. Buxbaum J.D., Koo E.H., Greengard P. (1993) Protein phosphorylation inhibits production of Alzheimer amyloid β/A4 peptide. *Proc. Natl. Acad. Sci. USA*, **90**: 9195–9198.

157. LeBlanc A.C., Koutroumanis M., Goodyer C.G. (1998) Protein kinase C activation increases release of secreted amyloid precursor protein without decreasing Aβ production in human primary neuron cultures. *J. Neurosci.*, **18**: 2907–2913.

158. Vassar R., Bennett B.D., Babu-Khan S., Kahn S., Mendiaz E.A., Denis P., Teplow D.B., Ross S., Amarante P., Loeloff R. *et al.* (1999) Beta-secretase cleavage of Alzheimer's amyloid precursor protein by the transmembrane aspartic protease BACE. *Science*, **286**: 735–741.

159. Saunders A.J., Kim T.-W., Tanzi R.E. (1999) BACE maps to chromosome 11 and a BACE homolog, BACE2, reside in the obligate Down syndrome region of chromosome 21. *Science*, **286**: 1255a.

160. Bennett B.D., Babu-Khan S., Loeloff R., Louis J.C., Curran E., Citron M., Vassar R. (2000) Expression analysis of BACE2 in brain and peripheral tissues. *J. Biol. Chem.*, **275**: 20 647–20 651.

161. Wong P.C., Zheng H., Chen H., Becher M.W., Sirinathsinghji D.J.S., Trumbauer M.E., Chen H.Y., Price D.L., Van der Ploeg L.H.T., Sisodia S.S. (1997) Presenilin 1 is required for Notch-1 DII1 expression in the paraxial mesoderm. *Nature*, **387**: 288–292.

162. Conlon R.A., Reaume A.G., Rossant J. (1995) Notch1 is required for the coordinate segmentation of somites. *Development*, **121**: 1533–1545.

163. De Strooper B., Annaert W., Cupers P., Saftig P., Craessaerts K., Mumm J.S., Schroeter E.H., Schrijvers V., Wolfe M.S., Ray W.J. *et al.* (1999) A presenilin-1-dependent gamma-secretase-like protease mediates release of Notch intracellular domain. *Nature*, **398**: 518–522.

164. De Strooper B., Saftig P., Craessaerts K., Vanderstichele H., Guhde G., Annaert W., Von Figura K., Van Leuven F. (1998) Deficiency of presenilin-1 inhibits the normal cleavage of amyloid precursor protein. *Nature*, **391**: 387–390.

165. Zhang Z.H., Nadeau P., Song W.H., Donoviel D., Yuan M.L., Bernstein A., Yankner B.A. (2000) Presenilins are required for γ-secretase cleavage of β-APP and transmembrane cleavage of Notch-1. *Nature Cell Biol.*, **2**: 463–465.

166. Yu G., Nishimura M., Arawaka S., Levitan D., Zhang L.L., Tandon A., Song Y.Q., Rogaeva E., Chen F.S., Kawaral T. *et al.* (2000) Nicastrin modulates presenilin-mediated notch/glp-1 signal transduction and βAPP processing. *Nature*, **407**: 48–54.

167. Hooper N.M., Turner A.J. (2000) Protein processing mechanisms: from angiotensin-converting enzyme to Alzheimer's disease. *Biochem. Soc. Trans.*, **28**: 441–446.

168. Nitsch R.M., Slack B.E., Wurtman R.J., Growdon J.H. (1992) Release of Alzheimer amyloid precursor derivatives stimulated by activation of muscarinic acetylcholine receptors. *Science*, **258**: 304–307.

169. DeLapp N., Wu S., Belagaje R., Johnstone E., Little S., Shannon H., Bymaster F., Calligaro D., Mitch C., Whitesitt C. *et al.* (1998) Effects of the M1 agonist xanomeline on processing of human β-amyloid precursor protein (FAD, Swedish mutant) transfected into Chinese hamster ovary-m1 cells. *Biochem. Biophys. Res. Commun.*, **244**: 156–160.

170. Chong Y.H., Suh Y.H. (1996) Amyloidogenic processing of Alzheimer's amyloid precursor protein in vitro and its modulation by metal ions and tacrine. *Life Sci.*, **59**: 545–557.

171. Lahiri D.K., Farlow M.R., Nurnberger J.I. Jr., Greig N.H. (1997) Effects of cholinesterase inhibitors on the secretion of beta-amyloid precursor protein in cell cultures. *Ann. N.Y. Acad. Sci.*, **826**: 416–421.

172. Mori F., Lai C.C., Fusi F., Giacobini E. (1995) Cholinesterase inhibitors increase secretion of APPs in rat brain cortex. *Neuroreport*, **6**: 633–636.

173. Nitsch R.M., Deng M., Tennis M., Schoenfeld D., Growdon J.H. (2000) The selective muscarinic M1 agonist AF102B decreases levels of total Aβ in cerebrospinal fluid of patients with Alzheimer's disease. *Ann. Neurol.*, **48**: 913–918.

174. Grundke Iqbal I., Iqbal K., Tung Y.C., Quinlan M., Wisniewski H.M., Binder L.I. (1986) Abnormal phosphorylation of the microtubule-associated protein tau (tau) in Alzheimer cytoskeletal pathology. *Proc. Natl. Acad. Sci. USA*, **83**: 4913–4917.

175. Spillantini M.G., Goedert M. (1998) Tau protein pathology in neurodegenerative diseases. *Trends Neurosci.*, **21**: 428–433.
176. Lovestone S., Reynolds C.H. (1997) The phosphorylation of tau: a critical stage in neurodevelopmental and neurodegenerative processes. *Neuroscience*, **78**: 309–324.
177. Mena R., Edwards P.C., Harrington C.R., Mukaetova-Ladinska E.B., Wischik C.M. (1996) Staging the pathological assembly of truncated tau protein into paired helical filaments in Alzheimer's disease. *Acta Neuropathol. (Berl.)*, **91**: 633–641.
178. Ishiguro K., Omori A., Sato K., Tomizawa K., Imahori K., Uchida T. (1991) A serine/threonine proline kinase activity is included in the tau protein kinase fraction forming a paired helical filament epitope. *Neurosci. Lett.*, **128**: 195–198.
179. Takahashi M., Tomizawa K., Ishiguro K., Sato K., Omori A., Sato S., Shiratsuchi A., Uchida T., Imahori K. (1991) A novel brain-specific 25 kDa protein (p25) is phosphorylated by a Ser/Thr-Pro kinase (TPK II) from tau protein kinase fractions. *FEBS Lett.*, **289**: 37–43.
180. Latimer D.A., Gallo J.-M., Lovestone S., Miller C.C.J., Reynolds C.H., Marquardt B., Stabel S., Woodgett J.R., Anderton B.H. (1995) Stimulation of MAP kinase by v-*raf* transformation of fibroblasts fails to induce hyperphosphorylation of transfected tau. *FEBS Lett.*, **365**: 42–46.
181. Lovestone S., Reynolds C.H., Latimer D., Davis D.R., Anderton B.H., Gallo J.-M., Hanger D., Mulot S., Marquardt B., Stabel S. et al. (1994) Alzheimer's disease-like phosphorylation of the microtubule-associated protein tau by glycogen synthase kinase-3 in transfected mammalian cells. *Curr. Biol.*, **4**: 1077–1086.
182. Ishiguro K., Shiratsuchi A., Sato S., Omori A., Arioka M., Kobayashi S., Uchida T., Imahori K. (1993) Glycogen synthase kinase 3β is identical to tau protein kinase I generating several epitopes of paired helical filaments. *FEBS Lett.*, **325**: 167–172.
183. Klein P.S., Melton D.A. (1996) A molecular mechanism for the effect of lithium on development. *Proc. Natl. Acad. Sci. USA*, **93**: 8455–8459.
184. Stambolic V., Ruel L., Woodgett J.R. (1996) Lithium inhibits glycogen synthase kinase-3 activity and mimics wingless signalling in intact cells. *Curr. Biol.*, **6**: 1664–1668.
185. Hong M., Chen D.C., Klein P.S., Lee V.M. (1997) Lithium reduces tau phosphorylation by inhibition of glycogen synthase kinase-3. *J. Biol. Chem.*, **272**: 25 326–25 332.
186. Lovestone S., Davis D.R., Webster M.-T., Kaech S., Brion J.-P., Matus A., Anderton B.H. (1999) Lithium reduces tau phosphorylation—effects in living cells and in neurons at therapeutic concentrations. *Biol. Psychiatry*, **45**: 995–1003.
187. Leroy K., Menu R., Conreur J.L., Dayanandan R., Lovestone S., Anderton B.H., Brion J.P. (2000) The function of the microtubule-associated protein tau is variably modulated by graded changes in glycogen synthase kinase-3β activity. *FEBS Lett.*, **465**: 34–38.
188. Hong M., Lee V.M.Y. (1997) Insulin and insulin-like growth factor-1 regulate tau phosphorylation in cultured human neurons. *J. Biol. Chem.*, **272**: 19 547–19 553.
189. Stewart R., Liolitsa D. (1999) Type 2 diabetes mellitus, cognitive impairment and dementia. *Diabet. Med.*, **16**: 93–112.

190. Solano D.C., Sironi M., Bonfini C., Solerte S.B., Govoni S., Racchi M. (2000) Insulin regulates soluble amyloid precursor protein release via phosphatidyl inositol 3 kinase-dependent pathway. *FASEB J.*, **14**: 1015–1022.

191. Buée L., Bussière T., Buée-Scherrer V., Delacourte A., Hof P.R. (2000) Tau protein isoforms, phosphorylation and role in neurodegenerative disorders. *Brain Res. Rev.*, **33**: 95–130.

192. Heutink P. (2000) Untangling tau-related dementia. *Hum. Mol. Genet.*, **9**: 979–986.

193. Grover A., Houlden H., Baker M., Adamson J., Lewis J., Prihar G., Pickering-Brown S., Duff K., Hutton M. (1999) 5′ splice site mutations in tau associated with the inherited dementia FTDP-17 affect a stem-loop structure that regulates alternative splicing of exon 10. *J. Biol. Chem.*, **274**: 15 134–15 143.

194. Hasegawa M., Smith M.J., Goedert M. (1998) Tau proteins with FTDP-17 mutations have a reduced ability to promote microtubule assembly. *FEBS Lett.*, **437**: 207–210.

195. Lewis J., McGowan E., Rockwood J., Melrose H., Nacharaju P., Van Slegtenhorst M., Gwinn-Hardy K., Paul M.M., Baker M., Yu X. *et al.* (2000) Neurofibrillary tangles, amyotrophy and progressive motor disturbance in mice expressing mutant (P301L) tau protein. *Nature Genet.*, **25**: 402–405.

196. Ishihara T., Hong M., Zhang B., Nakagawa Y., Lee M.K., Trojanowski J.Q., Lee V.M.Y. (1999) Age-dependent emergence and progression of a tauopathy in transgenic mice overexpressing the shortest human tau isoform. *Neuron*, **24**: 751–762.

197. Bales K.R., Verina T., Dodel R.C., Du Y.S., Altstiel L., Bender M., Hyslop P., Johnstone E.M., Little S.P., Cummins D.J. *et al.* (1997) Lack of apolipoprotein E dramatically reduces amyloid β-peptide deposition. *Nature Genet.*, **17**: 263–264.

198. Schmechel D.E., Saunders A.M., Strittmatter W.J., Crain B.J., Hulette C.M., Joo S.H., Pericak-Vance M.A., Goldgaber D., Roses A.D. (1993) Increased amyloid β-peptide deposition in cerebral cortex as a consequence of apolipoprotein E genotype in late-onset Alzheimer disease. *Proc. Natl. Acad. Sci. USA*, **90**: 9649–9653.

199. Strittmatter W.J., Weisgraber K.H., Huang D.Y., Dong L.-M., Salvesen G.S., Pericak-Vance M., Schmechel D., Saunders A.M., Goldgaber D., Roses A.D. (1993) Binding of human apolipoprotein E to synthetic amyloid β peptide: isoform-specific effects and implications for late-onset Alzheimer disease. *Proc. Natl. Acad. Sci. USA*, **90**: 8098–8102.

200. Strittmatter W.J., Saunders A.M., Goedert M., Weisgraber K.H., Dong L.M., Jakes R., Huang D.Y., Pericak-Vance M., Schmechel D., Roses A.D. (1994) Isoform-specific interactions of apolipoprotein E with microtubule-associated protein tau: implications for Alzheimer disease. *Proc. Natl. Acad. Sci. USA*, **91**: 11 183–11 186.

201. Huang D.Y., Goedert M., Jakes R., Weisgraber K.H., Garner C.C., Saunders A.M., Pericak-Vance M.A., Schmechel D.E., Roses A.D., Strittmatter W.J. (1994) Isoform-specific interactions of apolipoprotein E with the microtubule-associated protein MAP2c: implications for Alzheimer's disease. *Neurosci. Lett.*, **182**: 55–58.

202. Strittmatter W.J., Weisgraber K.H., Goedert M., Saunders A.M., Huang D., Corder E.H., Dong L.-M., Jakes R., Alberts M.J., Gilbert J.R. *et al.* (1994) Microtubule instability and paired helical filament formation in the Alzheimer disease brain are related to apolipoprotein E genotype. *Exp. Neurol.*, **125**: 163–171.

203. Nathan B.P., Bellosta S., Sanan D.A., Weisgraber K.H., Mahley R.W., Pitas R.E. (1994) Differential effects of apolipoproteins E3 and E4 on neuronal growth in vitro. *Science*, **264**: 850–852.
204. Nathan B.P., Chang K.C., Bellosta S., Brisch E., Ge N.F., Mahley R.W., Pitas R.E. (1995) The inhibitory effect of apolipoprotein E4 on neurite outgrowth is associated with microtubule depolymerization. *J. Biol. Chem.*, **270**: 19 791–19 799.
205. Giordano T., Bao Pan J., Monteggia L.M., Holzman T.F., Snyder S.W., Krafft G., Ghanbari H., Kowall N.W. (1994) Similarities between β amyloid peptides 1–40 and 40–1: effects on aggregation, toxicity *in vitro*, and injection in young and aged rats. *Exp. Neurol.*, **125**: 175–182.
206. Takashima A., Honda T., Yasutake K., Michel G., Murayama O., Murayama M., Ishiguro K., Yamaguchi H. (1998) Activation of tau protein kinase I glycogen synthase kinase-3β by amyloid β peptide (25–35) enhances phosphorylation of tau in hippocampal neurons. *Neurosci. Res.*, **31**: 317–323.
207. Wei H.F., Leeds P.R., Qian Y.N., Wei W.L., Chen R.W., Chuang D.M. (2000) β-amyloid peptide-induced death of PC 12 cells and cerebellar granule cell neurons is inhibited by long-term lithium treatment. *Eur. J. Pharmacol.*, **392**: 117–123.
208. Alvarez G., Muñoz-Montaño J.R., Satrústegui J., Avila J., Bogónez E., Díaz-Nido J. (1999) Lithium protects cultured neurons against β-amyloid-induced neurodegeneration. *FEBS Lett.*, **453**: 260–264.
209. Takashima A., Yamaguchi H., Noguchi K., Michel G., Ishiguro K., Sato K., Hoshino T., Hoshi M., Imahori K. (1995) Amyloid β peptide induces cytoplasmic accumulation of amyloid protein precursor via tau protein kinase I glycogen synthase kinase-3β in rat hippocampal neurons. *Neurosci. Lett.*, **198**: 83–86.
210. Lovestone S. (1997) Muscarinic therapies in Alzheimer's disease: from palliative therapies to disease modification. *Int. J. Psychiatry Clin. Practice*, **1**: 15–20.
211. Janus C., Pearson J., McLaurin J., Mathews P.M., Jiang Y., Schmidt S.D., Chishti M.A., Horne P., Heslin D., French J. *et al.* (2000) A beta peptide immunization reduces behavioural impairment and plaques in a model of Alzheimer's disease. *Nature*, **408**: 979–982.
212. Schenk D., Barbour R., Dunn W., Gordon G., Grajeda H., Guido T., Hu K., Huang J., Johnson-Wood K., Khan K. *et al.* (1999) Immunization with amyloid-beta attenuates Alzheimer-disease-like pathology in the PDAPP mouse. *Nature*, **400**: 173–177.

Index

ACE model, of disease liability 10–11
acute polymorphous psychosis, P300
    amplitude 144
addiction *see* substance abuse
Addison's disease 105
adenosinergic system 245–8
ADHD *see* attention deficit hyperactivity
    disorder
adoption studies 7, 8, 200
adrenal gland *see* HPA axis
adrenergic system *see* noradrenergic
    system
affective disorders
    adoption studies 7
    brain activity in 72, 80, 100–101
    brain electrical microstates in 148–9
    brain morphology 69, 184–5
    comorbidity in 12, 39, 47
    electrodermal activity in 150–51
    event-related potentials in 149–50
    eye movements in 150
    genetic component 43–4
    and glial cells 28
    hemispheric imbalance in 148, 150–51
    and the HPG axis 110–11
    molecular biology 39–44, 52
    neuroendocrinology 42–3
    neurotransmitter mechanisms 81–2
    pharmacological studies 44, 52
    qEEG characteristics 147–9
    twin studies 5, 6
    see also bipolar affective disorder;
        depression
aggression
    gene mapping 16
    see also antisocial behaviour
alcohol, blood tests for 50
alcoholism 7, 48–50
allelic association studies 14, 17–18, 19
Alzheimer's disease 287
    and apolipoprotein E 295–7, 299,
        305–6
    brain electrical microstates in 158

and CRF receptors 109
    genetic component 4, 15, 16, 20–21,
        292–3, 294–9
    genetic testing for 21, 22, 298, 299
    molecular biology 300–307
    neurochemistry 290–92
    neurofibrillary tangles in 288–9, 291,
        293, 300, 303–5, 306–7
    plaques in 287–8, 292, 296, 300–303,
        305, 306–308
    qEEG characteristics 156–8
    tissue remodelling in 35–6
    see also dementia
amygdala 212, 240–41
amygdalo-cingulo-hippocampal
    circuitry, and stress 215–16
amyloid cascade, in dementia 300,
    306–7
amyloid plaques *see* plaques
amyloid precursor protein *see* APP
amyloidopathies 289, 290
animal investigations 32–3
    in dementia 302, 305
    in panic disorder 248–9
    in schizophrenia 211–17
antalarmin, for anxiety disorders 47
anterior cingulate cortex, in
    schizophrenia 203–4, 216
antidepressants 40, 52, 109
antioxidants *see* free radicals
antipsychotic drugs 14, 82, 137, 198–9
antisocial behaviour 7, 11
    see also aggression
anxiety disorders
    biological research, history 237–8, 262
    brain activity in 72, 80
    comorbidity in 12, 45, 47
    electrodermal activity 154–6
    event-related potentials in 152–4
    eye movements in 155
    genetic component 11–12, 46, 262–4
    hemispheric imbalance in 152, 153,
        154–5

anxiety disorders (*cont.*)
 and the HPA axis 45, 46, 109, 154,
  251–3, 260–61
 molecular biology 45–6
 qEEG characteristics 151–2
 startle response 155–6, 259
 twin studies 11–12
 see also obsessive-compulsive
  disorder; panic disorder; stress
  disorders
apolipoprotein E, and Alzheimer's
 disease 295–7, 299, 305–6
APP, in dementia 36, 292–3, 297, 298,
 300–303, 304
arginine-vasopressin 112
attention deficit hyperactivity disorder
 cognitive dysfunction in 184
 gene mapping 14, 16
 and streptococcal infections 256
 twin studies 5, 6, 11
attentional deficit, in depression 184
autism 5, 6, 11, 13, 15, 183–4
autoimmune system *see*
 neuroimmunology
autosomal dominant dementias 292–4,
 298, 300
AVP *see* arginine-vasopressin

behaviour, environmental and genetic
 factors 4–5, 10–12
benzodiazepine receptors 74, 77, 81, 209
benzodiazepine-GABAergic
 system 249–50
biofeedback 156
bipolar affective disorder
 eye movements in 150
 GABA system in 208, 209
 and HPT axis abnormalities 101
 and omega-3 fatty acids 44
birth complications *see* perinatal
 problems
blood flow
 measurement 73, 74, 75, 77, 78, 79, 80,
  100–101
 in panic disorder 240
 in post-traumatic stress syndrome 258
 see also neurovascular coupling
brain
 volume, measurement of 66–7
 see also amygdala; hemispheric
  imbalance; hippocampus;

prefrontal cortex; headings
 beginning with neuro
brain electrical microstates 130–31
 in affective disorders 148–9
 in Alzheimer's disease 158
 in panic disorder 153
brain imaging 33
 see also computed tomography;
  computerized EEG tomography;
  emission tomography; low-
  resolution electromagnetic
  tomography; magnetic resonance
  imaging
brain morphology
 in affective disorders 69, 184–5
 in anxiety disorders 187, 240–41,
  254–5, 258
 in schizophrenia 63, 68–9, 137, 138,
  139–40, 201–5, 215–17
 see also neuronal loss; tissue
  remodelling
brain processes, coordination of 129–30,
 141–2
breathing *see* respiratory system
bulimia, twin studies 5, 6

caffeine, and panic disorder 245–8,
 252–3
candidate gene studies 13–14, 20
carbon dioxide *see* CO_2
cardiovascular activity 134
case-control matching, in genetic
 mapping 17–18
CCK *see* cholecystokinin
cell death *see* neuronal loss
cerebral blood flow *see* blood flow
cerebral glucose metabolism *see* glucose
 metabolism
childhood fatigue, twin studies 5, 6
childhood-onset schizophrenia 68, 79
cholecystokinin 250–51
cholinergic deficit, in dementia 290–91,
 292
clonidine, and panic disorder 244
CO_2 inhalation, and panic
 disorder 241–3
cocaine, effects 49
cognition
 and nicotine 39
 and substance abuse 47
cognitive ability, twin studies 5, 6–7, 11

cognitive disorders
  comorbidity in 34–5, 47
  molecular biology 34–9, 300–307
  see also dementia; psychoses;
    schizophrenia
cognitive dysfunction 182–3
  in attention-deficit hyperactivity
    disorder 184
  in autism 183–4
  in dementia 187–8
  in depression 184–5
  and hypothyroidism 99–100
  in obsessive-compulsive
    disorder 186–7
  in schizophrenia 185–6, 197–8
  in stress disorders 188–9, 259
coherence, in EEG 129, 141
comorbidity 29
  in anxiety disorders 11, 45, 47
  in cognitive disorders 34–5, 47
  in mood disorders 12, 39, 47
  in sleep disorders 50
  in substance abuse 47–8
computed tomography 60–63
computerized EEG tomography 130
control samples, in genetic mapping
  17–18
convergent functional genomics 33, 38
  in anxiety disorders 46
  in mood disorders 43–4
  in schizophrenia 38
  in sleep disorders 50–2
  in substance abuse 48–50
cortex *see* prefrontal cortex
cortico-striato-thalamo-cortical
  loops 216–17
corticotrophin-releasing factor (CRF) 47,
  92, 102–4, 106–9
corticotrophin-releasing hormone
  (CRH) 45, 46, 47
Cushing's syndrome 105

dementia
  APP in 36, 292–3, 297, 298, 300–303,
    304
  autosomal dominant 292–4, 298, 300
  cognitive dysfunction in 187–8
  event-related potentials 159
  genetic testing for 21, 22, 298–9
  genetics 292–9
  with Lewy bodies 289, 290

molecular biology of 34–6, 38–9,
  300–307
neurochemistry 290–92
see also Alzheimer's disease; vascular
  dementia
depression
  brain activity in 72, 80, 100–101
  brain morphology 69, 184–5
  cognitive dysfunction in 184–5
  effect on life events 12
  electrodermal activity in 150–51
  event-related potentials in 149–50
  and exercise 40–1
  and the hippocampus 40–1
  and the HPA axis 103, 105–9
  and the HPG axis 110–11
  and hypothyroidism 99–101
  and the pituitary-growth hormone
    axis 113–14
  qEEG characteristics 147–8
  transmitter mechanisms 81–2
  twin studies 5, 6, 11–12
  see also affective disorders
diagnostic testing *see* genetic testing
diffusion-weighted imaging 66
dimensional complexity 129–30, 141–2
dizygotic twins *see* twin studies
DNA pooling, in genetic mapping 18–19
DNA testing *see* genetic testing
dopamine
  in ADHD 14
  in schizophrenia 13–14, 36–8, 80–1,
    82, 199, 213–14, 219
  in substance abuse 47, 48
dopamine receptors, measurement 74,
  76, 77
dopamine transporters,
  measurement 74, 77
dorsolateral prefrontal cortex 204–5, 213
drug abuse *see* substance abuse
drugs *see* pharmacogenetics;
  pharmacological studies
dyskinesia *see* tardive dyskinesia
dyslexia, gene mapping 16

eating disorders
  molecular biology research 47–50
  see also bulimia
echo planar imaging 70–71
EEG *see* electroencephalography
electrodermal activity 133–4

electrodermal activity (*cont.*)
  in affective disorders 150–51
  in anxiety disorders 154–6
  in schizophrenia 146–7
electroencephalography 127–33
  quantitative analysis of *see* qEEG
emission tomography 72–8
  research findings 78–82, 100–101
end-organ damage *see* tissue
  remodelling
endocrinology *see* neuroendocrinology
environment, effects 4–5, 6, 10–12
epistasis 12–13
essential fatty acids *see* omega-3 fatty
  acids
estradiol, and mood disorders 42
ethics, of genetic testing 298–9
event-related desynchronization 128
event-related potentials 132–3
  in affective disorders 149–50
  in anxiety disorders 152–4
  in dementia 159
  in schizophrenia 142–5
exercise *see* physical activity
eye movements
  in affective disorders 150
  in anxiety disorders 155
  measurement of 134
  in schizophrenia 146, 147

familial advanced sleep phase
  syndrome 51
fascicle coherence 129
fear conditioning 212
  see also panic disorder
feedback *see* biofeedback; long-loop
  negative feedback; short-loop
  negative feedback
flumazenil, and panic disorder
  249–50
fMRI *see* functional magnetic resonance
  imaging
fragile X mental retardation, gene
  mapping 16
free radicals, and tardive dyskinesia
  38–9
frontal lobe dementias, genetics 293
functional magnetic resonance
  imaging 64, 69–72, 76

G proteins, in schizophrenia 37–8

galvanic skin response *see* electrodermal
  activity
gamma-aminobutyric acid (GABA)
  system 73, 203, 208–10, 218–19
  see also benzodiazepine-GABAergic
  system
gene expression 32, 33, 38
gene mapping 13–20
  see also convergent functional
  genomics; positional cloning
gene-environment interaction 4–5, 6, 12
gene-gene interactions 12–13
genes
  for affective disorders 43–4
  for alcoholism 48–9
  for anxiety disorders 11–12, 45–6,
    262–4
  for dementia 15, 16, 20–21, 292–9
  for Huntington's disease 15, 16, 294,
    295
  for obsessive-compulsive
    disorder 253–4
  for panic disorder 239–40, 243
  for post-traumatic stress
    disorder 257–8
  for schizophrenia 14, 16, 294
  see also psychogenes;
    psychosis-suppressor genes
genetic linkage detection 14–19, 21, 31,
  297
genetic testing 21–2
  ethics 298–9
genetics *see* inheritance;
  pharmacogenetics; psychiatric
  genetics
genotype-phenotype correlation 7–13,
  294, 296
glial cells, and mood disorders 30
glucocorticoid availability, effects 105–6
glucose metabolism
  in affective disorders 80, 100–101
  in panic disorder 240
  in schizophrenia 78–9
glutamate system, in
  schizophrenia 202–3, 210–11,
  214–15
gonads *see* HPG axis
gradient echo imaging *see* echo planar
  imaging
Graves' disease 101–2
growth hormone 42, 113–14, 244–5

hallucinations, qEEG
    characteristics 140–41
hemispheric imbalance
    in affective disorders 148, 150–51
    in anxiety disorders 152, 153, 154–5
    in schizophrenia 143, 144, 146–7
hemispheric influence 133–4
hippocampus
    and anxiety 46, 47
    and depression 40–1
    development, and maternal
        behaviour 35
    and panic disorder 240
    and post-traumatic stress
        syndrome 258
    and schizophrenia 202–3, 216
    see also amygdalo-cingulo-
        hippocampal circuitry
homosexuality, gene mapping 16
hormones 93–6, 97, 103, 104
    see also corticotrophin-releasing
        hormone; neuroendocrinology;
        noradrenergic system
HPA axis
    activity measurement 95–6
    and anxiety disorders 45, 46, 109, 154,
        251–3, 260–61
    and depression 103, 105–9
    effects of life events 108
    organization 102–4
HPG axis 109–11
HPT axis
    organization 96–8
    and psychiatric disorders 98–102
Huntington's disease
    genes for 15, 16, 294, 295
    genetic testing for 21, 298–9
hyperactivity see attention deficit
    hyperactivity disorder
hypercortisolism 105–6
hyperprolactinaemia 111
hyperthyroid states 101–2
hyperventilation, in panic disorder 241
hypothalamic-pituitary gonad axis see
    HPG axis
hypothalamic-pituitary-adrenal axis see
    HPA axis
hypothalamic-pituitary-end-organ
    axes 93–6
hypothalamic-pituitary-thyroid axis see
    HPT axis

hypothalamic-prolactin axis 111–12
hypothyroidism 42, 98–101

identical twins see twin studies
immunology see neuroimmunology
incomplete penetrance 7, 9, 299
infections, and psychiatric disorders 29,
    256–7
information processing deficits see
    cognitive dysfunction
inheritance, models 7–13
insomnia see sleep disorders
IQ see cognitive ability

lactate, and panic disorder 241, 242–3,
    249
Lewy bodies, in dementia 289, 290
life events
    effect of depression 12
    effect on HPA axis 108
limbic filtering, in schizophrenia 211–12
limbic lobe see amygdalo-cingulo-
    hippocampal circuitry
linkage detection see genetic linkage
    detection
lithium 38–9, 43, 304
long-loop negative feedback, of
    hormones 93, 94, 104
low-resolution electromagnetic
    tomography (LORETA) 131

magnetic resonance imaging 64–8
    research findings 68–9
    see also functional magnetic resonance
        imaging
male homosexuality, gene mapping 16
manic depressive disorder
    event-related potentials in 149, 150
    qEEG characteristics 148
    twin studies 5, 6
marijuana, effects 49
maternal behaviour, and hippocampal
    development 35
memory, and the prefrontal cortex 213
memory disorder
    in depression 184, 185
    in post-traumatic stress syndrome 259
microarray technology 30
modafinil 52
molecular biology 31–33
    of affective disorders 39–42, 50–51

molecular biology (*cont.*)
  of anxiety disorders 45–7
  of cognitive disorders 34–9, 300–307
  methodology 31–4
  of sleep disorders 50–53
  of substance abuse 47–50
molecular markers *see* peripheral
    molecular markers
monozygotic twins *see* twin studies
mood disorders *see* affective disorders
MRI *see* magnetic resonance imaging
myxoedema *see* hypothyroidism

narcolepsy 50–51, 52
natural experiments *see* adoption
    studies; twin studies
nerve growth factor, for dementia 39
neuroanatomy *see* brain morphology
neurochemistry
  of dementia 290–92
  of obsessive-compulsive
      disorder 255–6
  of panic disorder 244–51
  of post-traumatic stress disorder 260
  see also neurotransmitters
neurodevelopmental hypothesis, of
    schizophrenia 217–19
neuroendocrine axes *see*
    hypothalamic-pituitary-end-organ
    axes; pituitary-growth hormone axis
neuroendocrinology 91–3, 96
  and anxiety disorders 45, 46, 109, 154,
      250–53, 260–61
  and mood disorders 42–43, 103, 105–9
  see also hormones; noradrenergic
      system
neurofibrillary tangles, in Alzheimer's
    disease 288–9, 291, 293, 300, 303–5,
    306–7
neurohormones *see* hormones
neuroimmunology, in obsessive-
    compulsive disorder 256–7
neuroleptics *see* antipsychotic drugs
neuronal loss 206–7, 290–92
neuronal migration, in
    schizophrenia 217
neurophysiology 125–7
  of obsessive-compulsive disorder 255
  of panic disorder 241–4
  of post-traumatic stress disorder
      155–6, 259

  see also cardiovascular activity;
      electrodermal activity;
      electroencephalography; eye
      movements; startle response
neuroprotective agents *see* lithium
neuropsychology 181–2
  development of 182–3
  uses 189–90
  see also cognitive dysfunction
neurotransmitters 80–82
  loss, in dementia 290–92
  for schizophrenia 81, 208–11, 213–15,
      218–19
  see also dopamine; gamma-
      aminobutyric acid; glutamate
      system; serotonin; synaptic
      markers
neurovascular coupling 64, 69–70
nicotine, and cognition 39
noradrenergic system 244–5, 260
nuclear magnetic resonance *see* magnetic
    resonance imaging

obsessive-compulsive disorder
  brain morphology 187, 254–5
  cognitive dysfunction in 186–7
  event-related potentials in 152–3
  neurochemistry 255–6
  neurogenetics 253–4
  neuroimmunology 256–7
  neurophysiology 255
  qEEG characteristics 151–2
obstetrical complications *see* perinatal
    problems
odansetron 50
omega-3 fatty acids, and mood
    disorders 44
opiate receptors, measurement 77
oxidative stress *see* free radicals
oxytocin 112

PANDAS 256–7
panic disorder
  and the adenosinergic system 245–8
  and the benzodiazepine-GABAergic
      system 249–50
  brain electrical microstates in 153
  characteristics 239
  and cholecystokinin 250–51
  electrodermal activity in 154
  event-related potentials in 153

neuroanatomy 240–41
neuroendocrinology of 251–3
neurogenetics 239–40, 243
and the noradrenergic system 244–5
qEEG characteristics 152
and the respiratory system 241–3
and the serotonergic system 248–9
and sleep problems 243–4
penetrance 7, 9, 299
peptide hormones see hormones
perinatal problems, and
    schizophrenia 200, 201, 219
peripheral molecular markers 30–1, 35–6
personality, twin studies 5, 6–7, 11
PET see emission tomography
pharmacogenetics 21
pharmacological studies 33–4
    in ADHD 14
    in anxiety disorders 46
    in mood disorders 43–4, 52
    in schizophrenia 13–14, 37–8, 213–15
    in sleep disorders 51–52
    in substance abuse 49–50
    see also antidepressants; antipsychotic
        drugs; flumazenil
phenotype-genotype correlation see
    genotype-phenotype correlation
photic driving response, in
    schizophrenia 140
physical activity, and mood
    disorders 41–42
physiology see neurophysiology
pituitary see hypothalamic-pituitary
pituitary-growth hormone axis 113–14
plaques, in Alzheimer's disease 287–8,
    292, 296, 300–303, 305, 306–8
pneumoencephalography 60
positional cloning 14–19, 20–21
positron emission tomography see
    emission tomography
post-natal see perinatal
post-partum depression 111
post-traumatic stress disorder
    event-related potentials in 153–4
    and the HPA axis 109
    neuroanatomy 258
    neurochemistry 260
    neuroendocrinology 260–61
    neurogenetics 257–8
    neurophysiology 155–6, 259
pre-menstrual syndrome 110–11

pre-natal see perinatal
pre-pulse inhibition (PPI) 135, 145–6,
    211–12
predictive testing see genetic testing
prefrontal cortex 41, 204–5, 213
prolactin see hypothalamic-prolactin axis
psychiatric genetics, history 1–4
psychoanalysis, role 190
psychogenes 43
psychoses 36, 100, 136
    see also acute polymorphous
        psychosis; antipsychotic drugs;
        schizophrenia
psychosis-suppressor genes 43
psychostimulants 51–52
PTSD see post-traumatic stress disorder

qEEG 127–8, 130
    in affective disorders 147–9
    in Alzheimer's disease 156–8
    in anxiety disorders 151–2
    in schizophrenia 135–42

radiotracers see emission tomography
reading disabilities 11, 15, 16
recombination see genetic linkage
    detection
reelin, expression in schizophrenia
    217–18
region of interest (ROI)
    morphometry 66–7
respiratory system, and panic
    disorder 241–3
retroviruses, in psychiatric disorders 29

sample selection, in genetic
    mapping 17–18
schizophrenia
    adoption studies 8, 200
    animal investigations in 211–17
    brain activity in 71–2, 78–80, 135–42
    brain morphology 63, 68–9, 137, 138,
        139–40, 201–5, 215–17
    characteristics 197–8
    cognitive dysfunction in 185–6, 197–8
    electrodermal activity in 146–7
    epistasis in 12–13
    etiology 200–201, 217–19
    event-related potentials in 142–5
    eye movements in 146, 147
    gene mapping for 13–14, 15, 16, 17

schizophrenia (*cont.*)
genetic component 3, 8, 9, 11, 37, 136,
200–201, 294
genetic testing for 21–2
hemispheric imbalance 143, 144, 146–7
molecular biology 36–9
neurodevelopmental hypothesis
217–19
neuronal loss in 206–7
pharmacological studies 13–14, 38–9,
213–15
post-mortem studies 205–11
qEEG characteristics 135–42
sensory gating in 144–6
startle response 145–6, 211–12
subtypes, identification of 137–8
twin studies 2, 5, 6, 11, 12–13, 68–9,
136, 200, 202
see also antipsychotic drugs
sensory gating 144–6, 149, 212, 259
serotonergic system
and obsessive-compulsive
disorder 255–6
and panic disorder 248–9
and post-traumatic stress
syndrome 260
serotonin receptors
in affective disorders 81–2
measurement 77
in schizophrenia 14, 80, 82, 199
serotonin transporters,
measurement 74, 77
short-loop negative feedback, of
hormones 93, 94
sibling pairs, for gene mapping 17
single major locus model, of
penetrance 9
single photon emission tomography
(SPECT) *see* emission tomography
sleep disorders 50–52, 243–4, 255, 259
startle response
in anxiety disorders 155–6, 259
measurement of 134–5
in schizophrenia 145–6, 211–12
stereomorphometric studies, in
schizophrenia 206–7
stimulus intensity control, in
schizophrenia 143
stratification, in gene mapping 17–18
streptococcal infections, and psychiatric
disorders 256–7

stress
and the amygdalo-cingulo-
hippocampal circuitry 215–16
see also perinatal problems
stress disorders
cognitive dysfunction in 188–9,
259
see also post-traumatic stress disorder
striatum *see* cortico-striato-thalamo-
cortical loops
structural equation modelling 10
substance abuse 47–51
synaptic markers, in schizophrenia 211
synucleinopathies 289

tardive dyskinesia 38–9
tauopathies 289, 290, 293, 300,
303–5, 306
thalamus *see* cortico-striato-thalamo-
cortical loops
thyroid disorders 40–41, 98–102
see also HPT axis
tissue remodelling 30
in anxiety disorders 45–6
in cognitive disorders 35–6
in mood disorders 39–42
in sleep disorders 50
in substance abuse 47–8
see also brain morphology;
neurofibrillary tangles; neuronal
loss; plaques
tomography *see* computed tomography;
computerized EEG tomography;
emission tomography;
low-resolution electromagnetic
tomography; magnetic resonance
imaging
twin studies 2, 5–7, 10–13
of obsessive-compulsive disorder
254
of panic disorder 239
of schizophrenia 2, 5, 6, 11, 12–13,
68–9, 136, 200, 202

vascular dementia 158, 188
vasopressin *see* arginine-vasopressin
viruses *see* retroviruses
visual coherence 129

X-rays *see* computed tomography

yohimbine 244, 260

Acknowledgements

The Editors would like to thank Drs Paola Bucci, Umberto Volpe and Andrea Dell'Acqua of the Department of Psychiatry at the University of Naples, for their help in the processing of manuscripts.

This publication has been supported by an unrestricted educational grant from Eli Lilly, which is hereby gratefully acknowledged.